T0180805

Communications
in Computer and Information Science 2083

Editorial Board Members

Rationale

The CCIS series is devoted to the publication of proceedings of computer science conferences. Its aim is to efficiently disseminate original research results in informatics in printed and electronic form. While the focus is on publication of peer-reviewed full papers presenting mature work, inclusion of reviewed short papers reporting on work in progress is welcome, too. Besides globally relevant meetings with internationally representative program committees guaranteeing a strict peer-reviewing and paper selection process, conferences run by societies or of high regional or national relevance are also considered for publication.

Topics

The topical scope of CCIS spans the entire spectrum of informatics ranging from foundational topics in the theory of computing to information and communications science and technology and a broad variety of interdisciplinary application fields.

Information for Volume Editors and Authors

Publication in CCIS is free of charge. No royalties are paid, however, we offer registered conference participants temporary free access to the online version of the conference proceedings on SpringerLink (http://link.springer.com) by means of an http referrer from the conference website and/or a number of complimentary printed copies, as specified in the official acceptance email of the event.

CCIS proceedings can be published in time for distribution at conferences or as post-proceedings, and delivered in the form of printed books and/or electronically as USBs and/or e-content licenses for accessing proceedings at SpringerLink. Furthermore, CCIS proceedings are included in the CCIS electronic book series hosted in the SpringerLink digital library at http://link.springer.com/bookseries/7899. Conferences publishing in CCIS are allowed to use Online Conference Service (OCS) for managing the whole proceedings lifecycle (from submission and reviewing to preparing for publication) free of charge.

Publication process

The language of publication is exclusively English. Authors publishing in CCIS have to sign the Springer CCIS copyright transfer form, however, they are free to use their material published in CCIS for substantially changed, more elaborate subsequent publications elsewhere. For the preparation of the camera-ready papers/files, authors have to strictly adhere to the Springer CCIS Authors' Instructions and are strongly encouraged to use the CCIS LaTeX style files or templates.

Abstracting/Indexing

CCIS is abstracted/indexed in DBLP, Google Scholar, EI-Compendex, Mathematical Reviews, SCImago, Scopus. CCIS volumes are also submitted for the inclusion in ISI Proceedings.

How to start

To start the evaluation of your proposal for inclusion in the CCIS series, please send an e-mail to ccis@springer.com.

Mariella Särestöniemi · Pantea Keikhosrokiani ·
Daljeet Singh · Erkki Harjula · Aleksei Tiulpin ·
Miia Jansson · Minna Isomursu · Mark van Gils ·
Simo Saarakkala · Jarmo Reponen
Editors

Digital Health and Wireless Solutions

First Nordic Conference, NCDHWS 2024
Oulu, Finland, May 7–8, 2024
Proceedings, Part I

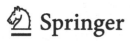 Springer

Editors

Mariella Särestöniemi
University of Oulu
Oulu, Finland

Pantea Keikhosrokiani
University of Oulu
Oulu, Finland

Daljeet Singh
University of Oulu
Oulu, Finland

Erkki Harjula
University of Oulu
Oulu, Finland

Aleksei Tiulpin
University of Oulu
Oulu, Finland

Miia Jansson
University of Oulu
Oulu, Finland

Minna Isomursu
University of Oulu
Oulu, Finland

Mark van Gils
University of Oulu
Tampere, Finland

Simo Saarakkala
University of Oulu
Oulu, Finland

Jarmo Reponen
University of Oulu
Oulu, Finland

ISSN 1865-0929   ISSN 1865-0937 (electronic)
Communications in Computer and Information Science
ISBN 978-3-031-59079-5   ISBN 978-3-031-59080-1 (eBook)
https://doi.org/10.1007/978-3-031-59080-1

This Springer imprint is published by the registered company Springer Nature Switzerland AG
The registered company address is: Gewerbestrasse 11, 6330 Cham, Switzerland

Paper in this product is recyclable.

Foreword

Digital transformation is reshaping healthcare tools, organizations, and operating models. The concept of digital health encompasses previously described electronic healthcare services, such as telemedicine or eHealth, augmented with advanced data processing and computing methods like artificial intelligence (AI). Broadly, digital health methods are believed to bring modern healthcare services to areas where they were previously unavailable. Similarly, advanced methods are seen to enable more precise diagnostics and treatments using collected digital health data. Additionally, advancements in monitoring healthcare quality and effectiveness are anticipated, along with progress in research and education through better secondary use of health information. The development of wireless technologies has brought healthcare services to users' mobile devices, allowing citizens to participate in their healthcare in unprecedented ways.

Finland has been one of the leading countries in digitalization within the European Union's DESI measurements for several years. Patient information systems in public healthcare have been solely electronic since 2007. Finland has also implemented a comprehensive national health data repository and exchange platform, KANTA, allowing citizens to access their own health information, too. Currently, every resident in Finland has an account in this national service, which proved its value especially during the COVID-19 pandemic.

Digital health is a timely research topic, particularly as Finland undergoes significant regional changes in the organization of health and social services. As part of this transformation, services are increasingly delivered through digital channels, with more responsibility given to citizens. Similar changes are underway to varying degrees in other Nordic countries. At the European level, the adoption of the EU's AI Act and the preparation of the European Health Data Space (EHDS) are significant. Addressing these challenges and opportunities requires not only advanced basic research and the development of methods and innovations but also applied research on treatment methods and digital care pathways, as well as research evaluating operations and expertise.

This Nordic Conference on Digital Health and Wireless Solutions (NCDHWS 2024) was organized by the Digital Health (DigiHealth) and 6G Enabled Sustainable Solutions (6GESS) research programs at the University of Oulu. These programs bring together multidisciplinary research activities in medical and health sciences, health economics, information, and sensor technology, as well as wireless communications. Our ambitious aim was to organize for the first time an international multidisciplinary conference providing an excellent opportunity for professionals, researchers, and industry leaders from different fields to discuss and share insights on the latest developments in digital health and related technology.

The host city Oulu is known for being at the forefront of technology innovation. It is a hub for research and development in the fields of digital health and wireless communications. Electronic health records, telemedicine and mobile health services have been in clinical use in the city for more than 25 years. There is active research aiming not only towards new territories like AI, novel sensor technology and edge computing, but also striving for scientific assessment of the impact of these innovations in real life.

The organization of this new type of multidisciplinary conference combining habits and customs of different fields would not have been possible without the hard work of many colleagues and experts who dedicated their time and expertise to make this conference successful. I would like to thank our multidisciplinary Organizing Committee, my co-chair Simo Saarakkala, and our coordinators Tuire Salonurmi and Sanna Tuomela for fruitful discussions and practical ideas shared in our regular meetings. Additionally, I would like to thank our Program Committee with International Reviewers and our Publication Chairs, both led by Mariella Särestöniemi for compiling excellent scientific content for the conference.

Furthermore, I would like to thank our excellent invited speakers for bringing their expertise in digital health and related technologies to the audience, and all our International Advisory Committee members for their kind assistance. I am grateful to Karoliina Paalimäki-Paakki for leading the Student Volunteer Committee and I would like to thank those student volunteers whose work with practical arrangements during the conference was invaluable. I would also like to thank our media team Katja Longhurst and Sallamaari Syrjä for maintaining our digital presence in various channels. My sincere thanks belong to Minna Komu for marketing the conference to companies and to Oulu University Hospital and to the Wellbeing Services County of North Ostrobothnia for supporting us in conference arrangements and providing a unique research environment. Finally, I would like to collectively thank all those who in various roles contributed to the success of NCDHWS 2024, either as an organizer or as a participant.

Oulu   Jarmo Reponen
May 2024

Preface

The Nordic Conference on Digital Health and Wireless Solutions (NCDHWS) is a new international multidisciplinary conference which brings together experts and professionals from different fields. Organization of such a conference necessitates the collaboration of multidisciplinary committees, jointly devising strategies to harmonize the diverse conference cultures from various fields. Thus, all the NCDHWS 2024 conference committees, including program committee chairs, organization committee, program committee, and international advisory committee, have representatives from several different fields of engineering, medicine, and health sciences. Additionally, altogether 27 different countries are represented in our committees, and even more different nationalities.

As an example of combining habits and customs of different fields in our conference organization, we accepted three different submission types: full papers (10–19 pages), short papers (6–9 pages) and abstracts (1–3). Full and short papers appear in the main text of the book and are indexed, whereas abstracts appear in the backmatter of the volumes. This first NCDHWS conference turned out to be successful: we received 100 submissions including 57 full papers, 11 short papers, and 32 abstracts. The review process for this conference was double-blind and our large program committee (i.e., international reviewer committee) consisted of 122 reviewers. For each full and short paper, we selected 3–5 reviewers and for abstracts 2–3 reviewers with suitable scientific background. OpenReview was used as the submission platform since it automatically checks for potential conflicts of interests for each reviewer. OpenReview also automatically ensures confidentiality by shielding program committee chairs from accessing evaluations of the papers where they are authors, and by shielding the identities of the reviewers of their own papers.

Reviewers were advised to score papers based on submission type using OpenReview's scoring table and to provide detailed comments to authors to improve the paper quality. OpenReview has an evaluation scale from 1–10 in which score 6 stands for "marginally above acceptance threshold". Additionally, OpenReviewer lets reviewers score their level of confidence. After the review process, the program committee chairs calculated for each paper the average score, weighted with the reviewers' confidence level, and made final decisions on the acceptance of the papers and their presentation type (oral/poster). Program committee chairs decided to accept all the papers reaching weighted average score 6, i.e., reaching the acceptance threshold level suggested by OpenReview scoring. Program committee chairs naturally did not handle reviewer assignments nor did they make final decisions on their own papers. From the submitted papers, 50 full papers and 7 short papers achieved OpenReview's score 6 and hence were accepted for the proceedings. All authors were requested to make corrections and improvements on their papers based on reviewers' comments before final camera-ready submission. For final versions, we carried out plagiarism checks with Turnitin and asked authors to take actions if the plagiarism scores were high.

This Springer proceedings consists of two volumes. Full and short papers appear in the main parts of the volumes ordered similarly to session themes of the conference. Abstracts appear in the back matters of both volumes following the same thematic session order. We would like to express our gratitude to the Springer Nature team who helped us with all practicalities in this book edition process.

Additionally, we would like to thank all the members of our committees: organization committee, program committee as well as international advisory committee, who altogether made the organization of this exciting multidisciplinary conference possible. We would like to greatly acknowledge the keynote and invited speakers who took time out from their busy schedules and traveled up to Oulu to give us inspiring talks on their research. Finally, we would like to express our sincere thanks to all the authors for choosing NCDHWS 2024 to present their research results. With all their interesting presentations combined with excellent invited speeches, this multidisciplinary gathering was successful and fruitful for new collaborations.

May 2024

Mariella Särestöniemi
Pantea Keikhosrokiani
Daljeet Singh
Erkki Harjula
Miia Jansson
Aleksei Tiulpin
Minna Isomursu
Mark van Gils
Simo Saarakkala
Jarmo Reponen

Organization

General Chairs (Conference President and Vice-president)

Jarmo Reponen   University of Oulu, Finland
Simo Saarakkala   University of Oulu, Finland

Program Committee Chairs

Mariella Särestöniemi (Chair)   University of Oulu, Finland
Erkki Harjula   University of Oulu, Finland
Minna Isomursu   University of Oulu, Finland
Miia Jansson   University of Oulu, Finland
Jarmo Reponen   University of Oulu, Finland
Aleksei Tiulpin   University of Oulu, Finland
Mark van Gils   University of Tampere, Finland

Publication Chairs

Mariella Särestöniemi   University of Oulu, Finland
Pantea Keikhosrokiani   University of Oulu, Finland
Daljeet Singh   University of Oulu, Finland

Organization Committee

Jarmo Reponen (Chair)   University of Oulu, Finland
Simo Saarakkala   University of Oulu, Finland
Erkki Harjula   University of Oulu, Finland
Matti Hämäläinen   University of Oulu, Finland
Minna Isomursu   University of Oulu, Finland
Miia Jansson   University of Oulu, Finland
Karoliina Paalimäki-Paakki   OAMK, Finland
Minna Komu   OuluHealth, Finland
Ari Pouttu   University of Oulu, Finland
Tuire Salonurmi   University of Oulu, Finland
Mariella Särestöniemi   University of Oulu, Finland

Jani Tikkanen   Pohde, Finland
Aleksei Tiulpin   University of Oulu, Finland
Sanna Tuomela   University of Oulu, Finland
Mark van Gils   University of Tampere, Finland

Program Committee

Ijaz Ahmad   VTT Research Centre, Finland
Outi Ahonen   Laurea Applied Science, Finland
Daria Alekseeva   Tampere University, Finland
Slawomir Ambroziak   Gdansk University of Technology, Poland
Daisuke Anzai   Nagoya Institute of Technology, Japan
Atakan Aral   Umeå University, Sweden
Aslak Aslaksen   Bergen University Hospital, Norway
Tunc Asuroglu   VTT Technical Research Centre of Finland,
                                   Finland
Robin Augustine   Uppsala University, Sweden
Kirsti E. Berntsen   Norwegian University of Science and Technology,
                                   Norway
Roberto Blanco   University of Turku, Finland
Kerryn Butler-Henderson   RMIT University, Australia
Stefano Caputi   University of Florence, Italy
Henry Carvajal   Universidad de Las Américas, Equador
Ioanna Chouvarda   Aristotle University of Thessaloniki, Greece
Omedev Dahia   Lovely Professional University, India
Nils Dahlström   University of Linköping, Sweden
Jeppe Eriksen   University of Aalborg, Denmark
Hany Ferdinando   University of Oulu, Finland
Pål Anders Floor   Norwegian University of Science and Technology,
                                   Norway
Mark van Gils   University of Tampere, Finland
Heidi Gilstad   Norwegian University of Science and Technology,
                                   Norway
Guido Giunti   Trinity College Dublin, Ireland
Casandra Grundstrom   Norwegian University of Science and Technology,
                                   Norway
Erkki Harjula   University of Oulu, Finland
Ying He   University of Sydney, Australia
Sari Heikkinen   Laurea University of Applied Sciences, Finland
Juuso Heikkinen   Oulu University Hospital, Finland
Helinä Heino   University of Oulu, Finland

Minna Hokka   Diaconia University of Applied Sciences, Finland
Syed Sajid Hussain   Norwegian University of Science and Technology,
                                 Norway
Piia Hyvämäki   Oulu University of Applied Sciences, Finland
Matti Hämäläinen   University of Oulu, Finland
Iiris Hörhammer   Aalto University, Finland
Milla Immonen   Lapland University of Applied Sciences, Finland
Minna Isomursu   University of Oulu, Finland
Antti Isosalo   University of Oulu, Finland
Miia Jansson   University of Oulu, Finland
Vesa Jormanainen   University of Helsinki, Finland
HemDutt Joshi   Thapar Institute of Engineering and Technology,
                                 India
Pirjo Kaakinen   University of Oulu, Finland
Kimmo Kansanen   Norwegian University of Science and Technology,
                                 Norway
Outi Kanste   Laurea University of Applied Sciences, Finland
Pasi Karppinen   University of Oulu, Finland
Jani Katisko   Oulu University Hospital, Finland
Kaisa Leena Kauppinen   University of Oulu, Finland
Pantea Keikhosrokiani   University of Oulu, Finland
Ali Khaleghi   Norwegian University of Science and Technology,
                                 Norway
Jussi Koivunen   Oulu University Hospital, Finland
Jorma Komulainen   University of Eastern Finland
Elina Kontio   Turku University of Applied Sciences, Finland
Juha Korpelainen   Oulu University Hospital, Finland
Hilkka Korpi   Oulu University of Applied Sciences, Finland
Tuomas Koskela   University of Tampere, Finland
Pirkko Kouri   Finnish Society of Telemedicine and eHealth,
                                 Finland
Narasimharao Kowlagi   University of Oulu, Finland
Elizabeth Krupinski   Emory University School of Medicine, USA
Sumit Kumar   Lovely Professional University, India
Rajeev Kumar   Chitkara University, India
Tanesh Kumar   Aalto University, Finland
Maria Kääriäinen   University of Oulu, Finland
Janne Lehtiranta   University of Turku, Finland
Ove Lintvedt   eHealth Research Center of Norway, Norway
Karen Livesay   RMIT University, Australia
Tinja Lääveri   Aalto University, Finland
Madhusanka Liyanage   University College Dublin, Ireland

Ratko Magjarevic	University of Zagreb, Croatia
Terence McSweeney	University of Oulu, Finland
Alexander Meaney	University of Helsinki, Finland
Kristina Mikkonen	University of Oulu, Finland
Pooja Mohanty	Norwegian University of Science and Technology, Norway
Ayan Mondal	Indian Institute of Technology Indore, India
Lorenzo Mucchi	University of Florence, Italy
Teemu Myllylä	University of Oulu, Finland
Mikko Nenonen	University of Oulu, Finland
Khanh Nguyen	University of Oulu, Finland
Huy Hoang Nguyen	University of Oulu, Finland
Anne Oikarinen	University of Oulu, Finland
Aleksandr Ometov	Tampere University, Finland
Diana Moya Osario	Linköping University, Sweden
Karoliina Paalimäki-Paakki	OAMK, Finland
Egor Panfilov	University of Oulu, Finland
Anagha P. Parkar	Haraldsplass Deaconess Hospital Bergen, Norway
Juha Partala	University of Oulu, Finland
Mauricio Perez	Uppsala University, Sweden
Teodora Popordanoska	KU Leuven, Belgium
Pawani Porambage	VTT Technical Research Centre of Finland, Finland
Tarja Pölkki	University of Oulu, Finland
Prabhat Ram	University of Oulu, Finland
Jarmo Reponen	University of Oulu, Finland
Peeter Ross	Technical University of Tallinn, Estonia
Heidi Ruotsalainen	University of Oulu, Finland
Simo Saarakkala	University of Oulu, Finland
Juha Salmitaival	Aalto University, Finland
Tuire Salonurmi	University of Oulu, Finland
Pedro Moreno Sanchez	University of Tampere, Finland
Daniel Pinto dos Santos	University Hospital of Cologne, Germany
Kaija Saranto	University of Eastern Finland, Finland
Kamran Sayrafian	National Institute of Standards and Technology, USA
Aleksi Schrey	University of Turku, Finland
Kamal Kumar Sharma	Ambala College of Engineering and Applied Research, India
Shallu Sharma	Bennett University, India
Charenjeet Singh	Lovely Professional University, India
Daljeet Singh	University of Oulu, Finland

Simone Soderi   IMT School for Advanced Studies, Italy
Ursula Sokolaj   Norwegian University of Science and Technology,
                                        Norway
Putra Sumari   Universiti Sains Malaysia, Malaysia
Mariella Särjestöniemi   University of Oulu, Finland
Atthapongse Taparugsanagorn   Asian Institute of Technology, Thailand
Jani Tikkanen   OYS - Oulun Yliopistollinen Sairaala, Finland
Aleksei Tiulpin   University of Oulu, Finland
Paulus Torkki   University of Helsinki, Finland
Johanna Uusimaa   University of Oulu, Finland
Gillian Vesty   RMIT University, Australia
Morten Villumsen   University of Aalborg, Denmark
Sidsel Villumsen   University of Aalborg, Denmark
Alpo Värri   University of Tampere, Finland
Fan Wang   University of Oulu, Finland
Handy Wicaksono   Petra Christian University, Indonesia
Lotta Ylinen   Tampere University, Finland
Cheah Yu-N   Universiti Sains Malaysia, Malaysia
Nasriah Zakaria   Al Maarefa University, Saudi Arabia

International Advisory Committee

Najeeb Al-Shorbaji   Middle East and North Africa Association of
                                        Health Informatics, Jordan
Slawomir Ambroziak   Gdansk University of Technology, Poland
Robin Augustine   Uppsala University, Sweden
Rimma Axelsson   Karolinska Institutet, Sweden
Paolo Bifulco   University "Federico II" of Naples, Italy
Matthew Blaschko   KU Leuven, Belgium
Bernd Blobel   University of Regensburg, Germany
Akshay Chaudhari   Stanford University, USA
Luis M. Correia   University of Lisbon IST, Portugal
Flavio Esposito   Saint Louis University, USA
Vahid Farrahi   TU Dortmund University, Germany
Michael Fuchsjäger   Medical University Graz, Austria
Hassan Ghazal   Moroccan Society for Telemedicine & eHealth
                                        (MSfTeH), Morocco
Michele Y. Griffith   International Society for Telemedicine and
                                        eHealth, USA
Casandra Grundstrom   NTNU, Norway
Ingfrid S. Haldorsen   Haukeland University Hospital, Norway

Manami Hori	Tokai University Europe, Japan
Vesa Jormanainen	Ministry of Social Affairs and Health, Finland
Dipak Kalra	European Institute for Innovation through Health Data, Belgium
Hiroshi Kondoh	Tottori University, Japan
Ilkka Korhonen	GE HealthCare Finland, Finland
Elisabeth Krupinski	Emory University School of Medicine, USA
S. Yunkap Kwankam	International Society for Telemedicine and eHealth, Switzerland
Claudia Lindner	University of Manchester, UK
Anthony Maeder	Flinders University, Australia
Janne Martikainen	University of Eastern Finland, Finland
Lorenzo Mucchi	University of Florence, Italy
Vasiliki Mylonopoulou	University of Gothenburg, Sweden
Miika Nieminen	University of Oulu, Finland
Jérôme Noally	Universitat Pompeu Fabra, Spain
Kaija Saranto	University of Eastern Finland, Finland
Kamran Sayrafian	National Institute of Standards and Technology, USA
Päivi Sillanaukee	Ministry of Social Affairs and Health, Finland
Stein Olav Skrøvseth	Norwegian Centre for E-health Research, Norway
Anthony Smith	University of Queensland, Australia
Rosanna Tarricone	Bocconi University, Italy
Paulus Torkki	University of Helsinki, Finland
Yoshito Tsushima	Gunma University, Japan
Peter van Ooijen	University Medical Center Groningen, Netherlands
Gillian Vesty	RMIT University, Australia
Johanna Viitanen	Aalto University, Finland

Contents – Part I

Digitalization in Health Education

Digital Health Innovations

Abstracts

Contents – Part II

Novel Sensors and Bioinformatics

Clinical Decision Support and Medical AI 2

Health Technology Assessment and Impact Evaluation

Wireless Technologies and Medical Devices

Abstracts

Remote Care and Health Connectivity Architectures in 6G Era

Expert Perspectives on Future 6G-Enabled Hospital Metaverse

Fan Wang[1] (ID), Risto Jurva[2](✉) (ID), Petri Ahokangas[1] (ID), Seppo Yrjölä[2,3] (ID),
and Marja Matinmikko-Blue[2,4] (ID)

[1] Martti Ahtisaari Institute, University of Oulu, 8000 Oulu, Finland
[2] Centre for Wireless Communications (CWC), University of Oulu, 8000 Oulu, Finland
jurva.risto@oulu.fi
[3] Nokia, Oulu, Finland
[4] Infotech, University of Oulu, 8000 Oulu, Finland

Abstract. This paper aims to understand the value-added services that the future 6G-enabled metaverse can and will bring to hospitals. This is important since most studies on 6G and the metaverse are heavily driven by technological solutions. Adopting a qualitative research approach, this paper collects experts' opinions on the usage scenarios of the 6G-enabled metaverse in hospitals. Six use cases within hospital contexts have been identified from open-ended interviews. The analysis of each case reveals that 6G, as a general-purpose technology, offers the necessary capabilities to support the development of the metaverse in hospitals. The metaverse-enabled services are expected to design future smart hospitals and improve work processes and resource allocation in hospitals, while also promoting preventive healthcare and training and enhancing the quality of care in emergency, treatment, and rehabilitation. Consequently, the development of both metaverse and 6G will progress in tandem, hand in hand, offering local services in hospitals. From a value perspective, this paper contributes to the development of the 6G and metaverse in the hospital vertical by understanding the needs, capabilities, and key values of the future 6G-enabled hospital metaverse.

Keywords: 6G · Metaverse · use cases · key values · hospital

1 Introduction

The hospital of future is digitally networked and closely connected to the digitalization of the health system [1]. The emergences of connected health, digital health, and mobile health result from the digital transformation of healthcare that reduces boundaries among health professionals, patients, devices, payers, upstream and downstream service providers, and other stakeholders [2]. In some scenarios, the focus is moving from clinical healthcare to home-based preventive healthcare or wellness covering a scale of daily well-being activities from mental, physical, and social aspects [3]. The preventive activities could be tailored to all age groups and levels of disabilities according to their health program.

M. Särestöniemi et al. (Eds.): NCDHWS 2024, CCIS 2083, pp. 3–20, 2024.
https://doi.org/10.1007/978-3-031-59080-1_1

With the development of industrial 4.0 and the sixth generation of Mobile Networks (6G), the envisioned future for intelligent health relies on a wireless-based healthcare network that enables real-time patient intervention, monitoring, and transformation into data-centric, intelligent, and automated processes in a virtual environment [3, 4]. However, the needs and key values (KVs) for 6G and metaverse in hospitals remain unclear. Therefore, our paper focuses on 6G and metaverse technologies in hospitals, and the potential to improve patient outcomes and create new opportunities for technological advancements in healthcare [4].

The 6G technology will be a disruption of wireless mobile communications enabling the development of services not seen before. The services are evolved by gathering data from numerous sources, analyzing it with AI, and sharing the refined data through various platforms and applications in various use cases of businesses. The 6G technology makes possible several new functionalities like sensing, positioning, and imaging [5]. Subsequently, the 6G enables large-scale metaverse implementation, which integrates the virtual world (digital twins and information) and the real world (objects) by creating a digital realm where people can interact with computer-generated environments and other users in real-time. The application of the metaverse integrates the virtual world and the real world, addressing the challenges of remote healthcare services caused by the absence of healthcare professionals at the location [6].

Most technology-focused academic research drives the development of 6G and Metaverse and its application in healthcare by focusing on vision, technical solutions, scenarios, and use cases. However, from a value-creation perspective, making the Metaverse real in a hospital context requires sensing, data connection, and physical and virtual models to enable interaction and exchange of information between the real and virtual world [7], thus involving multiple stakeholders to address a variety of needs.

In this study, the metaverse is seen as a critical application for deployment of the 6G network, and the 6G is observed to be a particularly important enabler for the metaverse development in healthcare. Viewing hospitals as ecosystems, the metaverse introduces an innovative approach to interaction within hospital environments. However, the development of 6G-enabled metaverse services, including aspects such as usage, expected outcomes, capability, constraints, key values, and impact in hospitals, has not yet been clarified in parallel with the development of 6G and metaverse technologies. Therefore, this paper focuses on the demand side to understand the future of 6G-enabled metaverse in hospitals and proposes two research questions as follows:

- How could 6G-enabled metaverse create value for future hospitals?
- What needs and use cases could be identified for future 6G-enabled hospital metaverse?

This paper aims to address stakeholder needs, requirements, constraints, and expected outcomes from the demand side, and KVs along with 6G and metaverse technology development. This approach will guide new technology development direction, allocate resources reasonably for better acceptance and adoption by stakeholders, and deliver the value that stakeholders hoped for the 6G-enabled Metaverse services.

2 Relevant Literature

2.1 Digitalization in Healthcare

Digitalization in healthcare refers to the socio-technological process of integrating digital technologies to improve and transform healthcare processes, services, and outcomes. The establishment of a connected, intelligent medical services environment with integrated sensing and intelligence capabilities relies on technologies, such as the Internet of Things, mobile internet, cloud computing, big data, and artificial intelligence. The purpose of digitalization is to improve patient care, healthcare delivery efficiency, and satisfaction, and advance medical treatment and research.

Health-related technologies have reformed medical healthcare in the areas of electronic health records (EHRs) that enable a doctor to manage a patient's medical information without accessing diverse systems [8]. Telemedicine provides remote healthcare services using ICT solutions for consultation, rehabilitation, and monitoring. Web-based digital services known as eHealth have rapidly developed to provide services such as e-prescription, e-referrals, and e-discharges. As increased use of mobile devices, such as smartphones, tablets, software and sensors, a new set of mobile health (mHealth) solutions has been developed to enable access to authorized data regardless of geographical location without the need to change devices [9, 10].

Digitalization improves the patient service process through digital platforms and self-services, such as online booking, self-symptom check, online chat, medical data access, and online prescription renewal. Digital tools have facilitated communication between patients and health professionals which saves cost and time. Digitalization has also empowered patients by granting access and management of their health and well-being through medical data access, digital care pathways, and commercially available apps that focus on health, diet, and exercise [11].

The outcomes of digitalization in healthcare are to integrate medical resources, optimize medical service processes, improve diagnostic and treatment efficiency, assist in clinical and hospital management decision-making, and achieve convenience in patient medical care, intelligent medical services, and refined hospital management. Facilitating by new technology, innovations, a connected infrastructure of medical devices, software applications, and health systems makes it possible for health professionals to care for patients anywhere, at any time, while empowering patients to take an active role in self-care and achieve preventive, predictive, personalized and participatory medicine [12, 13].

2.2 Wireless in Healthcare

The envisioned future 6G network is an integrated space-aerial-terrestrial network, encompassing interactions from device to terrestrial and satellite communications and driving the development of holographic-type communications, ubiquitous intelligence, tactile internet, multi-sense experience, and digital twin [18]. The goal of the future 6G network is to build a hyperconnected society where everyone and everything is connected [14]. The 6G goes beyond the 5G network in supporting tailored service provisioning, dynamic data exchange, and collaboration among objects, processes, people, and machines. The 6G will fulfill the requirements of diverse, dynamic, and locally tailored vertical applications that 5G cannot achieve due to stringent resource constraints [14].

The health industry has been identified as one of the vertical industries that can benefit from the 6G network [15]. The areas that can be supported by the 6G network include new local private networks, seamless robotic-assisted surgeries, telemedicine, emergency services, and the integration of interconnected devices for deep-body implants. The independent and uncoordinated subnetworks in hospitals require high reliability, determinism, and semi-autonomy in hospital contexts, e.g., to control robot arms and critical on-body devices [16], and local and indoor solutions. Therefore, medical wireless devices, machines, and sensors will require the 6G network for seamless connection, transmission, and processing of real-time health data [17, 18] in a secure and safe way of data exchange [19].

2.3 Metaverse in Healthcare

Metaverse has been defined by "*as a technology-mediated network of scalable and potentially interoperable extended reality environments merging the physical and virtual realities to provide experiences characterized by their level of immersiveness, environmental fidelity, and sociability*" [20]. The 3D-modelled virtual worlds and avatars connect the real world and users through augmented reality (AR), virtual reality (VR), and digital twins [21]. AR and VR offer improved 3D visualization and can be utilized repeatedly. This makes them ideal for various preoperative applications, such as training for young doctors and medical students [22], preoperative surgery planning, and remote monitoring. The combination of VR and AR allows geographically remote surgeons to guide surgeries by overlaying suggestions on their view through an AR system. Additionally, they enhance patient education through improved visualization [23]. AR/VR devices can also provide personalized therapeutic treatment and may apply to post-traumatic stress disorder (PTSD), anxiety and fear-related disorder (A&F), diseases of the nervous system (DNS), and pain management [24].

A digital twin makes a virtual replica of an object or system and receives updated data from the physical entity via real-time connection and may drive the healthcare revolution [25]. The concept of digital twins aims to simulate, diagnose, and predict outcomes using a digital replica, enabling the making of suitable decisions based on the results from the replica, which are then applied to the physical entity [26]. Digital twins are found to be useful for managing personal health by synchronizing data from various sensors and health registries in a timely manner [27, 28], and pre-surgery planning, and optimization of hospital facilities and inventory. Besides virtual replicas of objects and systems, the digital twin can be created from humans, which brings totally new aspects to the visioning of future healthcare [29].

2.4 Stakeholders and Key Values

Stakeholders play a crucial role in representing diverse demands and needs from both human and machine users specific to private and public organizations in the vertical healthcare industry. Meanwhile, different stakeholders will supply the resources and assets required to address a variety of needs, the provision of physical infrastructure (such as facilities and sites), equipment (including devices and networks), and data (content and context), all within the regulatory framework established by policymakers [30].

In the health service ecosystem, the five major groups of stakeholders have been classified as (1) Regulators who set regulatory guidelines; (2) Service providers are health professionals who provide services in hospitals, nursing homes, and extended homes. (3) Payers, statutory health insurance, private health insurance, and government agencies (4) Suppliers are the research organizations and technological companies that develop new products and services for treatments, and (5) Patients are the beneficiaries of the care [31]. The multiple stakeholders involved in a 6G ecosystem in the health industry include e.g. healthcare service providers, financial sources, telecommunication operators, mobile device providers, medical device providers, and users [32].

The goal of the future 6G network is to fulfill stakeholders' needs and requirements for creating value for individuals, organizations, businesses, and society through spectrum innovation and management [33, 34]. Value plays pivotal roles in showing and confirming the technology's capacity to meet stakeholder demands [32] and guide the development of technology in a more beneficial, ethical, and sustainable direction [35], particularly when adopting a service design thinking for the transformation of healthcare systems [36].Understanding needs and value from stakeholder perspectives on developing 6G and metaverse in hospitals further strengthens the value creation, benefiting not only businesses but also society [37]. It enables a shift from big tech to big democracy as well as delivers and captures the value of deploying 6G and metaverse in the future for sustainable healthcare and societal development.

[35] have developed a 6G visioning framework that enables stakeholders to communicate their needs, aims, and visions in future 6G development and ensure the successful innovation and commercialization of the future 6G network as society wants shown in Fig. 1.

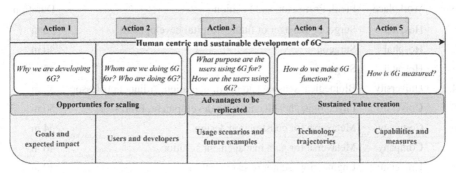

Fig. 1. Adapted from the 6G visioning framework in [35].

This framework addressed the essential questions to develop 6G from a human-centric and sustainability perspectives, such as: *"why we are doing 6G, who we are doing it for, who are doing it, what purposes users will use it for, how users will use it, how we will make 6G work and how we will measure"* [35]. In this paper, we will utilize the questions addressed in the framework proposed [35] to analyze our empirical inquiries in Sect. 3. The focus will be on the analysis of 6G-enabled metaverse use cases to understand stakeholders' needs, usage scenarios, technological capabilities, expected outcomes, impacts in local hospitals, and their importance in offering local 6G infrastructure setup and services.

3 Data and Materials

3.1 Research Approach

This study opted for a qualitative research method allowing us to explore the future envisioned Metaverse and wireless solutions and their application in a hospital context. Understanding the value of 6G and metaverse in-depth requires a conversation with different stakeholders to seek expertise in technology development [38].

For this study, we used a purposeful sampling strategy [39] by focusing on the experts who understand health technology and its development and adoption process in hospitals. Because this study is future-oriented, and the topics are not well-known for everyone, our sampling process needs to make sure that selected participants will be capable of sharing their expertise on the question asked and meet the aim of this study [40]. The experts invited consist of stakeholders involved in hospital operational processes, development functions, solution vendors, and service providers, including hospital managers, health professionals, developers, researchers, and company representatives. We anticipate that a diverse portfolio of experts will approach 6G and metaverse from different angles and perspectives, enabling our understanding of future 6G and metaverse in various areas of hospitals (Table 1).

Table 1. Data collection summary.

No.	Workplace	Field, Profession and Position	Duration
1	Hospital	Surgeon, manager of future hospital development	56 m
2	Hospital	Surgeon	40 m
3	Hospital	Surgeon	45 m
4	University	Biomedical sensing and instrumentation, Adjunct professor	52 m
5	University	Phycologist, health education development, Professor	50 m
6	Company	Metaverse for construction design	54 m
7	Company	Metaverse for pain management solution	46 m
8	University	Engineering, senior research fellow	30 m

We use open-ended questions as an interview strategy. Since 6G and metaverse are future-oriented technologies, the open-ended question allows interviewees to express their thoughts, experiences, and perspectives without being limited by predetermined response options. Open-ended questions provide an opportunity for interviews to shape the direction of the conversation and might lead to unexpected insights and uncover new information. The discussion topics fall into five themes: current digitalization situation in hospitals, 6G in hospitals, metaverse in hospitals, stakeholder, service, and infrastructure, as well as regulatory impacts.

To begin our data analysis, we initiated desk research, examining existing literature, documents, and transcripts. After a comprehensive study of the data, we observed that each interviewee had envisioned a use case based on their field of work and knowledge. These use cases correspond to each stage of the hospital care pathway, from emergency and treatment to rehabilitation. Additionally, there is a use case for building smart hospitals by applying 3D modeling now and integrating the metaverse in the future. We decided to describe and analyze these use cases to synthesize the key values of each case to explore the future 6G-enabled hospital metaverse.

3.2 Findings and Discussions

The Current Level of Digitalization. The discussions of the digitalization of hospitals, in general, indicated that a huge step was taken in the development and use of digital services and platforms during pandemics. Due to social distancing, people learned to use digital service portals, which advise maintaining well-being with personal actions and activities or guide self-diagnostics as preliminary care action. *"Individuals are progressively becoming accustomed to utilizing sensors and wearables to manage their well-being and acquire the skills to analyze health data for self-care". (Interviewee 4). Moreover,* many tasks like discussions with chat service, video consultancy, or renewing prescriptions happen now based on individuals' own activity.

Considering the digitalization of medical actions, *"the biggest benefits have been reached, in imaging and various analysis tasks when high data volumes can be analyzed and transferred in a minimum time." (Interviewee 4)* Imaging patients produce high volumes of data, which needs to be analyzed powerfully in a short time for diagnostics. Often, masses of data are sent to other locations, which assumes high data transfer capabilities. Another remarkable advantage of digitalization has been *"in the analysis of biosignals, where digitalization of analysis methods has enabled the detection and identification of some rare illnesses." (Interviewee 4).* Analysis and comparison of patient data with a vast amount of reference cohort data enables, e.g., to recognize deviations from normal trends of health data. More generally, the high increase in computing power making, e.g., real-time 3D video analyses, has been a crucial change in the patient care processes. For future improvement, doctors propose *"to develop a system which enables real-time situational awareness e.g. in urgent cases, when the operation room needs to be prepared for a patient arriving with an ambulance." (Interviewee 1).* The increase of edge computing capability of 5G and beyond technologies will help to achieve a real-time situational picture based on patient data. Subsequently, instead of processing high volumes of data in VR glasses, the data can be transferred wirelessly to the surrounding 6G network i.e. *"implementation of edge computing can be used for off-loading. The glasses' weight will be dramatically reduced, thus increasing the usability of the metaverse." (Interviewee 8).*

Another aspect where digitalization helps is the serious lack of professionals, specialists, and other resources, which even challenges the delivery of public health care services as statutory debts. This is further *"challenged by the demographics, which show the number of elderly to be in high growth, resulting in an increasing need for health services." (Interviewee 2)* Subsequently, some advancements are rather easy to develop like *"simple practical improvement would be to minimize the time used for manual data collection from patients being still today a frequently repeating activity, which has even caused cons in false medication due to human errors. (Interviewee 1)"* All this could be probably decreased by the integration of devices and instruments with improved data management processes, though, considering all the privacy rules. Moreover, developing data management practices by adopting increasingly more artificial intelligence technologies would help in the decision-making of operational patient processes.

Digitalization has considerably streamlined hospital workflows, enhancing the efficiency of clinical work. The digital care pathway not only reduces the time health professionals spend on filling out patient forms but also simplifies data retrieval. Appointment bookings can be effortlessly managed through digital protocols, while patient interactions, including pre-surgery preparations, can now be seamlessly conducted through mobile apps.

The Current Processes and Stakeholders. Typical stakeholders of hospital operational and development processes are based on both internal and external functions. Each organizational unit is the process owner of its special medical focus area or support function, and it needs to present plans and reasoning for its activity, procurement, and investments to the cost control function. When it comes to hospital patient care processes, the interviews revealed that there exists some room for development. Often the evaluations of processes are conducted internally, which often does not disclose all the process deficiencies. The hospital management oversees processes and needs to take action when shortages are detected. The process developers have co-operated with external specialists and researchers when targeting improvements.

Most of the medical units have specific devices and instruments, which are taken care of by the maintenance unit. This team is crucial to keeping the operations functional and in continuous completeness. Some of the processes, devices, and instruments are sensitive to environmental conditions like temperature or humidity, which need to be stable and constant. For that purpose, the hospital property management controls particular premises to maintain optimal circumstances of patient processes in various use cases. Through the patient care processes high volumes of data are generated constantly. Collection, protection, analysis, and safe sharing of data are assumed to have high-capacity computing and data transfer capabilities. The ICT department is responsible for operating, maintaining, and developing the data infrastructure. Moreover, various other support functions as stakeholders exist in the hospital. Logistics is responsible for the delivery of numerous things that are needed in the processes. Another support function is the security office to maintain overall security in the hospital premises.

Constraints. The constraints on digitalization and developing the 6G-enabled metaverse fall into different categories. Both the telecommunication and health industries are highly regulated. At the societal level, the current regulation appears bureaucratic and does not enable new businesses or innovations to enter hospitals due to the long clinical trial period and heavy process of preparation for certification and documentation, which is applied to medical innovations.

At the organizational level, the regulation of medical procurement also limits the potential for innovation adoption. Few resources with potentially insufficient competence are allocated to the purchase of future-oriented technology and equipment, such as the necessary VR glasses, or infrastructure for a virtual simulation environment. *"It took a long time for us to get permission from the research management group to buy more advanced and expensive VR and head glasses for our VR project." (Interviewee 5).* Safety for sensitive health data is obviously seen in hospitals. The interoperability among different technological solutions is not compatible, and collaboration between data-driven solutions is not sufficient, so innovation solutions are dead without sufficient investment from external investors.

At the individual level, technology resistance has been cited by most of the interviewees. Our empirical finding indicates that digitalization simplifies the processes of documenting, archiving, and searching for patient data, and it benefits the process of treatment. However, digitalization also increases the workload, e.g., time spent on inserting patient information into different systems. A common statement is that technology cannot replace human contact with patients. This is not the aim of developers either, but they are developing solutions for routine tasks e.g. to decrease time spent with computers when manually exporting and importing information between data systems. Also, remote or virtual consultation with doctors or nurses is often resisted by the customers. This can be potentially decreased when positive experiences about the virtual meetings are gained. A favourable experience can be e.g. quick digital appointment with the doctor on the next day instead of queueing for one week for a physical meeting with the professionals and the result of the consultation is the same in both cases. Many physical meetings could be replaced by virtual negotiations. Due to outdated infrastructure, errors often occur in documenting processes, sometimes, just simply because of e.g., *"the shortage of computer memory, or an unreliable network and bad connection" (Interviewee 3).* These administrative tasks prevent doctors from concentrating on treatment and clinical work.

Need for 6G and Metaverse in Hospital: Use Cases. Although the current digitalization has brought benefits to clinical treatment, processes, and services, further development is expected to improve the efficiency and effectiveness of clinical work. Considering the emerging technologies such as 6G and the Metaverse, detailed specifications or well-defined expectations are still lacking. However, based on our interviews, there is a strong demand for connecting physical objects, people, locations, and services to optimize work processes, which may lead to saving costs and improving the quality of care. Based on the interviewees' backgrounds and knowledge, they identified the use cases for the Metaverse and 6G.

Use Case 1 (Designing Smart Hospital). When constructing or renovating smart hospitals, 3D models can be generated within the metaverse to visualize prototypes and designs. This enables stakeholders to immerse themselves in the design phase, providing them with the ability to experience and convey their ideas. *"…to understand how to make that location work better. E.g., how to place certain operation models and blocks, see if there are enough spaces around them to be able to move around and how to place the different displays and devices there. Then maybe renovating a whole room for totally different use cases or new types of operations" (Interviewee 6).* This proactive approach helps in identifying design flaws and facilitates essential modifications.

The metaverse can be used to simulate various room configurations and dynamic aspects of hospitals, such as combining different rooms, to enhance planning and decision-making. *"Metaverse goes even one step further because you can actually go inside the space with other people and visualize the way how to utilize." (Interviewee 6).* The huge benefit of the metaverse is that simulates different situations in a faster way and brings more capabilities to enable you to move around to get a more realistic situation.

Metaverse simulates hospital capabilities and navigation e.g., covid 19 brought a huge number of patients into the hospital, metaverse can simulate the situation at the design stage by knowing the capabilities of the hospital and for building dynamics, like pop-up hospital rooms. Metaverse provides a higher-level understanding of the whole hospital building behaviors and environments by data coming from sensors at objects and people. *"You can track the patients and instruments, like fleet management." (Interviewee 6).* Data produced by sensors from the rooms in the hospital environment and its connection to the virtual environment gives a real understanding of the situation. *"They have glasses for data, obviously the same thing for real-time. And this way you can maybe much, much more efficiently kind of handle the situations. Inventories can be handled more efficiently by floating from many angles" (Interviewee 6).*

Use Case 2 (Improvement of Medical Workflow). A common use case involves the urgency of preparing for a critical surgical procedure, especially when there is preliminary information about a severely injured patient arriving via ambulance. *"When a patient is coming to an ambulance, it's a big mess in the hospital because they are calling to each other and we need to be prepared. It's coming, it's coming. And then where do we have free space and where are the needed instruments and equipment?" (Interviewee 1).* The efficient planning and coordination of essential medical devices, equipment, operation rooms, and estimated arrival time at various locations are crucial but often challenging to accomplish on short notice.

Use case 3 (Surgery Modeling). Some initial experiences about metaverse have been gathered, e.g., through 3D modeling of the skull, which is seen as a huge benefit in specific processes of diagnosing head-related illnesses. *"Doctors could be with VR glasses on with zero latency connection in real-time seeing how the operations work and capture the movement seeing what happening. With pictures from the machine, you cannot see and move." (Interviewee 7).* VR technologies, e.g. latest video device can get realistic images on VR that add value to telemedicine. The treatment will not solely rely on pictures and videos but allow doctors to see real situations in VR. Data safety and security are very important for metaverse usage in hospitals, *"I think the networks were closed so that you had black on service and hope on data handling inside of buildings." (Interviewee 2).* Therefore, the indoor and local network of 6G is needed.

Use Case 4 (Situational Awareness of Patients/Hospital - Mobility/Location/Navigating/Tracking). Remote monitoring of a patient in a remote location, e.g., at home, whose real-time vital data is available, and the doctor needs to make decisions for the care actions of local professionals beside the patient. *"Some visions foresee hospital beds at homes, increasing the need for situational awareness. The response will be much faster when we see this happening in real-time, e.g., by metaverse" (Interviewee*

7). 6G will enable the positioning of various objects. This can be utilized in prompt indoor navigation of personnel, patients, or visitors. With 6G capabilities, data is sent and processed in real time, allowing for immediate alarms if a critical event occurs. Tracking is essential to determine the locations of machines and equipment, as well as doctors and patients. Wireless solutions enable not only the mobility of patients and doctors but also allow machines and equipment to be positioned, tracked, and moved to the required locations. Instead of wasting time fetching instruments along long corridors, the personnel could call the autonomously navigating instruments to arrive in the operations room.

Use Case 5 (Pain Management and Mental Therapy). Experiments show good results in the treatment of chronic pain or mental illness with virtual technology like VR because with chronic conditions, patients are not willing to travel to the hospital all the time when they need to talk with doctors, particularly for some patients with serious illness and disabilities. *"Building services for those patients who are at home almost 24 h per day, would be a huge potential. In the metaverse, those people will be able to travel around the world and see different places, engaging in various activities, as technology advances and realism improves. It's beneficial for pain management and mental health."* *(Interviewee 7).*

Use Case 6 (Training and Education). Metaverse can provide training not only for health professionals but also for healthy individuals and patients. Metaverse supports preventive health and provides guidelines to prevent, reparation e.g., surgery in the virtual situation that can replace health care professionals for counseling. *"We should support healthy people to stay healthy…I think the metaverse is an excellent example of where we can encourage people to exercise, build virtual agents to be their friends, and guide them in their daily lives to improve their health"* *(Interviewee 5).*

The hospital-tested metaverse environment will guide prevention in the correct direction because the internet is full of information regarding diseases, but not all the information is valid and represents the true situation *"metaverse we can even develop these kinds of new tools of screening evidence, you know, making sure that what we present to our patients is correct information".*

For patient training, a similar example is also mentioned by Interviewee 7: *"(For first pregnancy), training for delivery is common in Finland. With metaverse, it can bring pregnant women to reality and get realistic ideas and understanding in the real, specific local hospital how things will be work and what kind of preparation would be and how the delivery will be done there."*

Education of new healthcare professionals in immersive environments supports learning of medical tasks and processes after which working in the real environment is more familiar without having worked there before. *"A good example is training in the automotive industry by VR, the accident rate dropped like 60% after training with VR solutions."* *(Interviewee 4).*

Analyzing KVs of Identified Use Cases. We apply the adapted 6G visioning framework by answering the fundamental questions of actions to be taken for building 6G future networks proposed by [35]. The related questions in [35] help to identify value addressed by use cases described in interviews. Since this study focuses on the healthcare context, the usage scenarios will be based on the hospital patient care pathways and their situational usage. The study results are presented in Table 2.

Table 2. Analysis of use cases: expected outcomes, usage scenarios, capabilities and impacts.

Use Cases	Expected Outcomes	Usage Scenarios	Capabilities	Impact
1 Designing smart hospital	*Why are we developing 6G?*	*What purpose are the users using 6G for? How are the users using 6G?*	*How do we make 6G function?*	What is the impact on future hospital)
	Hospital room usage optimization	Smart hospitals	Connectivity	Efficiency
	Matching and positioning hospital rooms, equipment, and human resources	Room positioning	Positioning	Saving
		Simulation of different combinations and purposes of uses of hospital rooms	Flexibility	Local services
		Development of processes	Mobility	
		Acquisition of instruments		
		Education		
2 Improvement of medical workflow	Patient Safety	Emergency	Mobility	Efficient usage of resources
	Hospital work process optimization	Moving wards	Tracing, Tracking, Navigating	Situational awareness
	Precise location	Location sharing	Sensing	
		Patient monitoring	Real-time data and computing	
3 Surgery modeling	Patient safety	Surgery process development	Flexibility	Sensing
	Patient monitoring	Remote surgery	Mobility	Data capabilities
	Decreasing errors		Information security & privacy	Wireless solutions
	Quick		Reliability	Local network
	Emergency response		Local services	Reliability

(*continued*)

Table 2. (*continued*)

Use Cases	Expected Outcomes	Usage Scenarios	Capabilities	Impact
4 Situational awareness	Remote monitoring, tracing, and tracking in local hospitals	Emergency	Real-time data	Sensing
	Moving wards	Ward transfer	Local services	Positioning
		Hospital transfer		Real-data capabilities
5 Pain management and mental therapy	Pain management	Rehabilitation	High-speed, Connectivity	Data capabilities
	Mental therapy			
6 Training and education	Preventive health and patient training	Accurate information	Simulation and visualization	Connectivity
	Research, training, and education	Education and hospital, nursing homes	Sustainability	Sustainability

The crucial link between the metaverse and 6G lies in real-time data connection and analysis, focusing on the effective utilization of diverse data sources such as patient information, environmental factors, sensors, and medical devices. In this context, connectivity facilitates connections among people, physical objects, and virtual realism through data. The illustrated use cases indicate that mobility is important in hospitals to connect patients, doctors, nurses, and needed medical equipment and machines, particularly during emergencies, and for remote patient monitoring. Mobility, e.g., mobility in ambulances and its connection to hospital environments, is critical to ensuring patient safety. Seamless data transmission across department boundaries will enhance mobility in ambulances, streamlining and seamlessly coordinating people, equipment, and facilities in a hospital environment, leading to situational awareness and more effective and timely responses to emergencies.

Situation awareness is one of the key values identified from use cases. To support situation awareness, a seamless wireless connection is required for real-time communication among different objects, e.g. sensors from patients, real-time data from medical instruments and equipment, and location and positioning of health staff. Flexibility allows optimized usage and combination of hospital wards and rooms without having to move around the equipment. Due to the sensitive medical and treatment data and safety operations, a secure, closed indoor network is needed to ensure the stability and safety of data.

Metaverse requires more reliable connections and faster data processing speeds to support the efficient exchange and collaboration of a large network of interconnected devices and sensors for hospitals. The fifth Generation (5G) communication network cannot meet the growing demands and requirements for metaverse use cases that require latency and reliability of short-packet transmission [41, 42]. Therefore, Six-Generation

(6G) Networks are expected to eliminate time and space barriers to optimize healthcare workflow [43] and meet the demand for seamless connectivity and ubiquitous intelligence [15]. The 6G is posited to support massive connectivity, empower AI and ML for real-time data analytics [44], and support the metaverse development for health practices and services with energy-efficient solutions.

Drawing from the use cases identified and analyzed, this paper has identified the key values and related capabilities, usage scenarios, and impact of 6G and metaverse in hospitals shown in Fig. 2.

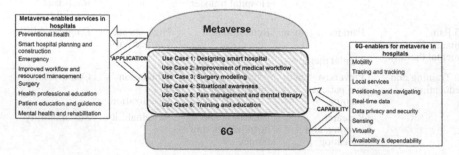

Fig. 2. Services, enablers, and use cases for 6G-enabled hospital metaverse.

The evolution of the metaverse will rely on the network of 6G as core infrastructure and services. 6G, as a general-purpose technology, offers the foundational platform and capability necessary for metaverse enabled services and its development [45] in hospitals. The 6G network alone, in the absence of metaverse as a practical application, would probably lack some key characteristics essential in the healthcare context. Thus, the metaverse, an emerging technology, is integrated within the 6G framework to unleash its capabilities contributing to each stage of the patient care pathway from emergency to rehabilitation. Consequently, the development of both metaverse and 6G will progress in tandem, hand in hand, offering local services in hospitals.

4 Conclusion

Technology advancement helps to develop hospital processes further and more effectively, leading to quality-of-care improvement and cost savings. The 5G and beyond or 6G technologies cannot bring any short-term solutions, but the challenging state of health care surely generates lots of expectations and requirements for the upcoming technologies under development. 6G is expected to play a significant role in telemedicine [46], remote surgery, fast processing of high data volumes, and other healthcare instruments and applications by providing ultra-reliable and low-latency connections for real-time medical procedures and diagnostics.

In the developing process of the 6G-enabled metaverse, it's important to consider key values, stakeholder needs, and healthcare regulations in the early stages of R&D technology projects to prevent future bottlenecks. The existing infrastructure, somewhat antiquated, faces challenges in meeting the demands of new technology, such as computer processing speed and memory capacity, and needs sufficient investment to build and renew the necessary infrastructure.

Understanding the needs and key values of the 6G-enabled metaverse will allow tailored solutions to their specific requirements, consequently diminishing healthcare professionals' resistance to the burdens of adopting new technology, including the associated training, and learning. Local services of 6G-enabled metaverse are needed, e.g. protecting patient-sensitive information and precise positioning of people and objects. The anticipated integration of 6G and metaverse technologies in hospital settings is predicted to create a demand for new roles distinct from the current stakeholders in the hospital. It's projected that the Information and Communications Technology (ICT) departments of hospitals, along with national Mobile Network Operators (MNOs), will not be solely responsible for managing the upcoming local 6G infrastructures. New businesses will emerge, but the current regulations that may slow down the process of healthcare innovation should be reformed to better support their emergence and development.

For managerial implication, the 6G-enabled metaverse should have: (1) support from the government and different organizations for funding; (2) an updated network to ensure connectivity and reliability; (3) investment in hardware and equipment that can fulfill metaverse requirements; (4) strong leadership from hospital management to support its development; (5) stakeholder engagement, especially from end-users, in the development process to guide the direction for building the 6G-enabled metaverse environment; and (6) regulations that do not hinder the development of using AI models and connectivity between different infrastructures for data.

Disclosure of Interests. The authors have no competing interests.

References

1. Cabanillas-Carbonell, M., Pérez-Martínez, J., Yáñez, J.A.: 5G technology in the digital transformation of healthcare, a systematic review. Sustainability (Basel, Switzerland) **15**, 3178 (2023). https://doi.org/10.3390/su15043178
2. Schiavone, F., Mancini, D., Leone, D., Lavorato, D.: Digital business models and ridesharing for value co-creation in healthcare: a multi-stakeholder ecosystem analysis. Technol. Forecast. Soc. Change. **166**, 120647 (2021). https://doi.org/10.1016/j.techfore.2021.120647
3. Kim, Y., Lee, S.: Energy-efficient wireless hospital sensor networking for remote patient monitoring. Inf. Sci. (N.Y.) **282**, 332–349 (2014). https://doi.org/10.1016/j.ins.2014.05.056
4. Wang, G., et al.: Development of metaverse for intelligent healthcare. Nat. Mach. Intell. **4**, 922–929 (2022). https://doi.org/10.1038/s42256-022-00549-6
5. Ahokangas, P., Aagaard, A.: The Changing World of Mobile Communications: 5G, 6G and the Future of Digital Services. Springer, Cham (2023)
6. Yang, D., et al.: Expert consensus on the metaverse in medicine. Clin. eHealth **5**, 1–9 (2022). https://doi.org/10.1016/J.CEH.2022.02.001

7. Qi, Q., et al.: Enabling technologies and tools for digital twin. J. Manuf. Syst. **58**, 3–21 (2021). https://doi.org/10.1016/j.jmsy.2019.10.001
8. Hansen, S., Baroody, A.J.: Beyond the boundaries of care: electronic health records and the changing practices of healthcare. Inf. Organ. **33**, 100477 (2023). https://doi.org/10.1016/j.infoandorg.2023.100477
9. Gagnon, M.-P., Ngangue, P., Payne-Gagnon, J., Desmartis, M.: M-Health adoption by healthcare professionals: a systematic review. J. Am. Med. Inform. Assoc. **23**, 212–220 (2016). https://doi.org/10.1093/jamia/ocv052
10. Lavallee, D.C., et al.: mHealth and patient generated health data: stakeholder perspectives on opportunities and barriers for transforming healthcare. mHealth **6** (2020). mHealth. (2019)
11. Canfell, O.J., Littlewood, R., Burton-Jones, A., Sullivan, C.: Digital health and precision prevention: shifting from disease-centred care to consumer-centred health. Aust. Health Rev. **46**, 279–283 (2022)
12. Hood, L., Flores, M.: A personal view on systems medicine and the emergence of proactive P4 medicine: predictive, preventive, personalized and participatory. N. Biotechnol. **29**, 613–624 (2012). https://doi.org/10.1016/J.NBT.2012.03.004
13. Hood, L., Auffray, C.: Participatory medicine: a driving force for revolutionizing healthcare. Genome Med. **5**, 110 (2013). https://doi.org/10.1186/gm514
14. Wang, X., Mei, J., Cui, S., Wang, C.-X., Shen, X.S.: Realizing 6G: the operational goals, enabling technologies of future networks, and value-oriented intelligent multi-dimensional multiple access. IEEE Netw. **37**, 10–17 (2023). https://doi.org/10.1109/MNET.001.2200429
15. Nekovee, M., Ayaz, F.: Vision, enabling technologies, and scenarios for a 6G-enabled internet of verticals (6G-IoV). Future Internet **15**, 57 (2023). https://doi.org/10.3390/fi15020057
16. Adeogun, R., Berardinelli, G., Mogensen, P.E.: Enhanced interference management for 6G in-X subnetworks. IEEE Access **10**, 45784–45798 (2022). https://doi.org/10.1109/ACCESS.2022.3170694
17. Janjua, M.B., Duranay, A.E., Arslan, H.: Role of wireless communication in healthcare system to cater disaster situations under 6G vision. Front. Commun. Netw. **1** (2020)
18. Serôdio, C., Cunha, J., Candela, G., Rodriguez, S., Sousa, X.R., Branco, F.: The 6G ecosystem as support for IoE and private networks: vision, requirements, and challenges. Future Internet **15**, 348 (2023). https://doi.org/10.3390/fi15110348
19. Berardinelli, G., et al.: Extreme communication in 6G: vision and challenges for 'in-X' subnetworks. IEEE Open J. Commun. Soc. **2**, 2516–2535 (2021). https://doi.org/10.1109/OJCOMS.2021.3121530
20. Giang Barrera, K., Shah, D.: Marketing in the metaverse: conceptual understanding, framework, and research agenda. J. Bus. Res. **155**, 113420 (2023). https://doi.org/10.1016/j.jbusres.2022.113420
21. Song, Y.-T., Qin, J.: Metaverse and personal healthcare. Procedia Comput. Sci. **210**, 189–197 (2022). https://doi.org/10.1016/j.procs.2022.10.136
22. Pinheiro Silva, T., Fernanda Andrade-Bortoletto, M., Queiroz Freitas, D., Oliveira-Santos, C., Mitsunari Takeshita, W.: Metaverse and oral and maxillofacial radiology: where do they meet? Eur. J. Radiol. **170**, 111210 (2023). https://doi.org/10.1016/j.ejrad.2023.111210
23. Ghaednia, H., et al.: Augmented and virtual reality in spine surgery, current applications and future potentials. Spine J. **21**, 1617–1625 (2021). https://doi.org/10.1016/J.SPINEE.2021.03.018
24. Liu, Z., Ren, L., Xiao, C., Zhang, K., Demian, P.: Virtual reality aided therapy towards health 4.0: a two-decade bibliometric analysis. Int. J. Environ. Res. Public Health **19**(3), 1525 (2022). https://doi.org/10.3390/IJERPH19031525
25. Khan, S., Arslan, T., Ratnarajah, T.: Digital twin perspective of fourth industrial and healthcare revolution. IEEE Access **10**, 25732–25754 (2022). https://doi.org/10.1109/ACCESS.2022.3156062

26. Kamel Boulos, M.N., Zhang, P.: Digital twins: from personalised medicine to precision public health. J. Pers. Med. **11**, 745 (2021). https://doi.org/10.3390/JPM11080745
27. Yang, D., Zhou, J., Song, Y., Sun, M., Bai, C.: Metaverse in medicine. Clin. eHealth **5**, 39–43 (2022). https://doi.org/10.1016/J.CEH.2022.04.002
28. Barricelli, B.R., Casiraghi, E., Gliozzo, J., Petrini, A., Valtolina, S.: Human digital twin for fitness management. IEEE Access **8**, 26637–26664 (2020). https://doi.org/10.1109/ACCESS.2020.2971576
29. Björnsson, B., et al.: Digital twins to personalize medicine. Genome Med. **12**, 4 (2019). https://doi.org/10.1186/s13073-019-0701-3
30. Latva-aho Kari, M.L.: Key Drivers and Research Challenges for 6G Ubiquitous Wireless Intelligence. University of Oulu, Oulu (2019)
31. Bessant, J., Künne, C., Möslein, K.: Opening Up Healthcare Innovation: Innovation Solutions for a 21st Century Healthcare System. Advanced Institute for Management Research (2012)
32. Yrjölä, S., Matinmikko-Blue, M., Ahokangas, P.: Developing 6G visions with stakeholder analysis of 6G ecosystem. In: 2023 Joint European Conference on Networks and Communications & 6G Summit (EuCNC/6G Summit), pp. 705–710. IEEE (2023)
33. Bouhafs, F., Raschellà, A., Mackay, M., den Hartog, F.: A spectrum management platform architecture to enable a sharing economy in 6G. Future Internet **14**, 309 (2022). https://doi.org/10.3390/fi14110309
34. Matinmikko-Blue, M., Yrjölä, S., Ahokangas, P., Hämmäinen, H.: Analysis of 5G spectrum awarding decisions: how do different countries consider emerging local 5G networks? Presented at the (2021)
35. Ahokangas, P., Matinmikko-Blue, M., Yrjölä, S.: Envisioning a future-proof global 6G from business, regulation, and technology perspectives. IEEE Commun. Mag. **61**, 72–78 (2022)
36. Vaz, N., Araujo, C.A.S.: Service design for the transformation of healthcare systems: a systematic review of literature. Health Serv. Manage Res. 09514848231194846 (2023). https://doi.org/10.1177/09514848231194846
37. Wikström, G.S.S.A.M.I.S.R.-A.G.G.B.S.O. Icon G.A.O. Icon D.P.H.M.-H.H.H.-S., Lund, D.: What societal values will 6G address? (2022)
38. Yrjola, S., Ahokangas, P., Matinmikko-Blue, M.: Value creation and capture from technology innovation in the 6G Era. IEEE Access **10**, 16299–16319 (2022). https://doi.org/10.1109/ACCESS.2022.3149590
39. Patton, M.Q.: Qualitative Research & Evaluation Methods. Sage, Thousand Oaks (2002)
40. Collingridge, D.S., Gantt, E.E.: The quality of qualitative research. Am. J. Med. Qual. **34**, 439–445 (2019). https://doi.org/10.1177/1062860619873187
41. Tang, F., Chen, X., Zhao, M., Kato, N.: The roadmap of communication and networking in 6G for the metaverse. IEEE Wirel. Commun. **30**, 72–81 (2023). https://doi.org/10.1109/MWC.019.2100721
42. Cao, J., et al.: Toward industrial metaverse: age of information, latency and reliability of short-packet transmission in 6G. IEEE Wirel. Commun. **30**, 40–47 (2023). https://doi.org/10.1109/MWC.2001.2200396
43. Giordani, M., Polese, M., Mezzavilla, M., Rangan, S., Zorzi, M.: Toward 6G networks: use cases and technologies. IEEE Commun. Mag. **58**, 55–61 (2020). https://doi.org/10.1109/MCOM.001.1900411
44. Bang, A., Kamal, K.K., Joshi, P., Bhatia, K.: 6G: the next giant leap for AI and ML. Procedia Comput. Sci. **218**, 310–317 (2023). https://doi.org/10.1016/j.procs.2023.01.013
45. Teece, D.J.: Profiting from innovation in the digital economy: enabling technologies, standards, and licensing models in the wireless world. Res. Policy **47**, 1367–1387 (2018). https://doi.org/10.1016/j.respol.2017.01.015
46. Shin, H., et al.: The future service scenarios of 6G telecommunications technology. Telecommun. Policy **48**(2), 102678 (2023). https://doi.org/10.1016/j.telpol.2023.102678

An LSTM Framework for the Effective Screening of Dementia for Deployment on Edge Devices

Bernard Wilkie[1]([✉]) [ID], Karla Muñoz Esquivel[1] [ID], and Jamie Roche[2] [ID]

[1] Department of Computing, Atlantic Technological University, Port Rd, Letterkenny F92 FC93, Co. Donegal, Ireland
bernardwilkie@gmail.com
[2] Department of Mechatronics, Atlantic Technological University, Sligo, Ash Lane, Co Sligo F91 YW50, Ireland

Abstract. Dementia is a series of neurodegenerative disorders that affect 1 in 4 people over the age of 80 and can greatly reduce the quality of life of those afflicted. Alzheimer's disease (AD) is the most common variation, accounting for roughly 60% of cases. The current financial cost of these diseases is an estimated $1.3 trillion per year. While treatments are available to help patients maintain their mental function and slow disease progression, many of those with AD are asymptomatic in the early stages, resulting in late diagnosis. The addition of the routine testing needed for an effective level of early diagnosis would put a costly burden on both patients and healthcare systems. This research proposes a novel framework for the modelling of dementia, designed for deployment in edge hardware. This work extracts a wide variety of thoroughly researched Electroencephalogram (EEG) features, and through extensive feature selection, model testing, tuning, and edge optimization, we propose two novel Long Short-Term Memory (LSTM) neural networks. The first, uses 4 EEG sensors and can classify AD and Frontotemporal Dementia from cognitively normal (CN) subjects. The second, requires 3 EEG sensors and can classify AD from CN subjects. This is achieved with optimisation that reduces the model size by $83\times$, latency by $3.7\times$, and performs with an accuracy of 98%. Comparative analysis with existing research shows this performance exceeds current less portable techniques. The deployment of this model in edge hardware could aid in routine testing, providing earlier diagnosis of dementia, reducing the strain on healthcare systems, and increasing the quality of life for those afflicted with the disease.

Keywords: Electroencephalogram · Dementia · Alzheimer's Disease · Frontotemporal Dementia · Machine Learning · Long Short-Term Memory · Deep Learning · Edge Deployment

1 Introduction

Dementia is defined as a series of disorders which progressively affects a person's cognitive abilities and is present in roughly 25% of those over the age of 80 [1]. The most common form is Alzheimer's disease (AD), representing roughly 60% of cases. This is

© The Author(s) 2024
M. Särestöniemi et al. (Eds.): NCDHWS 2024, CCIS 2083, pp. 21–37, 2024.
https://doi.org/10.1007/978-3-031-59080-1_2

followed by Frontotemporal (FTD) representing roughly 10% of cases [2]. The exact cause of FTD is not fully understood however AD is caused by the build of plaques around the posterior region of the brain that interfere with the electrical transmission between neurons [3]. Early stages of the disease can often be asymptomatic, leading to late diagnosis. While dementia is currently incurable, the efficacy of treatment that maintains mental function and slows the progression of the disease is greatly increased with early diagnosis [4].

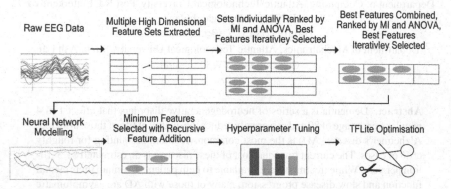

Fig. 1. Depicts the proposed Framework for Dementia Classification. Given raw Electroencephalogram (EEG) individually ranked features are extracted before being combined and iteratively selected. A tuned Neural Network is then optimised for EDGE operation using TensorFlow Lite.

The current state of the art for dementia diagnosis is a combination of Medical History and cognitive testing [5], Magnetic Resonance Imagery [5], Positron Emission Tomography (PET) scans [6], Cerebral Spinal Fluid [7], and the identification of specific biomarkers found during blood testing [8]. Collectively these diagnostic methods are effective, however, the overall cost and intrusive nature add increased pressure on the patient and the healthcare system.

This highlights the need for an accurate, easily accessible, automated solution for the routine screening of dementia in primary care centres, this would in-theory function as a triage system to refer patients for further testing. Advances in this field have the potential to reduce the load on healthcare systems, aid in early diagnoses of dementia and therefore enhance the quality of life for those afflicted.

This paper presents a model for dementia classification using Electroencephalogram (EEG) data. The framework, depicted in Fig. 1, is our process for feature extraction, dimensionality reduction, and modelling as designed for deployment in an edge device, minimizing electrodes, without sacrificing classification accuracy. The edge device acts as a routine testing platform for early dementia identification, releasing healthcare resources to enhance patients' quality of life.

The hypothesis, was to examine if a framework can be developed to produce a lightweight machine learning (ML) model designed for deployment in a minimal edge device with a view to mass routine patient screening and triage of potential dementia cases, this would be particularly beneficial in cases where a patient is asymptomatic or shows sign of Mild Cognitive Impairment (MCI). Cases could then be referred for further gold-standard screening in the effective diagnosis of dementia. The primary contributions of this research are in the framework for modelling dementia, the required electrode inputs and their features selected, and the Long Short-Term Memory (LSTM) architectures attained.

The rest of the paper is laid out as follows: Sect. 2 reports on the related work in the areas of diagnosis of dementia, feature selection, and Machine Learning (ML) models of dementia is covered. Section 3 details the research methodology used to build and evaluate this model, and its implementation. The results are analysed and discussed in the Sect. 4 and Sect. 5, respectively. Before concluding this work in Sect. 6.

2 Related Work

There is a wide variety of screening techniques used to assist in the diagnosis of dementia. Ranging from non-intrusive to intrusive methods, the journey to an accurate diagnosis usually begins in primary care centres with psychometric tests to detect a pattern of loss of skills and function. More recently, blood test biomarkers have shown to be objectively measurable characteristic used to indicate a pathogenic process to improve diagnostic accuracy [9]. However, in the absence of addition intrusive measures measure such as Cerebrospinal (CSF) fluid examination, and non-intrusive Positron Emission Tomography (PET), Computed Tomography (CT) and Magnetic Resonance Imaging (MRI), these techniques lack the holistic approach needed for an accurate and early diagnosis [10]. This section discusses the relevant related work reviewed in order to devise a novel approach for creating the proposed dementia model.

2.1 Psychometric Tests

Cognitive screening tools can provide a time-efficient and objective initial evaluation of cognitive function. For example, the Mini-Mental State Examination (MMSE) is a standardised clinical test used to assess a patient's cognitive impairment. It consists of eleven questions measuring the patient's abilities in orientation, concentration, and attention. The precise ranges are debated as factors such as age and education influence the cutoff. Cognitively normal (CN) generally receives a score between 27 and 30. The cutoff for MCI is normally in the range of 21 to 23, and the middle to late stage of cognitive decline receives scores lower than the MCI cutoff [11].

An alternative to MMSE, is the Addenbrooke's Cognitive Examination (ACE) [12]. The ACE assess six cognitive domains using 29 questions with a total 100-point test battery. The cutoff for MCI is 88, and the assessment technique is high reliability with a 93% sensitivity. Questions featured to Candidates include verbal analogies, arithmetic calculations, spatial relations number series puzzles, comprehension, and reading comprehension. Regardless of how well psychometric tests preform they should be considered as a component of a thorough assessment [13].

2.2 Medical Imaging

For a more holistic approach to diagnosing dementia, psychometric tests should be used in conjunction with Magnetic Resonance Imaging (MRI), Computed Tomography (CT), and Positron Emission Tomography (PET) scans. Authors in [14] researched the benefits of MRI and CT in diagnosing dementia. Their research showed CT imaging excelled in the identification cerebrovascular damage to the white matter of the brain, and MRI generated structural images of the brain can be used to study blood flow used in differentiating frontotemporal dementia.

In a similar vein researcher in [15] report on routine clinical use of hybrid PET/MR in patients with suspected dementia of patients in a memory clinic. The study revealed that a condensed hybrid PET/MRI protocol offers valuable supplementary information, significantly impacting clinical diagnosis and the management of patients in a considerable portion of cases, as compared to individual PET and CT scans. Evidently MRI, PET and CT scans are useful in detecting precursors to dementia, Alzheimer's disease, Frontotemporal cognitive decline [6].

2.3 Biochemical Markers

The financial implications and potential for creating congestion within an overburdened health system, should medical imaging be used as a primary tool for the diagnosis dementia, is great [14, 15]. Biochemical markers such as Cerebral Spinal Fluid, which is a protective liquid flowing around the brain and spinal cord, have proven to be a frugal approach to screen for dementia. Unfortunately, biochemical markers need to be extracted from the body through invasive test, that either involve a spinal tap, lumbar puncture, or blood tests. Analysis of the fluid can determine the presence of certain biomarkers indicating certain dementia diseases with an accuracy in excess of 80% [7].

Taking a different approach author in [16] combined data from four distinct cohorts to assess the positive and negative predictive values of an Alzheimer's disease (AD) blood test when applied in primary care settings. Utilising blood samples from 1329 participants, Random Forests analyses were employed to develop a blood screening tool. The tool demonstrated positive predictive values (PPV) and negative predictive values (NPV) of 0.81 and 0.95, respectively. For mild cognitive impairment, the PPV and NPV were 0.74 and 0.93, respectively.

Similarly, authors in [17] focused on the accumulation peroxidation of major phospholipids (e.g., phosphatidylcholine (PtdCho)) and degradation of antioxidative phospholipids (e.g., ethanolamine plasmalogen (PlsEtn)) in the brain. It was found that individuals with AD exhibited reduced levels of PlsEtn species in their plasma, particularly those containing the docosahexaenoic acid (DHA) component. Furthermore, patients with AD demonstrated lower PlsEtn levels and elevated PtdCho hydroperoxide (PCOOH) levels in their red blood cells (RBCs). In both AD and control blood samples, the levels of RBC PCOOH tend to align with plasma $A\beta40$ levels, and distinct correlations were observed between each PlsEtn species and plasma $A\beta$.

In consonant with the aforementioned findings' authors in [8] reviewed 50 studies comparing concentrations of $A\beta40$, $A\beta42$, t-tau, and YKL-40 in 7303 patients to established, that blood testing provides highly accurate results (93%) in detecting dementia, with β-amyloid and t-tau being key biomarkers. Despite their intrusive nature, biochemical markers as a screening tool for dementia have their benefits. Although screening tools are assessed based on their effectiveness in accurately discerning individuals with dementia from those without, the psychological distress caused by their intrusive nature is often overlooked [18]. An overview of the intrusive nature, cost, and portability, of dementia screening techniques using Biochemical Markers and Medical Imaging is shown in Table 1.

Table 1. An Overview of Diagnostic Methods.

Method	Invasive	Portable	Cost	Acc (%)
Spinal Fluid Test	Yes	No	Medium	80
MRI/CT/PET	No	No	High	89
Blood Test	Yes	No	Medium	93–95

2.4 Dementia Features and Modelling

Less intrusive, substantial more economical and more portable than medical imaging equipment is the EEG. An EEG is a measurement device that detects electrical signals generated from brain activity and is a popular choice for a variety of applications including brain monitoring, task automation via human-machine interfaces, and emotion detection. Standardised methods for electrode placement are set by the International Federation of Clinical Neurophysiology and include the 10-20 and 10-10 systems with 19 and 63 sensory electrodes, respectively.

Several time and frequency domain features are thoroughly researched in academic literature. Research from Staudinger and Polikar, and Puri et al. [19, 20] showed the efficacy of classifying dementia with signal complexity, entropy, and Hjorth Parameters. When analysing EEG data in the frequency domain, Spiegel and Renna [21] noted that cognitive impairment due to various mental diseases can be "characterized by decreased power and coherence in the alpha/beta frequency band while increased power and coherence in the delta/theta band".

Further research from Claudio Babilonia et al. [22] observed a particular correlation between AD patients and the posterior electrodes in the alpha frequency band. The performance of extracting power spectrum density features was also observed by Tavares et al. [23] and Alessandrini et al. [24]. Tavares et al. performed a backward wrapper method for feature selection to reduce dimensionality and testing with the best-performing models Linear Regression (LR) and Support Vector Machine (SVM). Alessandrini et al. applied Principal Component Analysis (PCA) to EEG data to reduce dimensionality and leveraged an LSTM to classify AD with an accuracy of 98%.

The use of PCA in research where the goal is the reduce the physical feature space would not be suitable as it would obfuscate the underlying sensor information however, the author's proposed architecture was used as a base template in the work with multiple

Table 2. An Overview of Dementia Classification Methods.

Authors	Electrodes	Method	Acc (%)
Tavares, G. *et al.* (2019) [23]	13	LR/SVM	97.1
Alessandrini, M. *et al.* (2022)[24]	16	LSTM	97.9
Puri. *et al.*(2022)[20]	6	SVM	97.5

variations tested for each network type. An overview of key comparative ML methods or models can be observed in Table 2.

In summary, the current gold standard method for diagnosing dementia involves access to healthcare staff and laboratory resources for analysing the blood samples, which in the current context of scarce and overloaded healthcare systems is not viable or functional. Therefore, the use of EEG signals in combination with an LSTM model for screening of dementia promises a suitable solution for this problem.

3 Methodology

This section centres on describing the dataset employed by this work and the series of steps involved in the creation of the framework used to attain the proposed dementia model.

3.1 Dataset

A dataset containing EEG recordings from 88 subjects was sourced from [25]. Of these, 36 were diagnosed with AD, 23 with FTD, and 29 were said to be CN subjects. Information on the results of a Mini-Mental State Exam was included for each subject, providing a score ranging from 30 to 0 relating to their individual cognitive decline. The original recordings were sourced from the Department of Neurology in the general hospital of Thessaloniki, Greece. The EEG used was a Nihon Kohden 2100 with 19 scalp electrodes (Fp1, Fp2, F7, F3, Fz, F4, F8, T3, C3, Cz, C4, T4, T5, P3, Pz, P4, T6, O1, and O2) and 2 reference electrodes (A1 and A2) according to the 10-20 international system. Clinical protocols were followed during the recording with each subject in the sitting position and their eyes closed. The average record time per subject was 13.5 min at a sampling frequency of 500 Hz, leading to a dataset with 35.6 million rows of information. Preprocessing steps for the dataset include a Butterworth band-pass filter of 0.5 Hz–45 Hz and were referenced to the A1 and A2 electrodes. Artifact removals were performed at the data source and included Artifact Subspace Reconstruction routine (ASR) and the RunICA algorithm for classifying eye and jaw artifacts via the automatic classification routine ICLabel.

3.2 Data Preprocessing

Data is segmented into training, validation, and test groups with a 60:20:20 random split based on subject identification numbers. This aids in building a more robust solution by ensuring none of the readings from a subject assigned to the training set are given to the testing model for inference. The dataset incorporates details such as age, gender, and severity. All efforts were made to ensure a fair distribution among test groups. Due to the limited sample size of 88 subjects, there is a potential for bias to permeate the framework, the authors implemented thorough measures to mitigate this risk. Keeping this in consideration, two binary classification models were developed using the dataset. The first will classify both FTD and AD from CN, and the second will classify AD from CN. A test set comprised of 19 subjects is reserved for the AD-FTD model, and a set of 12 subjects is reserved for AD only model.

Initial research suggested AD patients are more likely to be asymptomatic in the early stages of disease progression. The decision to build a separate model for AD and CN classification is made under the estimation that it would require less features, and therefore sensors, leading to a lower-cost platform that is more accessible.

3.3 Feature Extraction

A wide range of time and frequency domain features were extracted from the EEG data. The following is a summary of the 5 feature sets extracted at 2 and 4-s sampling windows.

- Statistics extracted included minimum, maximum, mean, range, standard deviation, energy, and autocorrelation. This set totals 133 features.
- The metric used to capture the tighter grouping of signal pairs is Mean Absolute Difference (MAD). This was extracted for each unique pair of sensors. This set totals 171 features.
- Hjorth Parameters extracted include Activity, Mobility and Complexity. This set totals 57 features.
- In calculating power spectrum densities, total, mean, and relative power (the sum of a frequency band relative to the sum of the power spectrum) are extracted. This is done using the Welsch method of deriving the mean of a series of Fast Fourier Transforms (FFT) to leverage the computational gains of the FFT when dealing with nonstationary signals [26]. This set totals 255 features.
- Cross Coherence is a statistical measure that measures the linear relationship between signal pairs at a specified frequency band [27]. This is calculated for each unique pair of sensors, at each frequency band. This set totals 855 features.

3.4 Initial Feature Selection

The goal of this research is to use the least number of features and therefore sensory electrodes. The most accurate method of selecting features would be to evaluate each feature pair, triple, and potentially higher-order combination until no more performance gains can be made. The total number of features extracted is 1,471, generating 1.1 million unique pairs for testing. As this is an inefficient use of time and computing, the least number of features for each category set was reduced by first ranking importance with Mutual Information (MI) [28], and iteratively testing and adding new features with benchmark models Support Vector Classifier (SVC) and K-Nearest Neighbour (KNN) [20] until no more accuracy gains can be made.

Features selected from the previous stage are then grouped and ranked with both MI and ANOVA. The process of testing and iteratively adding and retesting features until no more performance gains can be made is repeated. This provides a core number of features and the process of building the neural network models can begin.

3.5 Modelling

In building a performant Neural Network (NN) for the classification of dementia, a series of artificial neural networks were tested. This includes a simple sequential network known for its ability to model complex nonlinear relationships, a recurrent network which excels at capturing temporal information, and a more advanced type of recurrent network, the Long-Short Term Memory (LSTM) network, with the ability to maintain information over extended sequences. Once a performant model was chosen, model tunning with a large set of hyperparameters was performed.

3.6 Final Feature Selection and Optimisation

The tuned model is chosen as the testing metric for the remaining features. Features are scaled by removing the mean and scaling to unit variance. The process begins with testing each feature in isolation, then each feature pair, and each potentially higher-order combination until each model no longer classifies subjects incorrectly. The resulting set is the least number of features and therefore sensory electrodes required by the model to correctly classify the target label. Google's TensorFlow Lite (TFLite) library is leveraged to reduce model size and increase inference speed for edge deployment.

4   Results

This section presents results - graphs and tables - attained from executing each step depicted in the LSTM Framework, which was designed and followed as part of this work to create a model to classify dementia that will be deployed in an edge device. The scores and measurements attained help authors to make informed decisions at each step.

4.1   Feature Selection and Benchmark Results

The resulting reduction in dimensionality of the initial feature selection stage can be seen in Table 3. The modelling was sensitive to small changes, as such metrics Error Count and Mean Error were derived to produce more clarity into the underlying performance. Error Count refers to the number of test subjects incorrectly classified, and Mean Error refers to the mean unrounded prediction error.

Grouping previously selected features and ranking with ANOVA and MI before iteratively testing with SVC highlighted 57 features to be the least amount with the best performance. A confusion matrix of this result can be seen Fig. 2. The diagonal cells indicate true positives that are correctly classified. The off-diagonal cells indicate false positives that are incorrectly classified. The overall accuracy for the classifier was 0.93. The Precision and Recall were 0.94 and 0.84, respectively.

Table 3. Set Stage Feature Results.

Data	Method	Features Selected	Error Count	Mean Error	Acc (%)
Statistics	SVC	6	6	0.31	66
MAD	SVC	5	4	0.21	73
Hjorth	SVC	13	5	0.26	75
PSD	SVC	25	4	0.26	75
Coherence	KNN	24	5	0.26	71

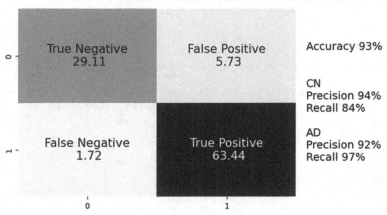

Fig. 2. The Confusion Matrix for the proposed framework trained and tested on the OpenNeuro dataset of 88 EEG recordings from: Alzheimer's disease, Frontotemporal dementia and Healthy subjects.

4.2 Initial Modelling Results

The results from building a simple sequential model showed a high mean error and a drop in accuracy compared to the SVC model. The recurrent model architecture of the base RNN and the LSTM showed a notable improvement in mean error and classification accuracy, an overview of which is provided in Table 4. A selection of hyperparameters tested is shown in Fig. 3, with time step and batch size both showing the best results from a value of 16.

4.3 Final Feature Selection

The success criteria for testing sets in higher order combination with the tuned LSTM was for the model to exceed 95% accuracy and no longer incorrectly classify any of the subjects. This was achieved for the AD-only models with 2 features and for the AD-FTD model with 3 features, Table 5 and Table 6 highlight the ranking of the feature sets. These findings mirror research from [21] and [22], with particular importance from posterior

Table 4. Initial Neural Network Model Results.

Method	Error Count	Mean Error	Acc (%)
SEQ	0.0	0.41	83
RNN	2.0	0.24	84
LSTM	0.0	0.09	91
LSTM Tuned	0.0	0.09	95

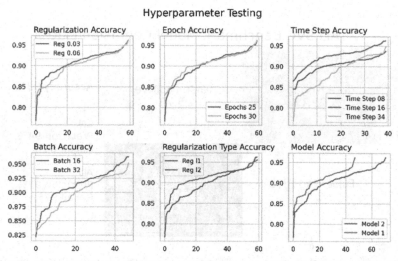

Fig. 3. Plot of Hyperparameter Results, showing the Regularization Accuracy, Epoch Accuracy, Time Step Accuracy, Batch Accuracy, Regularization Type Accuracy and Model Accuracy.

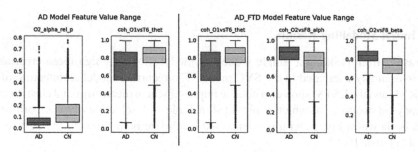

Fig. 4. Box Plot Value Distribution of Selected AD and AD_FTD Features After Removing the Mean and Scaling to Unit Variance.

electrodes on the alpha frequency band. Figure 4 shows the distribution of AD Model Feature Value Range and AD_FTD Model Feature Value Range, respectively.

Table 5. Alzheimer's Disease Model Feature Sets.

Features	Count	Error	Acc (%)
O2_alpha_rel_power, coh_O1vsT6_theta	0.0	0.305	98.1
coh_O1vsT6_theta, coh_O2vsF8_alpha	0.0	0.25	97.3
coh_O1vsT6_theta, coh_O2vsF8_beta	0.0	0.225	97
coh_C3vsT5_alpha, coh_O1vsT6_theta	0.0	0.245	95.4
Pz_alpha_rel_power, coh_O1vsT6_theta	0.0	0.3	95.2

Table 6. Alzheimer's Disease Frontotemporal Model Feature Sets.

Features	Count	Error	Acc (%)
coh_O1vsT6_theta, coh_O2vsF8_alpha, coh_O2vsF8_beta	0.0	0.190	97.5
coh_O1vsT6_theta, coh_O2vsF8_beta, coh_Fp1vsF3_delta	0.0	0.185	96.4
coh_O1vsT6_theta, coh_O2vsF8_beta, O2_delta_rel_power	0.0	0.205	96.3
coh_O1vsT6_theta, coh_O2vsF8_beta, coh_F3vsF8_delta	0.0	0.195	96.3
coh_O1vsT6_theta, coh_O2vsF8_beta, coh_O2vsT4_beta	0.0	0.210	96.3

Table 7. Inference, Sensor Count, Model Size

Model/Label	Sensors	Inference (s)	Size (KB)	Acc (%)
AD Model				
Standard	3	1.53	1,517	98.1
Lite	3	0.34	18	98.1
AD-FTD Model				
Standard	4	1.09	1,536	98.5
Lite	4	0.37	19	98.5

4.4 Inference and Architecture

Table 7 provides an overview of sensors required and optimisations gained from converting the standard TensorFlow model with TFLite. The lite version reduced inference speed by an average of 3.7×, and model size by 83× while maintaining prediction accuracy.

Table 8 provides the final training parameters of both models, and Fig. 5 highlights the architecture of the AD model. This is identical to the AD-FTD model with some adjustments to the parameters listed in Table 7. The Confusion Matrix for the AD model and the AD FTD model are shown in Fig. 6.

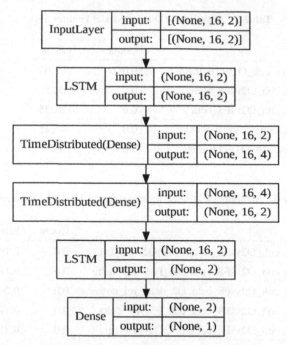

Fig. 5. LSTM RNN Model Architecture with Time Distributed Wrapper Applied to Dense Layers. A Time Step of 16 Leverages 16 Rows of Sequential Data per Single Output. Shape is in the Format of Batch, Time Step, Neurons. The Dense output is in the form of a Binary Sigmoid to Produce Either a CN or AD Result.

Table 8. Final Model Training Parameters

Parameter	AD Model	AD-FTD Model
Learning Rate	0.0005	0.001
Optimiser	Adam	Adam
Epochs	18	15
Shape	[2,4]	[3]
Batch Size	16	32
Activation	Elu	Elu
Times Step	16	32

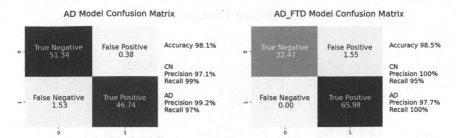

Fig. 6. From left to right, the Confusion Matrix for the Alzheimer's Disease Model, and the Alzheimer's Disease Frontotemporal Model, respectively.

5 Discussion

The research objectives was to design a performant neural network for the routine testing of dementia. By systematically extracting an extensive set of features, undergoing multiple meticulous feature selection phases, conducting model testing, and fine-tuning hyperparameters, this study introduces two innovative models designed for distinguishing between AD and CN, as well as AD-FTD and CN subjects. This was achieved with 3 and 4 sensory electrodes, respectively. This research also shows that through optimisations with TFLite, the models computational footprint is reduced without a trade-off of performance.

Table 9. Comparative Analysis

Authors	Label	Electrodes	Method	Acc (%)
Tavares, G. *et al.* (2019)	AD	13	LR/SVM	97.1
Alessandrini, M. *et al.* (2022)	AD	16	LSTM	97.9
Puri. *et al.*(2022)	AD	6	SVM	97.5
This Research	AD	3	LSTM	98.1
This Research	AD-FTD	4	LSTM	98.5

Comparative analysis with existing research [23, 24], and [20] shown in Table 9, highlights the proposed models hold, or evens exceed existing performance accuracy with a significant reduction in sensor requirement. Research from [29] and [30] put forward designs for miniaturized, portable EEG headbands. The electrode placement of these designs may then be adapted to mirror the sensor findings of this paper, which are highlighted in Fig. 7. The resulting device may then function as a lightweight, portable, and accessible platform for the monitoring or routine testing of dementia, reducing the load on healthcare systems, and increasing the quality of life for dementia patients.

Electrode Placement

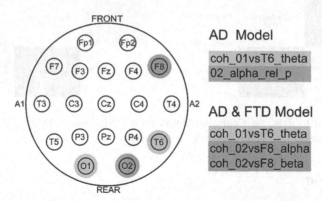

Fig. 7. Electrode Placement shows the required electrodes and their placement with respect to the 10-20 system

6 Conclusion

This research analysed the efficacy of a machine learning framework for the early detection of dementia using sensory EEG information. The findings demonstrated through careful and thorough feature selection and modelling, that a lightweight LSTM can predict the presence of AD and FTD from CN subjects with an accuracy of 98%. This can be achieved with optimisation that significantly reduces storage and inference speeds without sacrificing accuracy. Comparative analysis with existing research revealed that these proposed models require significantly fewer electrodes and provide performance accuracy comparable to or in excess of less-portable techniques currently researched. Future work can be devoted to creating a low-cost sensor platform, which will allow us to capture fresh data and re-test this model and approach. The resulting deployment holds the potential for developing a practical and accessible tool for the early detection of dementia, which could significantly impact healthcare systems, and patient outcomes.

Acknowledgments. The authors would like to acknowledge the work by Miltiadous et al. [25] for providing the dataset source that made this research possible.

Disclosure of Interests. The authors have no competing interest to declare that are relevant to the content of this article.

References

1. Lucca, U., et al.: Prevalence of dementia in the oldest old: the Monzino 80-plus population based study. Alzheimers Dement. **11**(3), 258-270.e3 (2015). https://doi.org/10.1016/J.JALZ.2014.05.1750
2. Chiu, M.J., Chen, T.F., Yip, P.K., Hua, M.S., Tang, L.Y.: Behavioral and psychologic symptoms in different types of dementia. J. Formos. Med. Assoc. **105**(7), 556–562 (2006). https://doi.org/10.1016/S0929-6646(09)60150-9
3. Baumann, B., et al.: Visualization of neuritic plaques in Alzheimer's disease by polarization-sensitive optical coherence microscopy. Sci. Rep. **7** (2017). https://doi.org/10.1038/SREP43477
4. Rasmussen, J., Langerman, H.: Alzheimer's disease – why we need early diagnosis. Degener. Neurol. Neuromuscul. Dis. **9**, 123 (2019). https://doi.org/10.2147/DNND.S228939
5. Mohammed, B.A., et al.: Multi-method analysis of medical records and MRI images for early diagnosis of dementia and Alzheimer's disease based on deep learning and hybrid methods. Electronics **10**(22), 2860 (2021). https://doi.org/10.3390/ELECTRONICS10222860
6. Oldan, J.D., Jewells, V.L., Pieper, B., Wong, T.Z.: Complete evaluation of dementia: PET and MRI correlation and diagnosis for the neuroradiologist. AJNR Am. J. Neuroradiol. **42**(6), 998 (2021). https://doi.org/10.3174/AJNR.A7079
7. Oudart, J.B., et al.: Incremental value of CSF biomarkers in clinically diagnosed AD and non-AD dementia. Front. Neurol. **11**, 560 (2020). https://doi.org/10.3389/FNEUR.2020.00560
8. Wilczyńska, K., Waszkiewicz, N.: Diagnostic utility of selected serum dementia biomarkers: Amyloid β-40, Amyloid β-42, Tau Protein, and YKL-40: a review. J. Clin. Med. **9**(11), 1–26 (2020). https://doi.org/10.3390/JCM9113452
9. Jack, C.R., et al.: A/T/N: an unbiased descriptive classification scheme for Alzheimer disease biomarkers. Neurology **87**(5), 539–547 (2016). https://doi.org/10.1212/WNL.0000000000002923
10. Ahmed, R.M., et al.: Biomarkers in dementia: clinical utility and new directions. J. Neurol. Neurosurg. Psychiatry **85**(12), 1426–1434 (2014). https://doi.org/10.1136/JNNP-2014-307662
11. O'Bryant, S.E., et al.: Detecting dementia with the mini-mental state examination in highly educated individuals. Arch. Neurol. **65**(7), 963–967 (2008). https://doi.org/10.1001/ARCHNEUR.65.7.963
12. Mathuranath, P.S., Nestor, P.J., Berrios, G.E., Rakowicz, W., Hodges, J.R.: A brief cognitive test battery to differentiate Alzheimer's disease and frontotemporal dementia. Neurology **55**(11), 1613–1620 (2000). https://doi.org/10.1212/01.WNL.0000434309.85312.19
13. Smith, G.E., Ivnik, R.J., Lucas, J.: Assessment techniques: tests, test batteries, norms, and methodological approaches. In: Textbook of Clinical Neuropsychology, pp. 38–57. Psychology Press (2008). https://psycnet.apa.org/record/2007-10435-004. Accessed 14 Dec 2023
14. Wahlund, L.O.: Structural brain imaging as a diagnostic tool in dementia, why and how? Psychiatry Res. Neuroimaging **306**, 111183 (2020). https://doi.org/10.1016/J.PSCYCHRESNS.2020.111183
15. Kaltoft, N.S., Marner, L., Larsen, V.A., Hasselbalch, S.G., Law, I., Henriksen, O.M.: Hybrid FDG PET/MRI vs. FDG PET and CT in patients with suspected dementia - A comparison of diagnostic yield and propagated influence on clinical diagnosis and patient management. PLoS One **14**(5), (2019). https://doi.org/10.1371/JOURNAL.PONE.0216409
16. O'Bryant, S.E., et al.: A blood screening test for Alzheimer's disease. Alzheimer's Dement. Diagnosis Assess. Dis. Monit. **3**, 83 (2016). https://doi.org/10.1016/J.DADM.2016.06.004

17. Yamashita, S., et al.: Alterations in the levels of Amyloid-β, phospholipid hydroperoxide, and plasmalogen in the blood of patients with Alzheimer's disease: possible interactions between Amyloid-β and these lipids. J. Alzheimer's Dis. **50**(2), 527–537 (2016). https://doi.org/10.3233/JAD-150640

18. Mehta, K.M., Fung, K.Z., Kistler, C.E., Chang, A., Walter, L.C.: Impact of cognitive impairment on screening mammography use in older US women. Am. J. Public Health **100**(10), 1917 (2010). https://doi.org/10.2105/AJPH.2008.158485

19. Staudinger, T., Polikar, R.: Analysis of complexity based EEG features for the diagnosis of Alzheimer's disease. Annual International Conference of the IEEE Engineering in Medicine and Biology Society, pp. 2033–2036 (2011). https://doi.org/10.1109/IEMBS.2011.6090374

20. Puri, D., Nalbalwar, S., Nandgaonkar, A., Kachare, P., Rajput, J., Wagh, A.: Alzheimer's disease detection using empirical mode decomposition and Hjorth parameters of EEG signal. In: International Conference on Decision Aid Science Application (DASA 2022), pp. 23–28 (2022). https://doi.org/10.1109/DASA54658.2022.9765111

21. Spiegel, A., Tonner, P.H., Renna, M.: Altered states of consciousness: processed EEG in mental disease. Best Pract. Res. Clin. Anaesthesiol. **20**(1), 57–67 (2006). https://doi.org/10.1016/J.BPA.2005.07.010

22. Babiloni, C., et al.: Resting-state posterior alpha rhythms are abnormal in subjective memory complaint seniors with preclinical Alzheimer's neuropathology and high education level: the INSIGHT-preAD study. Neurobiol. Aging **90**, 43–59 (2020). https://doi.org/10.1016/J.NEUROBIOLAGING.2020.01.012

23. Tavares, G., San-Martin, R., Ianof, J.N., Anghinah, R., Fraga, F.J.: Improvement in the automatic classification of Alzheimer's disease using EEG after feature selection. In: Proceedings of the IEEE International Conference on Systems, Man and Cybernetics, vol. 2019, pp. 1264–1269 (2019). https://doi.org/10.1109/SMC.2019.8914006

24. Alessandrini, M., Biagetti, G., Crippa, P., Falaschetti, L., Luzzi, S., Turchetti, C.: EEG-based Alzheimer's disease recognition using robust-PCA and LSTM recurrent neural network. Sensors (Basel) **22**(10), 3696 (2022). https://doi.org/10.3390/S22103696

25. Miltiadous, A., et al.: A dataset of 88 EEG recordings from: Alzheimer's disease, frontotemporal dementia and healthy subjects – OpenNeuro 17 February 2023. https://openneuro.org/datasets/ds004504/versions/1.0.2. Accessed 14 Dec 2023

26. Geng, D., Wang, C., Fu, Z., Zhang, Y., Yang, K., An, H.: Sleep EEG-based approach to detect mild cognitive impairment. Front. Aging Neurosci. **14** (2022). https://doi.org/10.3389/FNAGI.2022.865558/FULL

27. Jeong, H.T., Youn, Y.C., Sung, H.H., Kim, S.Y.: Power spectral changes of quantitative EEG in the subjective cognitive decline: comparison of community normal control groups. Neuropsychiatr. Dis. Treat. **17**, 2783 (2021). https://doi.org/10.2147/NDT.S320130

28. Vong, C., Theptit, T., Watcharakonpipat, V., Chanchotisatien, P., Laitrakun, S.: Comparison of feature selection and classification for human activity and fall recognition using smartphone sensors. In: International Conference on Digital Arts, Media and Technology, pp. 170–173 (2021). https://doi.org/10.1109/51128.2021.9425742

29. Kim, M., Yoo, S., Kim, C.: Miniaturization for wearable EEG systems: recording hardware and data processing. Biomed. Eng. Lett. **12**(3), 239–250 (2022). https://doi.org/10.1007/S13534-022-00232-0

30. Zhang, Q., et al.: A real-time wireless wearable electroencephalography system based on Support Vector Machine for encephalopathy daily monitoring. Int. J. Distrib. Sens. Netw. **14**(5), 155014771877956 (2018). https://doi.org/10.1177/1550147718779562

Adaptive Security in 6G for Sustainable Healthcare

Ijaz Ahmad[1]($\boxtimes$)(ID), Ijaz Ahmad[2](ID), and Erkki Harjula[1](ID)

[1] Centre for Wireless Communications, University of Oulu, Oulu, Finland
{ahmad.ijaz,erkki.harjula}@oulu.fi
[2] VTT Technical Research Centre of Finland, Espoo, Finland
ijaz.ahmad@vtt.fi

Abstract. 6G will fulfill the requirements of future digital healthcare systems through emerging decentralized computing and secure communications technologies. Digital healthcare solutions employ numerous low-power and resource-constrained connected things, such as the Internet of Medical Things (IoMT). However, the current digital healthcare solutions will face two major challenges. First, the proposed solutions are based on the traditional IoT-Cloud model that will experience latency and reliability challenges to meet the expectations and requirements of digital healthcare, while potentially inflicting heavy network load. Second, the existing digital healthcare solutions will face security challenges due to the inherent limitations of IoMT caused by the lack of resources for proper security in those devices. Therefore, in this research, we present a decentralized adaptive security architecture for the successful deployment of digital healthcare. The proposed architecture leverages the edge-cloud continuum to meet the performance, efficiency, and reliability requirements. It can adapt the security solution at run-time to meet the limited capacity of IoMT devices without compromising the security of critical data. Finally, the research outlines comprehensive methodologies for validating the proposed security architecture.

Keywords: 6G · Adaptive Security · Healthcare · Edge · Internet of Things

1 Introduction

6G is the next-generation wireless communication technology with promising unprecedented speed and low latency [1]. In addition to evolutionary improvements in performance to its predecessors, 6G will also include novel innovations such as convergence of computing, communication, and sensing [24]. It also supports better integration with AI/ML by enabling the extension of edge computing to the local level (further closer to UEs), and traditional mobile operator and customer organizations' communication infrastructures. It also facilitates the use of renewable energy sources, within and outside the network infrastructure, as well as it is envisaged to support quantum computing/communication

© The Author(s) 2024
M. Särestöniemi et al. (Eds.): NCDHWS 2024, CCIS 2083, pp. 38–47, 2024.
https://doi.org/10.1007/978-3-031-59080-1_3

requirements. IMT-2030 recommendations [1] comprise of novel capabilities such as artificial intelligence (AI) and sensing, ubiquitous connectivity, and integrated sensing which were not described in IMT-2020 (5G).

Digital healthcare applications, including decentralized clinical trials, mobile imaging, computer-assisted surgery, emergency response, and telemedicine, among many others, have considerable low-latency and stringent privacy requirements governed by regulatory authorities. In a digital healthcare solution, numerous connected things (IoMT) help in monitoring, processing, storing, and transmitting the patient's data. There is a need to protect the patient's data from potential exposure in full compliance with stricter regulatory and legislative requirements for privacy and security [23]. Conventional IoT-cloud setup faces the challenges of latency and exposure of sensitive data to a wider audience consisting of potentially hostile nodes.

The potential to process data at the network edge near the data source enables lower communication costs, reduced latency, enhanced efficiency, and increased system capacity for compute-intensive healthcare applications. In general, IoMT devices deployed in healthcare scenarios are resource-constrained and unable to sustain conventional heavyweight security solutions. Hence, there is a need to provide a context-aware and resource-efficient adaptable security architecture protecting sensitive information in dynamic network conditions, available resources, and evolving threat landscape. In this research, we propose an adaptive security architecture that leverages the potential emerging technologies such as distributed ledger technologies, zero-trust [9] security, differential privacy, and federated learning in a resource-constrained environment.

The rest of the paper is organized as follows: Sect. 2 describes the background and related work, and Sect. 3 presents our position statement. Section 4 provides robust evidence and reasoning to support our position and ensures our arguments are grounded in fact and logic. Section 5 comprises counterarguments and rebuttals, addressing the opposing perspectives hands-on, and Sect. 6 reflects on the discussions presented in the article.

2 Background and Related Work

2.1 Healthcare in 6G

The advancement of wireless communication networks has had a profound effect on the healthcare industry. The shift from 4G to 5G initiated a new era in digital healthcare [7], facilitating the emergence of the Intelligent Internet of Healthcare Things (IIoHT) or Internet of Medical Things (IoMT). This technology transition has created new possibilities in the healthcare sector, enhancing the efficiency, resilience, sustainability, affordability, and widespread availability of services. The expected shift to 6G is poised to profoundly transform healthcare [2,7]. 6G will be a comprehensive system that will combine sensors, mobile communications, and processing capacity to effectively link virtual and actual environments. In healthcare scenarios, this implies that, e.g., the vital signs of patients may be detected, analyzed, and transferred immediately over the 6G network. 6G is anticipated to enable physicians and nurses to collaborate in new ways by using advanced network features, such as augmented reality (AR) apps or telemedicine.

2.2   Security Challenges in IoMT

The start of the 21st century witnessed a broad shift of enterprises from local data centers to cloud infrastructure considering its flexibility and scalability, resulting in the expansion of the IoT ecosystem [14]. Lack of standardized protocols, limited security controls, and a focus on functionality over security has led to a wide range of vulnerabilities exploited in critical infamous security incidents notably Marai botnet [16], Stuxnet (2010), and Vastaamo health data breach [15]. Moreover, the use of 6G technology in the healthcare sector poses security and privacy concerns, particularly due to the sensitive nature of health data [23]. Furthermore, hostile attackers could compromise implantable medical devices (IMDs) [26] such as diabetic insulin pumps, internal heart defibrillators, and pacemakers, causing not only economic losses but endangering human lives. It is essential to tackle these challenges to effectively integrate healthcare based on 6G technology. Notwithstanding these barriers, the potential advantages of 6G in healthcare are vast, and it is anticipated that the technology will enable healthcare to be heavily reliant on AI and 6G communication technology.

2.3   Adaptive Security

Adaptive security indicates that security solutions may be adjusted on the fly to accommodate changing network conditions and evolving threats. Adaptive security helps protect healthcare services and data by encompassing mechanisms for prediction, detection, mitigation, and prevention of threats to privacy and security [20]. Existing approaches such as risk-based [8], Game-based [12], Requirements-driven [22], and event-driven [6] adaptive security models will be evaluated for edge-cloud continuum considering their applicability and adaptability.

2.4   Resource Efficient Healthcare Solutions in 6G

Sustainability is set as one of the new capabilities for IMT-2030 and security, privacy, and resilience as enhanced capabilities over the existing 5G (IMT-2020) [1]. Enhanced mMTC and uRLLC from 5G will pave the way for ubiquitous connectivity as an emerging use case in 6G that will call for robust and sustainable [11] security, privacy, and trust measures [24]. Conventional security measures and strategies use pre-set, manual methods to reduce risks and keep things safe in certain situations [5] at the cost of additional energy consumption resulting in larger energy footprints. The proposed adaptive security architecture will consider the available resources especially remaining energy while providing security in a healthcare scenario.

3   Position Statement

The development of the 6G and edge-cloud continuum will extend the widespread adoption of IoT in many delay-sensitive scenarios in healthcare [3]. Conventional stringent security mechanisms are resource-intensive and not flexible across the edge-cloud continuum. Hence, there is a need for context-aware adaptive security architecture considering the remaining energy, network dynamics, and evolving threat landscape. Adaptive security is a promising approach to address the rising security challenges by distributing security capabilities across the network, from local edge to MEC and ultimately to the cloud as illustrated in Fig. 1. The IoMT devices and the underlying network are monitored for security breaches from MEC (tier-2) in addition to computing delay-sensitive tasks that are too heavy for processing at the local edge. Local edge (tier-1) hosts lightweight cryptographic solutions with strict latency requirements, while delay-tolerant and computationally demanding security tasks are assigned to the cloud layer (tier-3). This enables adapting the security measures to the changing network conditions and the healthcare use-case requirements at run-time with no human intervention.

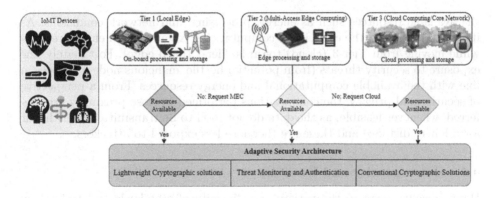

Fig. 1. Adaptive Security at Edge

4   Evidence and Reasoning

4.1   Performance and Efficiency

In many digital healthcare scenarios, the key requirements include the ability to communicate in real-time with no observable latency. One such example is emergency patient monitoring to communicate the patient's vitals from the incident site to the hospital. In such scenarios, secure communication is among the key features, in addition to performance and reliability. Adaptive security ensures that the communication is protected from potential disclosure while considering

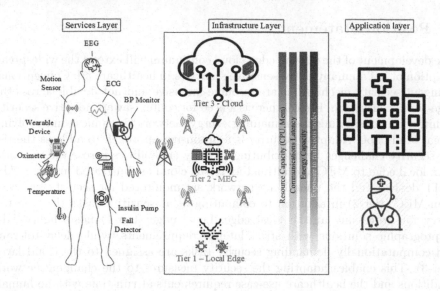

Fig. 2. Secure Digital Healthcare Architecture

the available resources such as energy, processing, and network conditions. As illustrated in Fig. 2, the capacity of computational resources and energy reduces while moving from Tier-3 (cloud) towards Tier-1 (local edge). Fortunately, the exposure to security threats (from potential hostile/malicious nodes) reduces in line with the available computational and energy resources. From a perspective of security and privacy, the computations performed in close proximity are preferred, whenever feasible, as the data do not need to be transmitted over the air for a longer distance and these are therefore less exposed to attackers.

4.2 Heterogeneity and Diversity

Heterogeneity refers to the variety and diversity of standards and technology included in medical devices. 6G networks are anticipated to facilitate a substantial volume of interconnected devices and transfer data of high intensity [17,21]. It is essential to tackle the diversity and range of IoMT devices to guarantee the security of 6G-enabled healthcare services and data. Traditional security solutions are inadequate in a diverse IoMT environment with a dynamic and evolving technological and threat landscape. The envisioned heterogeneity feature of future 6G networks increases the attack surface and may result in complex security challenges [25].

4.3 Technological Advancements

The IMT-2030 recommendations [1] have identified distributed ledger technologies (DLT such as blockchain), differential privacy, and federated learning as potential security technologies for achieving security and resilience in future 6G networks. Utilizing the potential of blockchain technology for authentication and securing healthcare data in a distributed manner with no or reduced reliance on centralized servers will improve the efficiency of the network. Similarly, with the breakthrough of Artificial Intelligence and Machine Learning based solutions can be developed for detecting and responding to threats efficiently in real-time.

4.4 Lightweight Cryptography

Security specialists at the National Institute of Standards and Technology (NIST) have declared a champion in their quest to identify a robust defender for data produced by resource-constrained devices. The triumphant contender, a set of cryptographic algorithms known as ASCON [10], has been recognized as NIST's standard for lightweight cryptography since February 2023. This helps in providing sustainable and affordable security in IoT-based resource-constrained devices whereby conventional heavyweight security solutions are considered as barriers to performance and survival.

4.5 Limited Exposure to Malicious Agents

By employing effective and adaptive security solutions across the edge-to-cloud continuum ensures the protection of sensitive data closer to the origin and thus reduces the geographical area of exposure to potential malicious agents. The widespread popularity and adoption of IoMT devices are continuously contributing to novel security threats and their complexities are increasing over time. The vulnerabilities in communication networks can be broken down into the core technologies and potential solutions can be looked into to achieve overall security [4]. Adaptive security ensures timely protection of data in a resource-constrained IoMT environment.

5 Counterarguments and Rebuttals

5.1 Complexity and Cost

Implementing adaptive security in 6G for sustainable healthcare could increase complexity and cost. Adaptive security is the ability to adapt to threats in real time and can potentially save costs associated with data breaches and system downtime. Recent research indicates that the long-term advantages of incorporating adaptive security in healthcare offered by 6G technology surpass these early obstacles of increased complexity and cost. The traditional approach of using a single security strategy is no longer suitable for 6G networks [24]. This is because there is a greater variation in device capabilities, energy conditions, service features, threats and vulnerabilities, and other attributes that change over time. Therefore, the selection and configuration of security strategies for 6G networks should be optimized flexibly and responsively. By using this adaptable strategy, it is possible to optimize resource use, which may result in a decrease in overall expenses over time.

5.2 Technology Maturity

6G technology is still in its infancy and it is too early to discuss its security aspects. IMT-2030 recommendation [1] describes 6G to be secure by design with the ability to continue operating in the presence of malicious agents and be able to recover from disruptive events. Recent research [19] suggests that the discussion and preparation for security concerns of 6G technology should begin without delay, even before the technology reaches full maturity. Instead, security issues should be included in the development process from the beginning. Implementing this strategy may facilitate the early detection and resolution of possible security vulnerabilities, resulting in the development of more resilient and secure 6G networks.

5.3 Privacy Concerns

Patient privacy is impacted by the increased connectivity and data sharing in 6G-enabled healthcare. 6G technology promises to make healthcare more efficient, robust, sustainable, and ubiquitous, yet increased communication raises patient privacy concerns [7,13]. Security and privacy concerns for 6G are being actively considered from the very beginning, with the identification of particular security requirements, highlighting of security challenges, and identification of gaps for future research. Moreover, emerging technologies such as DLTs and differential privacy are being explored as effective methods to significantly reduce the scale of attacks and personal data breaches [18]. Although privacy issues are present, the emphasis on adaptive security in 6G for sustainable healthcare is robust, guaranteeing the protection of patient data and the preservation of privacy.

6 Conclusion

The emergence of 6G technology has the potential to transform the healthcare industry. Nevertheless, the increased connectivity and data sharing that comes with 6G also present significant challenges in terms of security and privacy. This article has advocated for the indispensability of an adaptive security architecture in foreseeing the long-term viability of healthcare systems enabled by 6G technology. An architecture of this kind would not alone safeguard sensitive healthcare data but also guarantee the resilience and reliability of healthcare services in the presence of possible cyber hazards. Adaptive security can contribute to enhancing overall resource efficiency by deploying lightweight security solutions upon assessing the network dynamics and security requirements. We anticipate that this discussion will stimulate more investigation and advancement in this crucial field, facilitating the establishment of a secure and sustainable healthcare ecosystem supported by 6G technology. We plan to comprehensively analyze the results and evaluate the performance of the proposed architecture concerning energy and computation efficiency while dynamically responding to security and privacy threats considering the changing network conditions.

Acknowledgements. This research is supported by the Business Finland projects Tomohead (grant 8095/31/2022), Eware-6G (grant 8819/31/2022), Sunset-6G (grant 8682/31/2022), and the Research Council of Finland 6G Flagship program (grant number 346208).

References

1. Recommendation m.2160-0 (11/2023) framework and overall objectives of the future development of IMT for 2030 and beyond. Technical report. International Telecommunication Union (2023). https://www.itu.int/rec/R-REC-M.2160-0-202311-I/en
2. Abdellatif, A.A., Mohamed, A., Chiasserini, C.F., Tlili, M., Erbad, A.: Edge computing for smart health: context-aware approaches, opportunities, and challenges. IEEE Network **33**(3), 196–203 (2019). https://doi.org/10.1109/MNET.2019.1800083
3. Ahmad, I., et al.: Edge computing for critical environments: vision and existing solutions. arXiv preprint arXiv:2411.7567v1 (2023)
4. Ahmad, I., et al.: Communications security in industry X: a survey. IEEE Open J. Commun. Soc. **5**, 982–1025 (2024). https://doi.org/10.1109/OJCOMS.2024.3356076
5. Aman, W.: Assessing the feasibility of adaptive security models for the Internet of Things. In: Tryfonas, T. (ed.) Human Aspects of Information Security, Privacy, and Trust, HAS 2016. LNCS, vol. 9750, pp. 201–211. Springer, Cham (2016). https://doi.org/10.1007/978-3-319-39381-0_18
6. Aman, W., Snekkenes, E.: Event driven adaptive security in Internet of Things. In: Proceedings of the Eighth International Conference on Mobile Ubiquitous Computing, Systems, Services and Technologies (UBICOMM 2014), Rome, vol. 2428, pp. 7–15 (2014)
7. Batista, E., Lopez-Aguilar, P., Solanas, A.: Smart health in the 6G era: bringing security to future smart health services. IEEE Commun. Mag. 1–7 (2023). https://doi.org/10.1109/MCOM.019.2300122
8. Calvo, M., Beltrán, M.: A model for risk-based adaptive security controls. Comput. Secur. **115**, 102612 (2022). https://doi.org/10.1016/j.cose.2022.102612
9. Chen, X., Feng, W., Ge, N., Zhang, Y.: Zero trust architecture for 6G security. IEEE Netw. 1 (2023). https://doi.org/10.1109/MNET.2023.3326356
10. Dobraunig, C., Eichlseder, M., Mendel, F., Schläffer, M.: Ascon v1. 2: lightweight authenticated encryption and hashing. J. Cryptol. **34**, 1–42 (2021). https://doi.org/10.1007/s00145-021-09398-9
11. Halabi, T., Bellaiche, M., Fung, B.C.M.: Towards adaptive cybersecurity for green IoT. In: 2022 IEEE International Conference on Internet of Things and Intelligence Systems (IoTaIS), pp. 64–69 (2022). https://doi.org/10.1109/IoTaIS56727.2022.9975990
12. Hamdi, M., Abie, H.: Game-based adaptive security in the Internet of Things for eHealth. In: 2014 IEEE International Conference on Communications (ICC), pp. 920–925 (2014). https://doi.org/10.1109/ICC.2014.6883437
13. Kamal, M., Rashid, I., Iqbal, W., Siddiqui, M.H., Khan, S., Ahmad, I.: Privacy and security federated reference architecture for internet of things. Front. Inf. Technol. Electron. Eng. **24**(4), 481–508 (2023)

14. Kumar, J., et al.: Towards 6G-enabled edge-cloud continuum computing–initial assessment. In: Shaw, R.N., Paprzycki, M., Ghosh, A. (eds.) Advanced Communication and Intelligent Systems, pp. 1–15. Springer, Cham (2023). https://doi.org/10.1007/978-3-031-25088-0_1
15. Lindroos-Hovinheimo, S.: Serious cyberattack raises questions about QDPR application in Finland. Verfassungsblog (2020)
16. Margolis, J., Oh, T.T., Jadhav, S., Kim, Y.H., Kim, J.N.: An in-depth analysis of the Mirai botnet. In: 2017 International Conference on Software Security and Assurance (ICSSA), pp. 6–12 (2017). https://doi.org/10.1109/ICSSA.2017.12
17. Naseer, A., Khan, M.M., Arif, F., Iqbal, W., Ahmad, A., Ahmad, I.: An improved hybrid model for cardiovascular disease detection using machine learning in IoT. Exp. Syst. e13520 (2023). https://doi.org/10.1111/exsy.13520
18. Nguyen, V.L., Lin, P.C., Cheng, B.C., Hwang, R.H., Lin, Y.D.: Security and privacy for 6G: a survey on prospective technologies and challenges. IEEE Commun. Surv. Tutor. **23**(4), 2384–2428 (2021). https://doi.org/10.1109/COMST.2021.3108618
19. Porambage, P., Gür, G., Osorio, D.P.M., Liyanage, M., Gurtov, A., Ylianttila, M.: The roadmap to 6G security and privacy. IEEE Open J. Commun. Soc. **2**, 1094–1122 (2021). https://doi.org/10.1109/OJCOMS.2021.3078081
20. Porambage, P., Liyanage, M.: Security and Privacy Vision in 6G: A Comprehensive Guide. Wiley, New York (2023)
21. Pritika, Shanmugam, B., Azam, S.: Risk assessment of heterogeneous IOMT devices: a review. Technologies **11**(1), 31 (2023). https://doi.org/10.3390/technologies11010031
22. Salehie, M., Pasquale, L., Omoronyia, I., Ali, R., Nuseibeh, B.: Requirements-driven adaptive security: protecting variable assets at runtime. In: 2012 20th IEEE International Requirements Engineering Conference (RE), pp. 111–120 (2012). https://doi.org/10.1109/RE.2012.6345794
23. Shahid, J., Ahmad, R., Kiani, A.K., Ahmad, T., Saeed, S., Almuhaideb, A.M.: Data protection and privacy of the Internet of Healthcare Things (IOHTS). Appl. Sci. **12**(4), 1927 (2022). https://doi.org/10.3390/app12041927
24. Shen, S., Yu, C., Zhang, K., Ni, J., Ci, S.: Adaptive and dynamic security in AI-empowered 6G: from an energy efficiency perspective. IEEE Commun. Stand. Mag. **5**(3), 80–88 (2021). https://doi.org/10.1109/MCOMSTD.101.2000090
25. Ylianttila, M.: 6G white paper: research challenges for trust, security and privacy (2020)
26. Zhou, W., Jia, Y., Peng, A., Zhang, Y., Liu, P.: The effect of IoT new features on security and privacy: new threats, existing solutions, and challenges yet to be solved. IEEE Internet Things J. **6**(2), 1606–1616 (2019). https://doi.org/10.1109/JIOT.2018.2847733

Decentralized Pub/Sub Architecture for Real-Time Remote Patient Monitoring: A Feasibility Study

Kazi Nymul Haque(✉)[iD], Johirul Islam[iD], Ijaz Ahmad[iD], and Erkki Harjula[iD]

Centre for Wireless Communications, University of Oulu, Oulu, Finland
{kazi.haque,johirul.islam,ahmad.ijaz,erkki.harjula}@oulu.fi

Abstract. The confluence of the Internet of Things (IoT) within the healthcare sector, called Internet of Medical Things (IoMT), has ushered in a transformative approach to real-time patient monitoring. Traditional methods that typically involve the direct transmission of medical sensor data to the cloud, falter under the constraints of medical IoT devices. In response, Multi-access Edge Computing (MEC), as defined by the European Telecommunications Standards Institute (ETSI), brings forth an innovative solution by relocating computing resources closer to the origin of data. However, MEC alone does not fully address the exigencies of constrained medical IoTs in the realm of real-time monitoring. Our architecture advances the computing continuum by seamlessly integrating local edge computing for direct data capture, MEC for nuanced data processing, and cloud computing for the comprehensive synthesis and presentation of data. This synergy is further enhanced by the introduction of a robust message queue mechanism, assuring data resilience and uninterrupted data streaming during network disruptions. With a steadfast commitment to security, our system employs stringent measures to ensure the integrity and confidentiality of sensitive patient data during transmission. This architecture represents a significant leap in healthcare technology, emphasizing the criticality of patient safety, data security, and meticulous data management. The implications of this study are profound, indicating a trajectory for future exploration into the integration of sophisticated data types and AI-driven models to further refine patient monitoring and healthcare outcomes.

Keywords: IoT · IoMT · edge computing · cloud computing · patient monitoring · data security · container orchestration

1 Introduction

The burgeoning integration of the Internet of Things (IoT) and the Internet of Medical Things (IoMT) with edge and cloud computing technologies is catalyzing a paradigm shift in healthcare delivery. This synergy is pivotal in fostering real-time, efficient healthcare services, transcending the conventional limitations

ⓒ The Author(s) 2024
M. Särestöniemi et al. (Eds.): NCDHWS 2024, CCIS 2083, pp. 48–65, 2024.
https://doi.org/10.1007/978-3-031-59080-1_4

posed by the traditional IoT-cloud models. These models often struggle with challenges such as latency and bandwidth constraints, which are exacerbated by the dependency on distant cloud servers for data processing and analysis. Such constraints are particularly pronounced in healthcare applications, where real-time data processing and analysis are crucial for patient care [1].

Edge Computing (EC) emerges as a cornerstone in this architecture, mitigating latency by facilitating data processing closer to the data source. This proximity not only accelerates data processing but also bolsters data security-a critical consideration in healthcare applications. Furthermore, messaging queues play an indispensable role in orchestrating high-throughput data synchronization from a plethora of medical devices, ensuring seamless and reliable communication within the healthcare IoT ecosystem. This feature is instrumental in maintaining uninterrupted patient care, even amidst network disruptions [2].

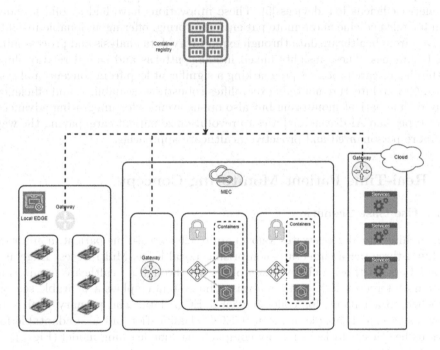

Fig. 1. Three-tier architecture integrating IoMT with edge and cloud computing

Our proposed three-tier architecture, depicted in Fig. 1, interfaces directly with medical sensors at the local edge, employs Multi-access Edge Computing (MEC) for comprehensive data processing, and utilizes cloud services to furnish healthcare professionals with holistic insights. This architecture, characterized by its modularity and scalability, leverages the prowess of microservices and containerization technologies such as Docker and Kubernetes, offering a superior alternative to traditional systems [3].

The advent of Artificial Intelligence (AI) and Machine Learning (ML) technologies heralds a new era in healthcare IoT, equipping it with sophisticated diagnostic and predictive analytics tools. These advancements facilitate improved patient outcomes and streamline healthcare operations by enabling informed, data-driven decision-making. However, the deployment of traditional AI/ML models at the edge is often hampered by computational complexities. This limitation underscores the significance of tiny machine learning models, which are tailor-made for on-device data processing, especially in critical care scenarios, ensuring the promptness of data analysis [4].

Security remains a cornerstone of our system, which adopts robust encryption and secure communication protocols to safeguard patient data, thereby ensuring compliance with healthcare regulations [7]. Our previous endeavors in IoMT have significantly contributed to enhancing user experience and technological innovation, spanning sensor integration [10], data analytics [6], and the development of energy-efficient IoT devices [5]. These innovations have laid a solid foundation for telemedicine and remote patient monitoring, offering actionable insights derived from healthcare data through exploratory data analysis and process mining techniques. These insights unveil hidden patterns and causal relationships within healthcare processes [9], marking a significant leap from conventional systems. Our architecture not only exemplifies robustness, scalability, and efficiency in real-time patient monitoring but also opens avenues for integrating advanced data types and AI-driven analytics to revolutionize patient care, paving the way for more personalized and proactive healthcare approaches.

2   Real-Time Patient Monitoring Concept

2.1   Use Case Scenario

Our architecture demonstrates a novel approach to real-time patient monitoring within a three-tier architecture, comprising Local Edge, Multi-Access Edge and Cloud tiers. In this article, we exemplify this through a healthcare monitoring system centered on ECG data analysis. The system employs a wearable sensor, attached to a patient, for collecting vital ECG data. The primary goal is to showcase a model capable of not just ECG classification but also adaptable for various healthcare tasks using any compact machine learning model (Fig. 2).

2.2   Service and Swarm Architecture

Our architecture is meticulously designed across three distinct tiers depicted in Fig. 3, each contributing significantly to the system's overall functionality. The Docker Swarm architecture of this system is defined within a specialized YAML file, which serves as the operational framework for deploying and orchestrating the containers across the Local Edge, MEC, and Cloud tiers. The YAML file is configured with precise instructions on where each container should be allocated, ensuring an organized and efficient deployment [11].

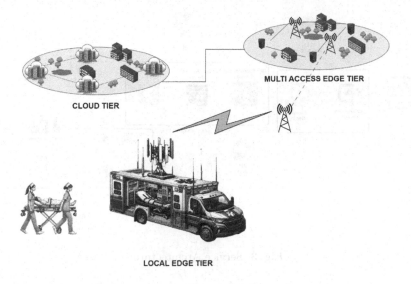

Fig. 2. Use case scenario

Local Edge (Raspberry Pi 4): At the Local Edge Level, which utilizes a Raspberry Pi device, the setup begins with the Acquisition Service that gathers critical ECG data from a IoMT sensor. Next, the Publishing Service steps in to send this health data along the pipeline, ensuring it's lined up for further processing. The Message Handling Service, crucial at this stage, manages this flow of information, keeping it organized and ready for further processing. The Local Edge tier is configured via a YAML file to deploy Docker containers for essential services. The Data Acquisition Service operates within the ADB container, capturing critical ECG data. The Data Publishing Service, running in the Publisher Container, manages the dissemination of the collected data. Lastly, the Messaging Queue Service within the RabbitMQ container orchestrates the queuing and secure transmission of messages.

Multi-access Edge (Virtual Machine): Moving to the Middle Tier, housed on a Virtual Machine, we have the Retrieval Service that picks up the health data for in-depth processing. A Standardization Service then prepares the data in a consistent format, which is crucial for accurate analysis. The Heartbeat Analysis Service, equipped with advanced algorithms, interprets the ECG data to classify and understand the received heart patterns. Following this, the Reporting Service disseminates these findings, paving the way for their final review and visualization. In the MEC tier the YAML file specifies the containers for advanced data handling. The Data Retrieval Service within the Consumer Container retrieves the queued data. The Data Standardization Service in the Normalizer Container ensures data uniformity, while the ECG Analysis Service within the ML Model Container performs the computational analysis. The Data Publishing Service in another Publisher Container then publishes the analyzed data for further processing.

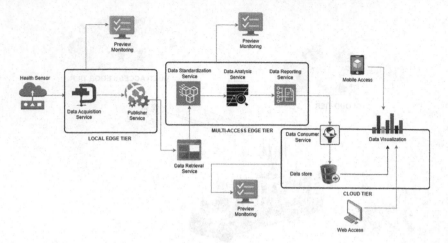

Fig. 3. Service Architecture

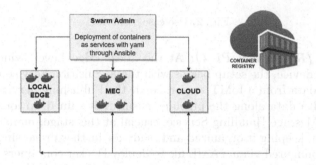

Fig. 4. Swarm Architecture

Cloud (Virtual Machine): Another Virtual Machine operates at the Cloud tier. Here, the Aggregation Service compiles all the ECG data and analytical results, creating a comprehensive dataset. The Visualization Service [9] then presents this information in an easy-to-understand format, which is essential for healthcare providers to monitor the patient's well-being effectively. The Cloud Tier is arranged in the YAML file to facilitate the final stages of data processing and visualization. The Data Aggregation Service, placed in the Consumer Container, compiles data from multiple sources. The Data Visualization Service, situated in the Grafana Container, converts this data into visual formats for effective monitoring. Figures 3 and 4 respectively shows the service and swarm architecture of our 3-tier model.

2.3   Message Queue Mechanism

In our system, the RabbitMQ container plays a crucial role in managing data during network disruptions [8] by temporarily queuing ECG data. This setup prevents data loss if the connection between the Local Edge and MEC tier is interrupted. Upon network restoration, RabbitMQ resumes normal operations, swiftly transmitting the stored data to the MEC for continued patient monitoring. This effective queueing and resumption process ensures complete data delivery and provides a robust buffer against network issues, significantly enhancing system reliability and efficiency.

2.4   RabbitMQ Security

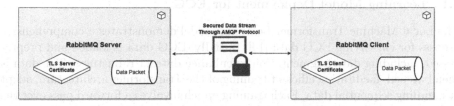

Fig. 5. Security Considerations

The need for security in data transmission is paramount, especially when dealing with sensitive healthcare data. To this end, the architecture employs Transport Layer Security (TLS) based certificates to establish a secure communication channel [12]. The RabbitMQ container at the Local Edge is fortified with a TLS server certificate. This setup ensures that all data leaving the edge device is encrypted, ensuring the confidentiality, node authentication, and integrity of the ECG data [13]. Both the MEC and Cloud layers are configured with TLS client certificates. These certificates validate the authenticity of the RabbitMQ server and establish a secure connection, ensuring that data received and transmitted by these tiers is protected from unauthorized access and tampering. Figure 5 shows the data packet streaming with AMQP protocol between RabbitMQ server and client with an encryption through TLS certificate.

3   Proof-of-Concept: Patient ECG Monitoring

Continuous electrocardiogram (ECG) monitoring is imperative for the early detection and monitoring of cardiac conditions. It enables healthcare professionals to track heart rhythm in real-time, facilitating prompt intervention in acute cardiac events and providing valuable data for long-term cardiovascular health management.

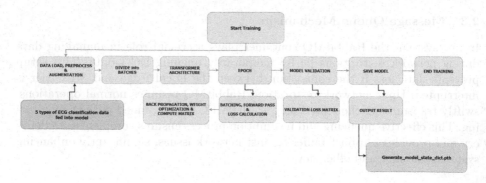

Fig. 6. Transformer Learning Architecture

3.1   Learning Model Deployment for ECG

The Local Machine Transformer Learning model demonstrates a comprehensive process for classifying ECG data [14]. Initially, ECG data is loaded and prepro-cessed, including data augmentation to enhance dataset robustness. The data is then batched, facilitating efficient training of the Transformer architecture, adept at handling sequential data. Each training epoch involves a forward pass over the dataset, generating predictions and calculating loss to inform the backpropaga-tion process, thereby optimizing the model's predictive accuracy. Concurrently, model validation tests its performance on unseen data, ensuring its applicability in real-world scenarios (Fig. 6).

Upon meeting training and validation criteria, the model's learned parame-ters are recorded in a `model_state_dict.pth` file, marking the training phase's completion. This structured approach not only converts raw medical data into actionable insights but also underscores the potential of such models in precise and timely cardiovascular diagnoses. This model's training was conducted uti-lizing ECG data sourced from Kaggle. While the accuracy achieved as depicted in Fig. 7 did not reach perfection, primarily due to the limited volume of data, the results are indicative of the model's potential. With a more substantial and varied dataset, it is anticipated that the model's accuracy would improve sig-nificantly. This prospect underscores the feasibility of integrating such a model into our three-tier architecture, where it could be fine-tuned and then deployed to broadcast its insights to the necessary channels within the system.

3.2   Technical Specifications

Hardware Specifications: Our proof-of-concept leverages a three-tiered Docker Swarm architecture, composed of Local Edge, MEC, and Cloud environments, to demonstrate a real-time patient monitoring system using ECG data collected via a Movesense sensor. The Local Edge is materialized by a Raspberry Pi 4 (RPi 4) Model B to efficiently handle initial data collection and queuing operations. It has a CPU with Broadcom BCM2711 CPU, Quad-core Cortex-A72 (ARM v8) 64-bit

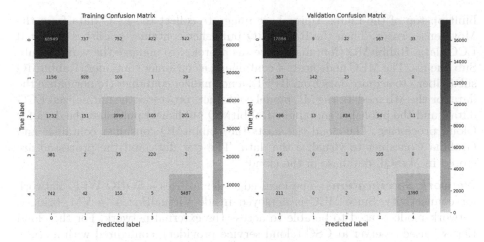

Fig. 7. Transformer Learning accuracy convolution matrix

SoC @ 1.5 GHz, Memory with 4 GB LPDDR4-3200 SDRAM. Storage is MicroSD card slot for loading operating system and data storage with 32 GB storage, with Gigabit Ethernet connectivity, 2 USB 3.0 ports and 2 USB 2.0 ports.

Table 1. Hardware and software specification

Services	Hardware	Build layer and scripts
ADB Container	Raspberry Pi 4 (Local Edge)	Alpine, Custom Scripts
Publisher Container		Python 3.8 slim, Custom Scripts
RabbitMQ Container		Official RabbitMQ Image
Consumer Container	Ubuntu x64 VM (VM1 at MEC)	Python 3.8 slim, Custom Scripts
Normalizer Container		
ML Model Container		Python 3.8 slim, Trained .pth
Publisher Container		Python 3.8 slim, Custom Scripts
Consumer Container	Ubuntu x64 VM (VM2 at Cloud)	Python 3.8 slim, Custom Scripts
MySQL Container		Official MySQL Image
Grafana Container		Official Grafana Image

The MEC and Cloud infrastructures are simulated using Virtual Machines (VMs), each with robust configurations to ensure seamless data processing and visualization. MEC and Cloud Nodes is deployed in virtual machine having Ubuntu (64-bit) OS. Each of the VMs has 2 GB RAM with 2 CPU cores having 25 GB storage which are interfaced through the bridged network adapters. The overall hardware configurations of the experimental setup are mentioned in the following Table 1.

Software Specifications: In our setup, the local edge (Raspberry Pi 4) is hosting the 3 related services as depicted in Table 1. The ADB Container is built on top of the Linux Alpine base image to collect the ECG data from the Movesense sensor. Then the RabbitMQ publisher container publishes collected ECG data. RabbitMQ Container serves as a broker to manage the various Pub-Sub queues. The MEC node hosts 4 containers, a consumer container (RabbitMQ subscriber - to acquire data from RPi 4), a normalizer container (to normalize the data for the ML model), the ML model container (processes the normalized ECG data), and the publisher container (RabbitMQ publisher) publishes the data for Cloud processing. The cloud tier hosts the RabbitMQ consumer container and Grafana Container to visualize the data. The raw data and the processed are stored in MySQL database in the cloud.

Network Specifications: The local edge tier utilizes a SOHO Wi-Fi network for connectivity. Since MEC is deployed inside VirtualBox as a VM, bridged network mode is used to be able to access the external network. For the cloud tier, we used a server at CSC (cloud service provider), configured with a static IP to allow only specific ingress and egress traffic from the local Edge and MEC tiers, enhancing security by rejecting packets from unauthorized IP addresses. This setup ensured a seamless and secure data flow across the tiers. Figure 8 shows the overall network topology of our architecture.

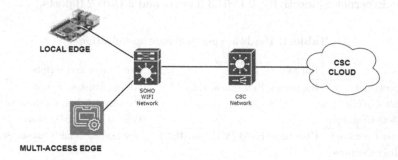

Fig. 8. Network Topology

3.3   Nanoservice Deployment

During this experiment, we considered multiple approaches to configure the setup. These include *Bare metal* installations, where necessary libraries and packages are installed directly onto hardware without involving any virtualization. Alternatively, the necessary libraries and packages can be configured in a virtualized environment using either an official docker image or a multi-stage docker build. A detailed comparison of the image size is provided in Table 2.

   We experimented using the original docker build in a virtualized environment since training the ML model takes long in multi-stage docker environment [20]. In the proposed architecture, all the containerized services are orchestrated through the Docker Swarm that ensures balanced service distribution across all tiers (local edge, MEC, cloud) for scalability and robustness as depicted in Fig. 9. Docker Swarm's configuration and its service deployment is discussed in Sect. 2.2.

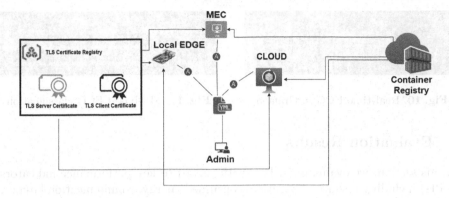

Fig. 9. Container Orchestration with security Features

Table 2. Estimated Docker Image Sizes

Container	Original Size	Bare Metal	Multi-Stage Build
adb_container	13.5 MB	153 MB	23 MB
publisher-image	111 MB	251 MB	108 MB
consumer-image (MEC)	134 MB	328 MB	123 MB
consumer-image (Cloud)	136 MB	323 MB	118 MB
normalizer-image	263 MB	422 MB	213 MB
ML-model-image	5.09 GB	5.6 GB	2.98 GB

3.4 Data Storage and Visualization

The consumer container (at the cloud layer) stores the data into MySQL database as soon as it receives the raw data from the local edge and ML post-processed data from the MEC. For healthcare professionals to understand and react the data has to be visualized effectively and timely. The proposed architecture leverages the robustness of MySQL and Grafana containers within the cloud infrastructure. This combination is pivotal for effective data handling and visualization. Specifically, MySQL serves as persistent storage of both raw ECG data and the processed results. This approach effectively bridges the gap between raw data collection and actionable healthcare insights. Grafana's visualization proficiency is clearly demonstrated in Fig. 10 and Fig. 11, where it effectively renders ECG signals and their classifications in an accessible manner. These visualizations offer real-time insights, enabling healthcare professionals to swiftly identify and act upon cardiac irregularities, which is vital for timely clinical intervention.

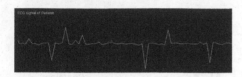

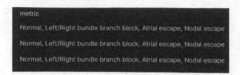

Fig. 10. Real-time ECG in Grafana   **Fig. 11.** ML-based ECG classification

4 Evaluation Results

In this section, we evaluate our PoC with regard to key performance indicators (KPIs) including resource utilization, consumed energy, communication latency, resilience and robustness along with other delay components. It is important to note that in our experiment, both the MEC and cloud tiers are intentionally configured with constrained resources to simulate a real-world scenario where system resources may be limited. Despite these constraints, our architecture is designed to manage these resources efficiently. This uniform configuration also allows us to explore the system's scalability and adaptability, ensuring that it can handle varying loads and still perform optimally. For instance, our configuration reflects a more conservative resource allocation, while a realistic setup would typically endow the cloud layer with abundant resources to handle intensive computational tasks, which can be considered in extending this experiment for the future. This approach enables us to test the system's robustness under constrained conditions, mirroring potential real-life scenarios where resource optimization is essential. Here is a detailed breakdown of each evaluation metric (KPIs).

4.1 Resource Utilization

CPU and Memory Consumption: In the experiment, we measure the CPU and memory consumption to monitor the resource utilization. Linux-native *htop* command provides real-time insights into the CPU and memory usage across the tiers [17]. The local edge (Raspberry Pi) equipped with lower resource capacity, shows a higher percentage of CPU and memory utilization. The resource utilization as presented in Fig. 12 shows a lower utilization for MEC and Cloud but it is mainly due to the greater resource capacity these have.

Network Utilization: The bar chart in Fig. 13 shows network utilization across the tiers by evaluating the impact of network disruptions on data transmission. During disruptions, the Local Edge maintains its network utilization, implying resilient local processing. When normal conditions are restored, there's a marked increase in network traffic from the Local Edge to the MEC and subsequently to the Cloud, indicating a rapid catch-up of data transfer to process the accumulated information. This demonstrates the system's capacity to handle interruptions and quickly restore efficient data flow, which is essential for consistent real-time monitoring services. Section 4.5 of the article provides a detailed discussion of this aspect.

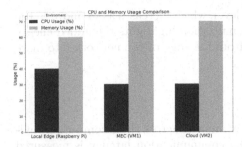
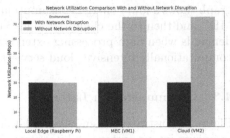

Fig. 12. CPU and Memory consumption   **Fig. 13.** Network utilization

Storage Optimization: Figure 14 shows a comparative view of storage usage across the three-tier architecture. It shows the Raspberry Pi (Local Edge) with moderate storage usage, which is significantly less than the VM1 (MEC) and VM2 (Cloud) tiers. The latter two demonstrate higher storage usage, with the cloud tier requiring the most storage space. This reflects the varying storage demands and capacities of each tier within our patient monitoring system.

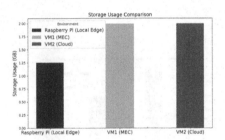
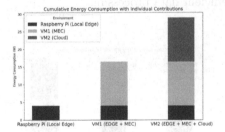

Fig. 14. Storage usage   **Fig. 15.** Cumulative Energy consumption

4.2 Computational Energy Consumption

Energy consumption was measured across the tiers using specialized tools. For the local tier (Raspberry Pi), energy usage is correlated with its operating temperature, which was monitored using the *vcgencmd* command-line utility, indicating an average consumption of around 7–8 W at full load [18]. For the MEC and cloud tiers, the energy use was directly gauged using the *turbostat* tool, which provides precise power metrics for Intel-based CPU cores [19]. We also calculated cumulative energy consumption by combining tier utilization to determine our architecture's overall energy footprint.

The bar graph depicted in Fig. 15 illustrates the cumulative energy consumption across the tiers of our proposed patient monitoring architecture, with each tier's energy usage visually stacked. For the local edge tier (Raspberry Pi), the graph shows a lower energy consumption level, which increases as we move to the MEC and then to the cloud tier. This visualization highlights the added energy demands when data processing extends from the edge of the network into more computationally intensive cloud services.

4.3 Communication Latency

Figure 16 illustrates the cumulative latency impacts across three computing environments in our system architecture. The communication latency is measured from the data origin at the Movesense sensor to the cloud tier. We employed the 'traceroute' utility to map the communication routes and identify sources of delay. The latency from the sensor to the Raspberry Pi, representing the local edge computing layer, is depicted in the first column. We then computed the latency for the Mobile Edge Computing (MEC) environment by adding the latency from the Raspberry Pi to the MEC tier. Finally, the cloud latency includes the latency from the MEC to the cloud tier. This tiered approach to latency measurement allows us to compare transmission times [15] from the sensor to the Local Edge, MEC, and Cloud comprehensively, highlighting the importance of optimization at each stage to minimize total system latency. Such optimization is critical for real-time patient monitoring systems that rely on efficient data processing.

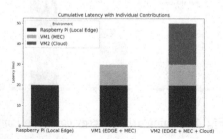

Fig. 16. Communication Latency   **Fig. 17.** Other Delays

4.4 Other Delay Components

Figure 17 present the comparative analysis of setup, runtime, and computational delays across three different environments: Local Edge, MEC, and Cloud. The setup delay is measured by the time it takes for system components to initialize and become ready for operation, as gauged by the profiling tool 'GProf'. Runtime delay encompasses the time span from the creation of data to its full processing, which is monitored via precise timestamps. The computational delay reflects the duration of processing computational tasks, captured through logging timestamps before and after task execution.

Table 3. Evaluation KPIs for Three-Tier Architecture

KPI	RPi (Local Edge)	VM1 (MEC)	VM2 (Cloud)
Latency (ms)	10–30	5–15	15–25
Setup Delay (s)	30–60	20–40	20–40
Runtime Delay (ms)	100–300	50–200	50–200
Computational Delay (ms)	200–500	100–400	100–400
CPU Usage (%)	40–70	30–60	30–60
Memory Usage (%)	60–90	70–90	70–90
Disk Usage (GB)	0.5–2	1–3	1–3
Network Throughput (Mbps)	10–50	50–100	50–100
Energy Consumption (W)	3–5	10–15	10–15

Contrary to the initial description, Table 3 indicates that while the Local Edge exhibits the highest average setup delay, the Cloud environment demonstrates the highest variability in setup delays. Runtime and computational delays [16], however, are generally higher in the Cloud environment, confirming that initiation and execution at the Local Edge are quicker, but computational tasks are more time-consuming in the Cloud. This comparison underscores the trade-offs between the immediacy of local processing and the intensive computational capabilities of the Cloud. In our test setup, the Local Edge exhibited higher setup delays due to resource constraints, while the Cloud, allocated lower resources for this specific test, showed medium setup times. However, in real-world applications, the Cloud is typically provisioned with ample resources, which would significantly reduce its setup delay compared to the Local Edge and MEC environments.

4.5 Resilience and Robustness

We evaluate the resilience and robustness of the proposed architecture by changing the network conditions. We simulated network disruptions between the local edge and MEC tier to evaluate the queue mechanism's resilience within the ECG monitoring scenario. The goal was to assess the capability of RabbitMQ container to manage data during such interruptions effectively. During tests on network disruption resilience, the RabbitMQ queue's performance was rigorously tested by simulating a disconnection of the local edge from the rest of the network infrastructure. Such situation can occur in real-life when, e.g., an ambulance transporting monitored patient goes temporarily outside the network coverage. With the MEC's consumer container deactivated, vital signs data was queued at the local edge, testing the queue's capacity. Upon connection re-establishment, the smooth processing of queued data confirmed the system's robustness in maintaining data continuity during outages, demonstrating the queue's effective management and the system's resilience.

In testing RabbitMQ's robustness, we confirmed the system's resilience against network disruptions - an essential feature for healthcare monitoring. The queue capably handled large loads and maintained data integrity, proving its reliability. Our architecture's adaptability was highlighted as it efficiently managed data flow during interruptions. The plot depicted in Fig. 18 illustrates the queue's behavior over time, showing data accumulation during disconnection and rapid recovery upon reconnection, reflecting the system's preparedness for real-world challenges.

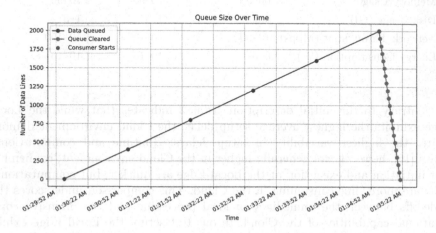

Fig. 18. Queue Behavior and Data Processing after Network Restoration

5   Discussion

5.1   Key Findings

Resilience and Robustness: Our study validates the efficiency of a Raspberry Pi, MEC, and Cloud VMs-based system for edge computing, with RabbitMQ proving resilient in managing data during network disruptions, ensuring uninterrupted patient monitoring.

Reduced Latency: Data analytics with a tier closer to the patient (MEC) contributes to reducing the latency and performance of the data analytics algorithm and the healthcare staff can know the situation timely.

Resource Utilization: The three-tier architecture enables us the efficient utilization of resources across the swarm of cluster nodes (i.e., local edge, MEC and cloud nodes) in a distributed manner.

Enhanced Security: Distributing the data acquisition to the local edge and applying ML techniques at the MEC helps enhance the security of the architecture since the data is not exposed to a wider audience. TLS security measures safeguarded data transmission, a critical aspect of patient privacy. MySQL and

Grafana integration in the Cloud tier facilitated real-time ECG signal analysis, improving clinical decision-making.

Realtime Remote Monitoring: Our three-tier architecture outperforms traditional cloud-IoT systems in scalability and real-time processing, with Docker Swarm containerization offering a significant advancement over inflexible centralized designs. Enhanced data visualization and alerting mechanisms could notably improve patient care, especially in telemedicine.

The findings encourage further advancements in container-based architectures and data analytics integration in healthcare settings. Future work may explore the inclusion of more complex data and AI-driven models for a more personalized approach to patient healthcare.

5.2 Limitations and Future Work

Our architecture presents a promising avenue for enhancing healthcare monitoring. However, addressing its limitations is crucial for continuing the progress. The current system efficiently manages data throughput, yet scaling to accommodate larger datasets and user loads is essential.

We have implemented SSL certificates for security, with no performance evaluation for post-TLS deployment and its impact, highlighting a gap for future study. Security improvements are planned, with a transition to Kubernetes clusters to leverage robust security features. [21] and best practices. Future efforts will refine system configurations, ensuring enhanced security and management of deployments in complex healthcare IoT environments.

Achieving energy efficiency, especially for edge devices, remains a challenge, with future work aimed at optimizing consumption for sustainability. Upcoming expansions include image-based data analytics, utilizing deep learning models like CNNs, U-Nets [22], and GANs [23] for advanced medical image analysis.

6 Conclusion

This work showcases a successful integration of IoT and IoMT with edge and cloud computing, forming a robust three-tier architecture for enhanced real-time patient monitoring. The proposed system merges local edge computing, MEC, and cloud computing to optimize healthcare data processing and insights extraction. At the local edge, rapid data acquisition and processing are achieved with no observable latency, while the MEC layer employs sophisticated models for deeper health data analysis. In the cloud, an advanced visualization service presents both raw and processed data, aiding medical decision-making and enhancing monitoring efficiency. The system utilizes Docker containers to create isolated environments for running applications, ensuring modular and scalable patient data processing. This setup streamlines updates and maintenance, crucial for real-time patient monitoring in hospital settings. This research marks a significant advancement in healthcare IoT, demonstrating the transformative potential of technology in patient care. Future research will aim at system optimization, integrating more complex data, employing adaptive security, and deploying AI models for further improvements in patient monitoring and healthcare technology overall.

Acknowledgements. This research is supported by the Business Finland projects Tomohead (grant 8095/31/2022), Eware-6G (grant 8819/31/2022), and the Research Council of Finland 6G Flagship program (grant number 346208).

References

1. Islam, J., Harjula, E., Kumar, T., Karhula, P., Ylianttila, M.: Docker enabled virtualized nanoservices for local IoT edge networks. In: 2019 IEEE Conference on Standards for Communications and Networking (CSCN), pp. 1–7. IEEE (2019)
2. Xie, Z., Ji, C., Xu, L., Xia, M., Cao, H.: Towards an optimized distributed message queue system for AIoT edge computing: a reinforcement learning approach. Sensors **23**(12), 5447 (2023). https://doi.org/10.3390/s23125447
3. Singh, V., Peddoju, S.K.: Container-based microservice architecture for cloud applications. In: 2017 International Conference on Computing, Communication and Automation (ICCCA), pp. 847–852. IEEE (2017)
4. Lin, J., Zhu, L., Chen, W.-M., Wang, W.-C., Han, S.: Tiny machine learning: progress and futures [Feature]. IEEE Circ. Syst. Mag. **23**(3), 8–34 (Third quarter 2023). https://doi.org/10.1109/MCAS.2023.3302182
5. Harjula, E., Kumar, T., Islam, J., Kovacevic, I.: Distributed network and service architecture for future digital healthcare. Finnish J. eHealth eWelfare **14**(1), 6–18 (2022). https://doi.org/10.23996/fjhw.111777
6. Isosalo, A., et al.: Local edge computing for radiological image reconstruction and computer-assisted detection: a feasibility study. Finnish J. EHealth EWelfare **15**(1), 52–66 (2023). https://doi.org/10.23996/fjhw.122647
7. Obaid, O.I., Salman, S.A.B.: Security and privacy in IoT-based healthcare systems: a review. Mesopotamian J. Comput. Sci. **2022**, 29–40 (2023). https://doi.org/10.58496/MJCSC/2022/007
8. Madhu, M.P., Dixit, S.: Distributing messages using RabbitMQ with advanced message exchanges. Int. J. Res. Stud. Comput. Sci. Eng. (IJRSCSE) **6**(2), 24–28 (2019). https://doi.org/10.20431/2349-4859.0602004
9. Manoj, M.V., Prashanth, B.S., Shastry, K.A., Sneha, H.R.: Healthcare data visualization. Artif. Intell. Inf. Manage. Healthc. Perspect. **88**, 179–211 (2021). https://doi.org/10.1007/978-981-16-0415-7_9
10. Leppänen, T., et al.: Mobile agents for integration of Internet of Things and wireless sensor networks. In: 2013 IEEE International Conference on Systems, Man, and Cybernetics (SMC), pp. 14–21. IEEE (2013)
11. Marathe, N., Gandhi, A., Shah, J.M.: Docker Swarm and Kubernetes in cloud computing environment. In: 2019 International Conference on Trends in Electronics and Informatics (ICOEI), pp. 179–184 (2019)
12. Chen, F.: Data transmission security in computer network communication. J. Phys. Conf. Ser. **1881**(4), 042014 (2021). https://doi.org/10.1088/1742-6596/1881/4/042014
13. Maatkamp, M.W.H.: Unidirectional secure information transfer via RabbitMQ. M.Sc. thesis, School of Computer Science and Informatics, University College Dublin, supervised by Dr. Martin van Delden and Dr. Nhien An Le Khac, December 2015. https://doi.org/10.13140/RG.2.1.1412.0720

14. Che, C., Zhang, P., Zhu, M., et al.: Constrained transformer network for ECG signal processing and arrhythmia classification. BMC Med. Inform. Decis. Making **21**, 184 (2021). https://doi.org/10.1186/s12911-021-01546-2

15. Adebiyi, A.A., John, S.N., Ndujuiba, C.: Analytical derivation of latency in computer networks. Br. J. Math. Comput. Sci. **4**(24), 3476–3488 (2014). https://doi.org/10.9734/BJMCS/2014/10770

16. Ramaswamy, R., Weng, N., Wolf, T.: Characterizing network processing delay. In: 2004 IEEE Global Telecommunications Conference (GLOBECOM), pp. 1629–1634. IEEE (2004)

17. Venkatraman, A., Pandey, V., Plale, B., Shei, S.-S.: Benchmarking effort of virtual machines on multicore machines. Technical report, Indiana University (2007). https://help.luddy.indiana.edu/techreports/TRNNN.cgi?trnum=TR654. Accessed 3 Mar 2024

18. Bekaroo, G., Santokhee, A.: Power consumption of the Raspberry Pi: a comparative analysis. In: 2016 IEEE International Conference on Emerging Technologies and Innovative Business Practices for the Transformation of Societies (EmergiTech), pp. 361–366. IEEE (2016)

19. Alqurashi, F.S., Al-Hashimi, M.: An experimental approach to estimation of the energy cost of dynamic branch prediction in an Intel high-performance processor. Computers 2023 **12**, 139 (2023). https://doi.org/10.3390/computers12070139

20. Badisa, N., Grandhi, J.K., Kallam, L., Bulla, S.: Efficient Docker Image Optimization using Multi-stage Builds and Nginx for Enhanced Application Deployment. Naveen Badisa Lab, August 2023. License CC BY 4.0. https://doi.org/10.21203/rs.3.rs-3276965/v1

21. Shamim, M.S.I., Bhuiyan, F.A., Rahman, A.: XI commandments of Kubernetes security: a systematization of knowledge related to Kubernetes security practices. In: 2020 IEEE Secure Development (SecDev), pp. 58–64. IEEE (2020)

22. Ronneberger, O., Fischer, P., Brox, T.: U-Net: convolutional networks for biomedical image segmentation. In: Navab, N., Hornegger, J., Wells, W., Frangi, A. (eds.) Medical Image Computing and Computer-Assisted Intervention - MICCAI 2015. LNCS, vol. 9351, pp. 234–241. Springer, Cham (2015). https://doi.org/10.1007/978-3-319-24574-4_28

23. Guo, Y., Wang, H., Fan, Y., Li, S., Xu, M.: Super-resolution image reconstruction based on self-calibrated convolutional GAN. https://doi.org/10.48550/arXiv.2106.05545

Preliminary Study on Wellbeing and Healthcare Services Needs in Japan and Finland for Telehealth Solutions Based on Dwelling

Jaakko Hyry[1]([✉]) (iD), Pasi Karppinen[2], Takumi Kobayashi[1],
and Daisuke Anzai[1] (iD)

[1] Graduate School of Engineering, Nagoya Institute of Technology,
Nagoya 466-8555, Japan
hyry.jaakko@nitech.ac.jp
[2] University of Oulu, Pentti Kaiteran katu 1, 90570 Oulu, Finland

Abstract. The Japanese and Finnish healthcare systems have several longstanding challenges from the scattered data in storing databases due to location sensitivity and sometimes unequal services for their users. In addition to the data itself, location plays another role for the citizens living in urban or rural areas. They suffer from different well-being outcomes as stress and sedentary lifestyles have presented negative impacts on the urban dwellers. As remote work and technological solutions have become more common, in this conceptual research, we explore the general healthcare and living area challenges and how to make services more equal to everyone. We also discuss the possible telehealth solutions and how, for example, wearable body sensors' use could offer improvements to the availability and accessibility of healthcare services.

Keywords: Healthcare · Telehealth · Telemedicine · Remote health · Wearable devices · Rural · Digital divide · Remote work

1 Introduction

"Leave no one behind" is the core principle of the UN Agenda 2030 [1] as it is crucial for institutions to possess the capability to guide and harness digital technologies inclusively and equitably. The digital divide is most pronounced in rural and remote areas due to the inequality in connectivity [2]. Additionally, the capacity to collaborate effectively with the private sector and other entities to promote the public interest is equally important [1].

While technology is advancing towards more capable and complex solutions to ease every day lives, digital health services in the EU, and specifically in Finland and Japan face similar growing issues; How to get the relevant services equally to everyone regardless of dwelling? An issue for people living in rural areas is not only poor connectivity, but also that they do not have access to

M. Särestöniemi et al. (Eds.): NCDHWS 2024, CCIS 2083, pp. 66–78, 2024.
https://doi.org/10.1007/978-3-031-59080-1_5

the same services offered in larger, concentrated cities [3]. This is not limited to regular citizens but also for people with disabilities [4] and presents an equality problem where your location affects your health outcome. These services which often require physical mobility, such as emergency services, or a health assessment, are needed especially for the older population. This is due to the tendency of the younger generations to move away from rural areas. This phenomenon skews the age demographics even more towards older population in rural areas and it has already been an economic and sustainability concern in Japan [5], and there is a need for more eHealth services due to the increased amount of age related diseases [6]. We focus on Japan and Finland due to the existing research collaboration between the countries and having experience in their healthcare systems and assistance efforts for the elderly, including creating mobile services [7], safety guidance [8] and telecommunication [9] and medication guidance [10]. The still existing problems need further collaboration, focus outside of single solutions and on the broader problems in healthcare. The researchers have access to institutions, researchers and materials from both countries to ease this process. It is worthy of note, that some of the examples mentioned in this study are derived from these real-world experiences of the researchers in both countries, having access to local news sources, and from interactions with researchers and doctors, also during Covid-19. They act as illustrations on how e.g. the Japanese healthcare system works in a daily life albeit from somewhat subjective point of view. As a smaller population country, Finland can implement healthcare solutions faster, which can also be later implemented on a smaller scale in Japan. This ongoing exchange of efforts has so far been shown beneficial, but in the future the scope should be extended as several European countries have shown to have good eHealth structures. As an example, 27 EU countries have 100% electronic medical records (eMR) structures compared to Japan's 45% [11]. As such, we want to see why the Japanese healthcare progress is slower compared to Finland and if we can have answers for them through this study.

The general problem is however how to deliver services for the rural elderly populations. In Japan some prefectures have attracted families and younger generations to move to the rural areas as they seek a more quiet life and a better place to raise their kids [12]. This is indicative of the stress people experience in larger cities. Supporting this notion is the evidence of people having greater likelihood of mental illnesses in larger cities even with better access to healthcare services [13] to rural. Looking at the mental well-being of individuals, there is evidence that having access to greener environments positively affects mental health [14]. Regarding physical health, the positive benefits of green environments also exists for children's respiratory resilience [16]. For this to happen studies are needed on how healthcare services are currently provided, and how they differ between various dwelling areas. In addition, how to offer better access to digitally enhanced future healthcare for mental and physical well-being.

As an example, a recent 6G-project in Finland, aims to reach UN's sustainable goals by using future technology to create new services for smart cities and is also doing these in collaboration with Japan [17]. These UN sustainable goals aim to offer healthcare for all parties regardless of age and economic status [18] and can be seen as a future problem alleviating effort. In this conceptual paper we first look into two relatively similar countries in terms of their social structures and the distribution of population in rural and urban areas, but also the differences the implementation of their digital health structures. We look into how the two countries could benefit from sharing solutions and data in an efficient way. We begin by discussing the challenges in telehealth to point out the problems and what basic needs for example administrative or educational should be done when offering them. Then we delve into wearable sensors for vital health tracking and why they should be used. Finally we discuss a singular example technologies could address, stress and mental health issues among citizens and healthcare staff especially in Japan. Lastly we propose future work in regards to a broader study on existing solutions and new technologies.

2 Population and Healthcare System Structures

2.1 Country Structures

To understand the problems within the two countries, we need to look at how differently they are structured. Japan has a population of 125 million people living in an area of 378 000 km^2 and 91.9% of this population is concentrated in the bigger cities [19,20] because the exodus of people from rural areas keeps continuing. This is especially evident in mountainous areas and remote islands [21]. The median age in the country is at about 48 years old and currently the amount of elderly population is the largest in the world. This is because the amount of people over the age of 65 has increased from 7.1% in 1970 to 26.6% by 2015 [22]. Finland on the other hand, has a population of only 5.5 million in a fairly similar sized area of 338 400 km^2 [23] while 72.3% of the population lives in urban areas. From this total, the amount of citizens over the age of 65 is 23.1% and similarly to Japan this number is also increasing. While the population densities of the two countries are quite different, with Finland having 18 people per sq.km compared to Japan's 338 per sq.km, the two countries suffer from increased physical and monetary burdens to the healthcare system as the amount of medical care needed increases with age. This is evident with the working aged population not being able to support the growing needs of the rising amount of elderly as the population imbalance divide expands.

2.2 Healthcare Data Structures

While Japan and Finland share similar healthcare structures, with both offering general hospital and clinics on a municipal level, the Japanese healthcare data is more scattered between various institutions. In other words, each clinic and hospital has their own Electronic Medical Records (EMR) implementation for storing patient records and the method for creating a systematic transfer from old paper records into digital versions differs based on the size of the hospital. As of 2022, about 73,3% of the Japanese hospitals used EMR's and 57.8% are connected to an external network [24]. This would enable sharing of health records with other hospitals but the low rate of implementation is a hindering factor. One concern is of data theft within the institutions. This presents a problem of accessibility for patients own data, as they needs to request it themselves if they wish to combine health reports or share health history with other clinicians. This was a bigger issue when Japan lacked a social security number system in the past. Recently a more digital society for administrative purposes with a new My Number Card system with a social security number was created in 2015, also used for filing taxes, health insurance and clinical visits. Initially, My Number Card had a penetration rate of only 15.5% as of March 2020 [25]. This was a societal issue as Japan had been slow in adopting other digital services in general and only in recent years has implemented e.g. mobile payments, which even though have grown hugely, are scattered like the healthcare service into different company provided systems and services. However, due to the low adoption rates, the Japanese government decided on giving a large monetary incentive for new registrants of the My Number Card, so the user base has now grown into 73% as of December 2023 [27]. However, the card implementation for sharing health data at clinics is still underway and many rely on the old ID registrations. This in turn makes the government's goal for digital transformation, again more difficult [26]. The lack of features slows implementation when the desired data is not always available when creating telehealth solutions.

Finland's health system has relied on social security numbers for decades for individual identification. It also has a largely decentralised healthcare administration, with multiple funding sources, and three channels for statutory services in first-contact care: the municipal system, the national health insurance system, and the occupational health care offered for employees. The core of the system is done by local municipalities who finance the primary and specialised care. This system runs fairly well, but can have long wait times due to lack of healthcare workers [28]. Compared to Japan, Finland has created a unified database for a lot of its medical data, patients clinical visits and also for digital receipts delivery. This current system is called MyKanta used by 3.5 million citizens [29] from the total population of 5.5 million. It gathers all of the necessary medical data for individual citizens to check using their own secure, online bank login credentials or separate digital certificate cards. Citizens can also opt-in/-out of data sharing in MyKanta for medical studies or between institutions if they so choose to. MyKanta medication receipts can also be used in selected countries within the EU [30], so sharing has been made more open compared to the Japanese equivalent EMRs. This enables Finnish medical institutions to more easily predict patient needs for future healthcare, and to study the data as a whole for general population predictions. It is also a legislative issue as data privacy is a common concern around the globe.

3   Telehealth Solutions and Challenges

Creation of digital systems has been a target for both countries for a long time. The Finnish Society for Telemedicine and eHealth was already founded in 1995 and has produced the first electronic tools, like the e-prescription, e-referrals and e-consultation over the years [31]. As such the Finland's societal goal has been to promote health through telecommunications and to share knowledge within the health care communities. With this the country already has a solid basis on some existing telehealth adaptations. Finland has also invested in the Healthcare Information Technology education for healthcare professional to better understand the role of technology needed in the healthcare sector. As of 1998, there has already been video consultation for psychiatry available for patients [32] and a study made in 2006 showed that 3 out of 4 patients in general practice could be diagnosed reliably via remote work [33], which clearly reduces the load on caretakers and also removes the need for patients to travel to get diagnosed.

Japan has studied telemedicine solutions also for more than 20 years, and the research community has seen the discrepancy in delivering health to rural areas as an important factor. However, the bulk of these studies are written in Japanese and there is a lack of systematic reviews on the Japanese telemedicine studies as pointed out in [34], so these findings, which the international community might find important, do not easily reach that audience. While an extensive review is needed, Japanese journals has already looked into doctor-patient diagnosis using digital tools, studied effectiveness of telemedicine, management of diseases like diabetes or heart failure and studied elderly care, but a more comprehensive approach is needed. Japan and Finland have both also started to focus on one of the more important factors related to the economy, the implementation of telemedicine that will help save huge costs in healthcare. But, there is a need to do a literature review on the existing studies to understand the extent, so we can start creating more precise solutions to the problems. While at a basic level telehealth can help with the diagnosis and communication issues quite readily, there are still procedures which so far can not be easily done remotely, such as, radiology for example. It requires the x-rays done with a professional healthcare staff and to have some larger equipment, or to have an on-location hospital required for other treatments. A study [35] addressing telehealth challenges highlights the following common problems, primarily related to human factors:

- **Staff training:** Training the staff for telehealth is a challenge as some nurses fear that telehealth makes them redundant or contrary to the goal would increase the workload instead of reducing it.
- **Project management:** A dedicated project manager is needed to ensure that implementation of telehealth projects stay within the allotted time restraints as the amount of staff time to carry out telehealth work was often underestimated.
- **Patient and staff support:** Choosing the correct patients for telehealth procedures is important as some are reluctant to use the process. Training the patient in the use of telehealth is as equally important as the staff as some diseases require specialized equipment.
- **Technology:** When delivering telehealth, the compatibility for the patients existing networks is needed. This is also a factor when considering rural areas, which might not have the necessary networks to achieve data speeds needed

for some newer technologies. Setup, calibration and maintenance of needed equipment is also crucial.

- **Local partnership:** To successfully implement telehealth solutions, local authorities should be included in the process so that they understand what are the goals of the concepts.
- **Funding:** Most telehealth projects lack long-term funding, so to be able to implement more successful projects, multi-year funding should be secured.
- **Strategic planning:** A long-term plan is recommended for a successful implementation as it takes time to complete.

These are points which are also reflected in [38] and [36] as various layers of the digital divide. They are also common in areas outside of this divide, as for example the introduction of new methods into a work environment is often met with resistance from the older workforce accustomed to the existing, learned ways. What we can speculate is that there are similarities to other existing worries present in a working environment, e.g. the fear of new technologies. The oft result in a refusal to learn, to use or to be exposed to anything new which would require re-learning [37]. As such effective implementation requires a solid plan from the implementing agency from the ground level (patients, nurses, doctors) to the higher level (administrators, engineers) to cover all of the stages of uncertainty. A steady construction of layers to support the low, middle and high level activities is needed. As an example, the training, comprehension and sharing of the tasks, pre-planning, having adequate funding and following through on a plan. Additionally it is important to make sure that all parties, especially the local authorities who need to actually use the system for a long period, to understand the overarching goal cohesively.

4 Sensor Technologies and Health

The rise of wearable body sensors, such as the Apple Watch [39], Oura Ring [40], and Dexcom sensor [41], has introduced a wealth of health data that can significantly benefit telehealth. These technologies can now monitor a user's heart rate variability (HRV), sleep quality, various exercise types, and even glucose levels. The introduction of these sensor technologies opens up possibilities for preventative healthcare. Instead of periodic check-ups, healthcare staff can now access relevant health data directly from wearable devices. Predictive assessments based on continuous user data or aggregated data from multiple individuals can influence health outcomes by identifying potential issues early on. While this do not replace the need for comprehensive check-ups, it aids in lifestyle advice and timely interventions, particularly for sedentary lifestyle problems.

For the elderly, wearable sensors, like smart sensors, can detect events such as sudden falls and prompt assistance, enhancing safety [42]. The use of wearable sensors can contribute to reducing inequality in healthcare access by reaching a broader audience, offering predictive and preventative medical services regardless of location. It enables healthcare institutions to allocate resources efficiently, predicting when and where they are needed for individuals, based on sensor data. However, the challenge lies in effectively reaching users in rural areas, even though the use of sensors can potentially reduce the need for frequent doctor visits. While developing better telehealth treatment methods from tracking data is crucial, the primary goal of sensor data remains the prevention of medical issues. We propose an extensive look into what exact existing equipment could be used for vital data tracking, which commercial sensor data is reliable enough for medical use or are they interpretive data for estimations only. Or is there need to create totally new sensors for each situation. As there are a variety of existing sensors available, it would be logical to start first with the existing solutions as a basis. Also, for any medical implementation due to strict device guidelines e.g. regarding health and radio frequency interference, the use of any existing solution would reduce the costs of implementations as it is one of the burdens for societies and even more in the future. If we look at even Wifi implementations in hospitals, we can already use the pre-existing network to track equipment, people and even respiratory rates without changes into the structure [43], so we hope to discover the same for existing wearable sensors effective use in healthcare.

Notably, while wearable sensors offer real-time advantages, consideration should also be given to the use of external digital sensors integrated into the environment. For instance, an implanted sensor in a commonly used location like a toilet could provide processed health data from multiple users without requiring individual effort or changes in routines. Wearable sensors are just one aspect of the broader picture, and this study initially focuses on them due to their flexibility in data collection.

Over the years and across various projects, visits to nursing homes in Finland and Japan, both in urban and rural areas, aimed to comprehend the caregiving processes, the elderly's daily lives, and their physical or mental challenges. Observations revealed that many solutions did not utilize technological aids, relying instead on paper and pen guides or calendars for reminders, especially in cases of dementia. While these manual methods were effective, they required physical presence for updates. Teleassistance could potentially replace certain tasks or personnel, allowing digital solutions to streamline updates and reduce the time spent on routine tasks. This becomes particularly crucial in addressing the shortage of nursing staff, a prevalent issue in the current aging population, as highlighted in various studies.

5   Physical and Mental Health Based on Dwelling

As stated earlier in [14], mental health is affected by the dwelling area of individuals as there are more prevalence of mental issues in the urban areas. Additionally, sedentary lifestyles are often related to office work and present themselves as various diseases; obesity, decreases cardiac output and systemic blood flow, and elevated chronic inflammation caused by this sedentary behaviour and are risk factors for cancer [44]. As these basic physical and mental declines happen, we can argue that moving from an urban area to a rural location would increase the overall health outcomes of people. This is not only a positive for adults getting these diseases, but other positive effects are for children with respiratory issues as improvements happen if they interact more with nature. General studies have shown that air quality, increase in exercise, stress reduction and social cohesion increase from contact with nature. These also affect general well-being of individuals [45] and provide better future health prognosis. It is suggests that moving to a rural area should be considered for individuals with a high stress work or sedentary lifestyle diseases, if possible. The positives of rural areas is due to Covid-19 presenting new and interesting developments regarding remote work in companies. Due to the isolation periods, employees had to stay at home and perform duties remotely. This meant companies had to adjust from on-location to a hybrid or fully remote and it helped create a more telework style living. Because of it, employees are now facing a new reality where they can choose where to work from and are not tied to commuting depending on the work. This makes rural areas more attractive due to the space they can offer [46] and because of the aforementioned positive effect on the mental and physical health compared to an urban environment. This would suggest that in the future there might be a bigger influx of people choosing rural living instead of urban centers. It also insinuates that telehealth plays an important role as the services are needed for people of all ages and the current centralisation of services to cities need to be reconsidered.

During Covid-19, the hospitals suffered from overworking problems, such as stress, as the staff needed to respond to the pandemic wave of new patients. While severe patients needed to be taken care of at hospitals, the less severe were isolating at home. In Japan these were followed up by daily phone and/or video calls to inquire the symptoms and the general health of a covid patient. The pandemic created a sudden need to deal with an influx of telehealth diagnosis but soon new applications need to replace the video and phone calls. This was to reduce the workload for the nurses by having patients create self reporting through teleservices, instead of one-to-one nurse calls. Both patients and citizens suffered from the effect of stress, while the former was due to the amount of work, the latter were due to isolation issues. Stress is a significant factor in overall well-being, and there's a growing feasibility in using smart devices to measure stress levels. Heart rate variability (HVR) has been identified as a reliable predictor for stress based on data obtained from the Apple Watch [47]. Moreover, smartwatches have proven to be effective tools in predicting COVID-19 infections, especially when combined with self-reported symptoms [48]. This underscores the potential utility of sensor devices in rural areas, as the data they provide can contribute to the early detection of both mental and physical health deterioration.

6 Proposed Future Research

To identify current challenges perceived by medical professionals and the preferences of healthcare recipients regarding improvements in healthcare services. The following efforts needed to be made. To gain a comprehensive understanding of how telehealth can be improved in Finland and Japan, and how new technology can be designed, an examination on the current technological landscape in both countries for both urban and rural areas is essential. This involves conducting a systematic review of existing literature, particularly focusing on Japanese publications not available in other languages. Additionally, surveys targeting medical institutions and citizens in urban and rural settings should be conducted.

The comprehensive research approach includes literature reviews, qualitative and quantitative interviews, observations, and questionnaire surveys. The objective is to gather a dataset from both countries that can uncover unique, shared, or unidentified problems in telehealth.

To establish a solid foundation, the proposed steps include: 1) detailed comparison of Finnish and Japanese services, 2) identification of existing telehealth services, and 3) exploration of ways to create new or enhance existing eHealth systems. With a focus on improving individual well-being, additional steps involve: 4) enhancing physical and mental well-being for all individuals through these systems, and 5) increasing inclusivity, social connectivity, and reducing the digital divide. Based on the data results, there is an opportunity to formulate a broader system's design guideline for developing eHealth services. This guideline, depicted in Fig. 1, could serve as a basis for government policymakers. A less-explored avenue involves conducting a comparative study on how urban and rural living impacts mental and physical health. This includes investigating if there are optimal dwelling locations near urban areas and this kind of study could facilitate better access to urban medical care while benefiting from the natural advantages of rural living.

7   Discussion

The core principle of the UN Agenda 2030, "Leave no one behind," underscores the importance of guiding and harnessing digital technologies inclusively. The digital divide, most pronounced in rural areas, raises challenges in providing equitable access to healthcare services. This paper explored the shared issues faced by the EU, Finland, and Japan, focusing on delivering relevant services to all, irrespective of dwelling. Examination of the demographic structures of Japan and Finland reveals distinctive challenges posed by an aging population and increasing healthcare demands. Disparities in population density contribute to heightened burdens on healthcare systems, necessitating innovative approaches to address the rising needs of the elderly in rural areas. Comparing healthcare data structures in Japan and Finland, the study highlights the differences in data accessibility and privacy concerns. While Finland boasts a unified database system (MyKanta), Japan faces challenges in implementing Electronic Medical Records (EMRs) due to concerns about data theft and slow digital service adoption. However, there are privacy related issues in collecting healthcare data, so consideration on how legislation and privacy for one's own health data is maintained is needed when dealing with sensitive data. Finland is already fairly advanced in this area from the use of e.g. MyData [49,50], which is a non-profit solution on maintaining data privacy and ownership of it by the citizens. Both countries have a history of studying telehealth solutions,

Phase 1 - Identify:
- General Healthcare & eHealth services
- Cities vs. rural areas service structures
- Medical staff problem points & needs (survey)
- Service users problem points & needs (survey)

Phase 2 - Analyse:
- Deliverables: What are the commonalities?
- What are the differences?
- What are the improvement points?

Phase 3 - Conceptualise:
- Deliverables: A guideline for designing a service system for Finland and Japan
- Future design and research approaches

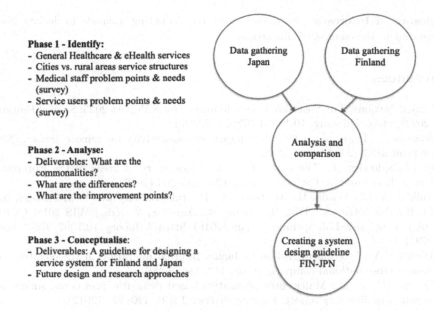

Fig. 1. The research phases of the future work

stressing the importance of leveraging technology for healthcare improvements. Challenges identified include staff training, project management, patient and staff support, technology compatibility, local partnerships, funding, and strategic planning. The COVID-19 pandemic and the rise of remote work present opportunities for the increased adoption of telehealth services. Wearable devices and sensor technologies offer potential solutions for monitoring health metrics and providing real-time data. The study underscores the significance of sensor technologies in predicting and preventing health issues, especially for the elderly population. The paper proposes a comprehensive research plan, including a systematic literature review, surveys for medical institutions and residents, and the creation of design guidelines for eHealth services. The aim is to gather data on existing technologies, identify unique problems, and develop solutions to increase inclusivity and well-being. Collaboration, knowledge sharing, and a holistic approach are highlighted as essential for addressing multifaceted challenges and opportunities in the implementation of digital health services. The importance of international collaboration in developing and testing telehealth services is also highlighted. In conclusion, this research contributes to the understanding of telehealth challenges and solutions in Finland and Japan, offering insights for future improvements in healthcare systems, with a focus on inclusivity and well-being in times of the digital divide.

Acknowledgments. This research and development work was supported in part by the MIC/SCOPE (grant number JP225006004) and by the Scandinavia-Japan Sasakawa Foundation grant.

Disclosure of Interests. The authors have no competing interests to declare that are relevant to the content of this article.

References

1. United Nations: The Sustainable Development Goals Report 2023: Special Edition (2023). https://doi.org/10.18356/9789210024914
2. Saarnisaari, H., et al.: A 6G white paper on connectivity for remote areas. arXiv preprint arXiv:2004.14699 (2020)
3. Kos-Łabędowicz, J.: The issue of digital divide in rural areas of the European Union. Ekonomiczne Problemy Usług **126**, 195–204 (2017)
4. Tuikka, A.-M., Vesala, H., Teittinen, A.: Digital disability divide in Finland. In: Li, H., Pálsdóttir, Á., Trill, R., Suomi, R., Amelina, Y. (eds.) WIS 2018. CCIS, vol. 907, pp. 162–173. Springer, Cham (2018). https://doi.org/10.1007/978-3-319-97931-1_13
5. Ishikawa, Y.: Internal migration in Japan. Internal migration in the countries of Asia: a cross-national comparison, pp. 113–136 (2020)
6. Ikejima, C., et al.: Multicentre population-based dementia prevalence survey in Japan: a preliminary report. Psychogeriatrics **12**(2), 120–123 (2012)
7. Pulli, P., et al.: Design and development of mobile services platform for senior citizens. In: 2007 IEEE International Technology Management Conference (ICE), pp. 1–8. IEEE (2007)
8. Pulli, P., et al.: Mobile augmented teleguidance-based safety navigation concept for senior citizens. In: 2nd International Conference on Applied and Theoretical Information Systems Research (2nd. ATISR2012), pp. 1–9 (2012)
9. Yamamoto, G., et al.: Grid-pattern indicating interface for ambient assisted living. In: Proceedings of International Conference on Disability, Virtual Reality and Associated Technologies, pp. 405–408 (2014)
10. Hyry, J., et al.: Design of assistive tabletop projector-camera system for the elderly with cognitive and motor skill impairments. ITE Trans. Media Technol. Appl. **5**(2), 57–66 (2017)
11. Slawomirski, L., et al.: Progress on implementing and using electronic health record systems: developments in OECD countries as of 2021 (2021)
12. Obikwelu, F.E., Ikegami, K., Tsuruta, T.: Factors of urban-rural migration and socio-economic condition of I-turn migrants in rural Japan. J. Asian Rural Stud. **1**(1), 70–80 (2017)
13. Gruebner, O., Rapp, M.A., Adli, M., Kluge, U., Galea, S., Heinz, A.: Cities and mental health. Dtsch. Arztebl. Int. **114**(8), 121 (2017)
14. Siah, C.J.R., Kua, E.H., Goh, Y.S.S.: The impact of restorative green environment on mental health of big cities and the role of mental health professionals. Curr. Opin. Psychiatry **35**(3), 186–191 (2022)
15. Cole, M.B., Lee, E.K., Davoust, M., Carey, K., Kim, J.: Comparison of visit rates before vs after telehealth expansion among patients with mental health diagnoses treated at federally qualified health centers. JAMA Netw. Open. **5**(11), e2242059 (2022). https://doi.org/10.1001/jamanetworkopen.2022.42059
16. Parmes, E., et al.: Influence of residential land cover on childhood allergic and respiratory symptoms and diseases: evidence from 9 European cohorts. Environ. Res. **183**, 108953 (2020)

17. Matinmikko-Blue, M., et al.: White paper on 6G drivers and the UN SDGs. arXiv preprint arXiv:2004.14695 (2020)
18. United Nations: The Sustainable Development Goals Report 2019 (2019). https://unstats.un.org/sdgs/report/2019/. Referenced 11 Jan 2024
19. United Nations Statistics Division Website (2023). http://data.un.org/Data.aspx?q=JAPAN+population+age&d=POP&f=tableCode:22;countryCode:392. Referenced 11 Jan 2024
20. United Nations, Department of Economic and Social Affairs, Population Division (2019b). World urbanization prospects: The 2018 revision (ST/ESA/SER.A/420). United Nations. https://population.un.org/wup/Publications/Files/WUP2018-Report.pdf
21. Center for Research and Promotion of Japanese Islands: Statistical yearbook of Japanese islands 2017. Center for Research and Promotion of Japanese Islands (J) (2019)
22. Fukawa, T.: Elderly population projection and their health expenditure prospects in Japan. Mod. Econ. **8**(11), 1258 (2017)
23. Statistics Finland Website (2021). https://pxdata.stat.fi/PxWeb/pxweb/en/StatFin/StatFin__vaerak/statfin_vaerak_pxt_11ra.px/table/tableViewLayout1/. Referenced 13 Jan 2024
24. Takeshita, K., Takao, H., Imoto, S., Murayama, Y.: Improvement of the Japanese healthcare data system for the effective management of patients with COVID-19: a national survey. Int. J. Med. Informatics **162**, 104752 (2022)
25. Ogawa, A., Akai, N.: Determinants of penetration rate of "Identify Number Card" in Japan (No. 21J002). Osaka School of International Public Policy, Osaka University (2021)
26. Tomura, N., et al.: Construction of the E-Government case study of Japan and Estonia. Int. J. Appl. Inf. Manage. **1**(3), 145–151 (2021)
27. Ministry of Internal Affairs and Communications (MIC), Regarding the issuance and number of My Number cards held, December 2023. (In Japanese). https://www.soumu.go.jp/main_content/000921347.pdf. Referenced 24 Jan 2024
28. Keskimaki, I., et al.: Finland: health system review. Health Syst. Transit. **21**(2), 1–166 (2019)
29. MyKanta: About MyKanta services. https://www.kanta.fi/en/about-kanta-services. Referenced 11 Jan 2024
30. Kanta.fi webpage. https://www.kanta.fi/en/buying-prescription-medicines-abroad. Accessed 2 Mar 2024
31. Reponen, J.: Finnish society of telemedicine. J. Telemed. Telecare **11**(1), 51 (2005)
32. Mielonen, M.L., Ohinmaa, A., Moring, J., Isohanni, M.: The use of videoconferencing for telepsychiatry in Finland. J. Telemed. Telecare **4**(3), 125–131 (1998)
33. Timonen, O.: The teleconsultation in general practice. A randomized, controlled study of a remote consultation experiment using a videoconferencing system. Int. J. Circumpolar Health **63**(3), 289–290 (2004)
34. Akiyama, M., Yoo, B.K.: A systematic review of the economic evaluation of telemedicine in Japan. J. Prev. Med. Public Health **49**(4), 183 (2016)
35. Joseph, V., West, R.M., Shickle, D., Keen, J., Clamp, S.: Key challenges in the development and implementation of telehealth projects. J. Telemed. Telecare **17**(2), 71–77 (2011)
36. Robinson, L., et al.: Digital inequalities 2.0: legacy inequalities in the information age. First Monday **25**(7) (2020)

37. Scholkmann, A.B.: Resistance to (digital) change: individual, systemic and learning-related perspectives. Digital transformation of learning organizations, pp. 219–236 (2021)
38. Robinson, L., et al.: Digital inequalities 3.0: emergent inequalities in the information age. First Monday **25**(7) (2020)
39. Seshadri, D.R., et al.: Accuracy of Apple Watch for detection of atrial fibrillation. Circulation **141**(8), 702–703 (2020)
40. Altini, M., Kinnunen, H.: The promise of sleep: a multi-sensor approach for accurate sleep stage detection using the Oura ring. Sensors **21**(13), 4302 (2021)
41. Guillot, F.H., et al.: Accuracy of the Dexcom G6 glucose sensor during aerobic, resistance, and interval exercise in adults with type 1 diabetes. Biosensors **10**(10), 138 (2020)
42. González-Cañete, F.J., Casilari, E.: A feasibility study of the use of smartwatches in wearable fall detection systems. Sensors **21**(6), 2254 (2021)
43. Ge, Y., et al.: Contactless WiFi sensing and monitoring for future healthcare-emerging trends, challenges, and opportunities. IEEE Rev. Biomed. Eng. **16**, 171–191 (2022)
44. Park, J.H., Moon, J.H., Kim, H.J., Kong, M.H., Oh, Y.H.: Sedentary lifestyle: overview of updated evidence of potential health risks. Korean J. Family Med. **41**(6), 365 (2020)
45. Coventry, P.A.: Nature-Based Outdoor Activities for Mental and Physical Health: Systematic Review and Meta-analysis. Population Health (2021)
46. Phillipson, J., et al.: The COVID-19 pandemic and its implications for rural economies. Sustainability **12**(10), 3973 (2020)
47. Hernando, D., Roca, S., Sancho, J., Alesanco, Ä., Bailón, R.: Validation of the apple watch for heart rate variability measurements during relax and mental stress in healthy subjects. Sensors **18**(8), 2619 (2018)
48. Zhu, T., Watkinson, P., Clifton, D.A.: Smartwatch data help detect COVID-19. Nat. Biomed. Eng. **4**(12), 1125–1127 (2020)
49. Koivumäki, T., Pekkarinen, S., Lappi, M., Väisänen, J., Juntunen, J., Pikkarainen, M.: Consumer adoption of future MyData-based preventive eHealth services: an acceptance model and survey study. J. Med. Internet Res. **19**(12), e429 (2017)
50. Wang, F., Karppinen, P., Ahokangas, P.: Exploring factors influencing actor engagement in MyData health platform: a case study from Finland (2023)

User Experience and Citizen Data

Dynamics in Entry and Exit Registrations in a 14-Year Follow-Up of Nationwide Electronic Prescription and Patient Data Repository Services in Finland

Vesa Jormanainen[1,2](✉) (iD)

[1] Faculty of Medicine, Doctoral School of Health Sciences, Doctoral Programme in Population Health, University of Helsinki, P.O. Box 63, 00014 Helsinki, Finland
vesa.jormanainen@gov.fi
[2] Ministry of Social Affairs and Health, Clients and Services in Healthcare and Social Welfare, P.O. Box 33, 00023 Helsinki, Finland

Abstract. There exist a need to carry out further research in order to describe implementation and adoption of nationwide healthcare information systems. This research aimed to follow-up in a 14-year period (2010–2023) of public and private healthcare service organizations' entries to and exits from the centralized electronic Prescription and Patient Data Repository Services in Finland. Our material comes from the official Social Welfare and Healthcare Organization Registry (*SOTE-organisaatiorekisteri*), which is part of the national Code Server and the Kanta Services. Registry data were extracted in an excel file format in 3 January 2024. Outcomes were continuous registration of services or registered exist from the services. We found profound dynamics in the registry data. In the nationwide Prescription Services, the registered organizations provided altogether 8,884 follow-up years, during which in 2010–2023 there were in total 1,530 healthcare service organization entries and 553 exits from the national services, whereas 977 organizations had the national services in production in 2023. In Patient Data Repository Services, the registered organizations provided altogether 7,692 follow-up years, during which in 2011–2023 there were totally 1,980 healthcare service organization entries and 494 exits from the national services, whereas 1,486 organizations had the national services in production in 2023. No effects of Covid-19 epidemic were observed. Permanent legislation may explain many of the peak numbers observed in this research. Effects of the structural reform to reorganize healthcare, social welfare and rescue services to wellbeing services counties starting January 2023 were observed in this registry research on public healthcare service organizations.

Keywords: Long-term follow-up · National healthcare data systems · Kanta Services · Finland

M. Särestöniemi et al. (Eds.): NCDHWS 2024, CCIS 2083, pp. 81–92, 2024.
https://doi.org/10.1007/978-3-031-59080-1_6

1 Introduction

Healthcare is both complex and hierarchical, characterized by interrelated subsystems, and social, characterized by formal structures and elementary units [1–5]. Most healthcare reforms are not properly followed-up, and their outcomes are rarely evaluated [6]. The demand for healthcare system and service reforms is compelling, and often there is little choice but to implement complex information and communication technology on a large, often nationwide scale [7, 8]. Clearly, there exist a need to carry out further research in order to describe implementation and adoption of nationwide healthcare information systems.

Health information exchange (HIE) is the electronic transfer of patient data and health information between healthcare providers or institutions regionally, nationally and internationally between different information systems [5, 9–11]. HIE systems assist healthcare organizations in collecting, processing and disseminating electronic information internally and in their environment [12]. An electronic health record system (EHR) is an electronic collection of health-related data concerning one subject of care – the patient. It provides clinical data [13, 14] and a longitudinal record of information in computer processible form across practices and specialists in real time [15]. An EHR can include an organized web-based patient portal allowing patients independent access to their own data. However, only a small number of nationwide implementations of shared patient-accessible EHRs have been launched in OECD countries, including that of Finland [5, 16–18].

Health information systems (HIS) integrate the data collection, processing, reporting, and use of the information necessary for improving health service effectiveness and efficiency through better management. Comprehensive HIS implementation is risky [19–21]. Implementing a new nationwide HIS is a megaproject: large-scale, complex and costly, taking many years to develop and build, involving multiple public and private stakeholders and impacting millions of people [20, 22, 23].

Finnish patient records became electronic in phases during the 1970s [24, 25]. Finland's first large-scale health information development programme in healthcare and social welfare services was the Satakunta Macro Pilot regional programme, which ran in Western Finland in 1998–2001 [26]. In primary healthcare, the prevalence of electronic patient records was 50% in 1998, and 50% in municipal primary healthcare hospitals in 2002; by contrast, the figure was 100% by 2007 [27]. By 2007, all central and university hospitals had electronic patient records, electronic image repositories and laboratory systems in place [28]. In 15 June 2001, the Ministry of Social Affairs and Health (STM) proposed that the Social Insurance Institution of Finland (Kela) together with the Finnish Medicines Agency (Fimea) begin assessing the requirements for developing electronic prescriptions in Finland [29].

Large-scale implementation of nationwide HIS services is a rather novel research theme, the concepts and definitions of which are still to be established. Thus far, no comprehensive review of the empirical research literature has been performed for strategies for electronic health implementation [30].

The World Health Organization (WHO) has recently introduced the term 'digital health', which is the systematic application of information and communications technologies, computer science, and data to support informed decision-making by individuals, the health workforce, and data systems, to strengthen resilience to disease and improve health and wellness [31–33]. The health system challenges can be grouped into nine overarching categories: information, availability, quality, acceptability, utilization, efficiency, cost, accountability, and equity [33]. Digital health application is the software, information and communications technology systems or health communication channels that deliver or execute the digital health intervention and health content.

The follow-up data from May 2010 to December 2018 provided the first observations on the increasing availability of the nationwide Kanta Services in Finland [34]. However, there were no means to observe the services separately by public or private healthcare service organizations. This research aimed to extend the follow-up from January 2019 to December 2023, and thus, in order to cover a 14-year period (2010–2023) of healthcare data processing in the centralized electronic Prescription and Patient Data Repository Services. During the study period, two major events took place in Finland, e.g. the Covid-19 epidemic (starting March 2020) and the major re-organization of healthcare, social welfare and rescue services (starting January 2023). The objective of this research was to document if these major events had any impacts on healthcare organizations' entries to and exits from two nationwide Kanta information services.

2   Material and Methods

2.1   Nationwide Kanta Services in Finland

The Kanta Services is the name of Finland's nationwide centralized, shared, and integrated electronic data system services. The main national Kanta Services were introduced in phases in 2010–2018. The Kanta Services form a unique service concept and entity comprising My Kanta Pages, Prescription Services, a Pharmaceutical Database, a Patient Data Repository, the archiving of old patient data, a client-data archive for social welfare services, the sharing of medical certificates, the Kelain online prescription service and the Kanta client test service [34]. The Finnish national legislation on Kanta Services came into effect in 2007.

2.2   Material

The Finnish Institute for Health and Welfare (THL) maintains the official Social Welfare and Healthcare Organization Registry (*SOTE-organisaatiorekisteri*), which is accessible for everybody via internet. The registry is part of the national Code Server [https://koo distopalvelu.kanta.fi/codeserver/], and the Kanta Services. In this official registry, data on public and private organizations are compiled from social welfare and healthcare service providers and their service units. The registry data are used for registration and release of electronic prescriptions, patient and customer documents in the healthcare Kanta Services. The THL (specifications) and the social welfare and healthcare service providers (data) together are responsible to maintain the registry up-to-date and data correct. The Kela provides dates of the registered entries and exits in the registry.

2.3 Methods

Full registry data were extracted in an excel file format in 3 January 2024. The full registry contained originally 44 columns (variables) and 121 018 rows (organization issues). Officially registered dates of entries to and exits from the Prescription and Patient Data Repository Services were identified by public and private sector organizations, respectively. The registry only contained data on organizations, not on medication dispensing community pharmacies or prescribing professionals (e.g., physicians, dentists or nurses).

Outcomes were continuous registration of the services or registered exist from the services.

3 Results

3.1 Prescription Services

In total 252 entries to the nationwide Prescription Services among public healthcare service provider organizations took place in 2010–2023, out of which largest numbers around 2011–2013 with the highest peak number (n = 113) in 2012 (Table 1). In 2022–2023, numbers were higher than in previous years. In total 169 exits from the nationwide Prescription Services among public organizations took place in 2010–2023, out of which the largest numbers in 2016, 2019 and 2023 with the highest peak number (n = 118) in 2023. The number of organizations that had Prescription Services in production rose to 133 from 2010 to 2013 stabilizing to level 170–181 in 2014–2022. In 2023, 23 public organizations entered and 118 public organizations left the Prescription Services, and 83 organizations had the services in production.

In total 1,302 entries to the nationwide Prescription Services among private healthcare organizations took place 2010–2023, out of which largest numbers in 2014 and 2016–2017 with the highest peak numbers (Table 1). In 2014, there were also more entries than in other years. In total 384 exits in the nationwide Prescription Services among private healthcare service organizations in 2010–2023, out of which the highest number (n = 71) in 2019. The number of private organizations that had Prescription Services in production rose to 52 from 2012 to 2014 stabilizing to level 37–71 in 2015–2023. In 2023, 56 private organizations entered and 55 organizations left the Prescription Services, and 198 organizations had the services in production.

In 2010–2023, in total 1,530 organization entries and 553 exits took place in the nationwide Prescription Service, and 977 organizations had the Prescription Services in production in 2023.

3.2 Patient Data Repository Services

In total 247 entries to the nationwide Patient Data Repository Services among public healthcare service organizations took place in 2011–2023, out of which largest numbers around 2014–2015 and 2023 with the highest peak number (n = 128) in 2014 (Table 2). In total 161 exits from the Patient Data Repository Services among public healthcare organizations took place in 2011–2023. The number of public sector organizations that had the services in production rose to 144 from 2011 to 2014 stabilizing to level 169–191

Table 1. Prescription Services: annual number of organization entries, exits and in production of nationwide electronic Prescription Services by public and private healthcare service organizations in 2010–2023 in Finland.

| | Prescription Services | | | | | | | | |
| | Public | | | Private | | | All | | |
Year	Entry	Exit	Production	Entry	Exit	Production	Entry	Exit	Production
2010	1	0	1	2	0	2	0	0	0
2011	22	0	23	0	0	2	1	0	1
2012	113	3	133	0	0	2	113	3	111
2013	43	2	174	33	0	35	76	2	185
2014	6	2	178	181	6	210	187	8	364
2015	7	4	181	32	6	236	39	10	393
2016	14	18	177	335	28	543	349	46	696
2017	5	2	180	327	21	849	332	23	1005
2018	1	2	179	87	52	884	88	54	1039
2019	1	10	170	68	71	881	69	81	1027
2020	1	1	170	56	46	891	57	47	1037
2021	0	0	170	61	62	890	61	62	1036
2022	15	7	178	64	37	917	79	44	1071
2023	23	118	83	56	55	918	79	173	977
	252	169		1302	384		1530	553	

in 2015–2022. In 2023, 23 organizations entered to and 118 organizations left the Patient Data Repository Services, and 86 organizations had the services in production.

In total 1,733 entries to the nationwide Patient Data Repository Services among private healthcare organizations took place in 2010–2023, out of which largest numbers in 2014 and 2016–2017 with the highest peak numbers (Table 2). In 2014, there were also more entries than in other years. In total 384 exits from the Patient Data Repository Services among private healthcare service organizations took place in 2010–2023, out of which the highest number (n = 71) in 2019. The number of organizations that had Patient Data Repository Services in production rose to 812 from 2016 to 2018, and had an increasing trend thereafter. In 2023, 224 organizations entered to and 70 organizations left the Patient Data Repository Services, and 1,400 organizations had the services in production.

In 2011–2023, in total 1,980 organization entered to and 494 left the nationwide Patient Data Repository Services among private healthcare service organizations. Altogether 1,486 organizations had the nationwide Patient Data Repository Services in production in 2023.

In Patient Data Repository Services, the registered organizations provided altogether 7,692.1 follow-up years, out of which 2,372.8 years from the exit group and 5,557.9 years from the continuous group.

Table 2. Patient Data Repository Services: annual number of organization entries, exits and in production of nationwide Patient Data Repository Services by public and private healthcare service organizations in 2010–2023 in Finland.

	Patient Data Repository Services								
	Public			Private			All		
Year	Entry	Exit	Production	Entry	Exit	Production	Entry	Exit	Production
2010	0	0	0	0	0	0	0	0	0
2011	1	0	1	0	0	0	1	0	1
2012	14	1	14	0	0	0	14	1	14
2013	2	0	16	0	0	0	2	0	16
2014	128	0	144	0	0	0	128	0	144
2015	49	2	191	0	0	0	49	2	191
2016	2	18	175	78	2	76	80	20	251
2017	6	2	179	205	4	277	211	6	456
2018	1	1	179	553	18	812	554	19	991
2019	1	10	170	200	53	959	201	63	1129
2020	1	2	169	144	56	1047	145	58	1216
2021	2	0	171	161	72	1136	163	72	1307
2022	17	7	181	168	58	1246	185	65	1427
2023	23	118	86	224	70	1400	247	188	1486
	247	161		1733	333		1980	494	

4 Discussion

Based on literature, the current research is a rather rare study reporting detailed data on national level implementation of two large-scale healthcare centralized services in a 14-year time span in Finland by using a unique official database that contained data on organization entry and exit dates by public or private healthcare service providers in 2010–2023 in Finland. In this study, we report the first time healthcare private sector organizations' entries to and exits from two nationwide services in Finland.

We found profound dynamics among public and private healthcare organizations in the registry data. In the nationwide Prescription Services, 1530 healthcare organizations entered to and 553 left the national services, whereas 977 organizations had the national services in production in 2023. In Patient Data Repository Services, 1980 healthcare organization entered to and 494 left the national services, whereas 1486 organizations had the national services in production in 2023.

Permanent legislation may explain many of the number peaks observed in this research. For example in Prescription Services, the centralized Prescription Centre services were launched in mid-May 2010. The target date for pharmacies to adopt the Prescription services was set by end-March 2012, whereas it was by end-March 2013 for public primary healthcare providers. Private healthcare providers were divided in two phases based on their annual prescription volume: the target date was end-December 2014 for healthcare providers who had more than 5,000 prescriptions annually, whereas the target date was end-December 2016 for the rest of private healthcare service providers. These legally set target dates explain rather well the cumulative effects of the observations shown in Table 1. Similar observations in Patient Data Repository Services are found in Table 2. Especially in the Patient Data Repository Services, there were healthcare service organizations' entries and exits before the services were launched in early-November 2013. These exists and entries were due to development (2011) and a 'sliding' to the services by common registries in 2012.

In Finland, the responsibility for organizing healthcare, social welfare and rescue services was transferred from municipalities and joint municipal authorities to wellbeing services counties on 1 January 2023 [35]. Today there are 21 wellbeing services counties. The region of Uusimaa is divided into four wellbeing services counties. The City of Helsinki continues to be responsible for organizing healthcare, social welfare and rescue services. The HUS Group is responsible for demanding specialized healthcare duties separately laid down by law. This major reform – the largest in Finland since the World War II – may well explain observed effects on healthcare service organizations in 2022–2023 in this research.

In this registry study, neither in the Prescription Services nor in the Patient Data Repository Services on healthcare service organizations' service entry or exit time series revealed any specific effects due to Covid-19 epidemic in Finland.

Most of the literature on change, reforms and transformations in healthcare describes initiatives typically performed by a single healthcare organization or by one service alone [36]. Literature suggests that the success of a large-system transformation depends on local history, and, in particular, the role of the physicians appears to be crucial to healthcare transformations.

Transformational change (e.g. implementation of a nationwide HIS or infrastructure) involves significant and fundamental systemic change in an organization's working methods, requiring changes in structure, culture and management [37, 38]. The transformational change of organizations is usually required for successful implementation of a large-scale HIS or HIE. However, successful transformational change programmes are rarely replicated in another setting [15]. Moreover, large-scale transformation health system processes usually involve possible tensions between bottom-up and top-down approaches [37].

The large investments required for HISs and HIEs have driven demand for effective monitoring of the resulting adoption, use and impact [39]. Longitudinal monitoring can provide valuable feedback on underlying policies and highlight the complex nature of monitoring and the assessment of implementation (and adoption). Establishing an evidence base for health information policies, trends and developments may involve utilizing transparent, published and continuous monitoring and assessments.

In a recent study in Denmark and Finland, implementations of a new commercial data system was analyzed by documents including user surveys, assessment reports, material from project partners, and research papers [40]. The Danish and Finnish implementations were still troubled five and three years, respectively, after the first go-live. In Denmark, the business case and implementation processes have been sharply criticized. The correction of usability problems and unstable system integrations have been slow, the time required to perform common clinical tasks has increased, and 32% of the users remain dissatisfied or very dissatisfied with the system. In Finland, the physicians' and nurses' experience improved technical performance but inferior usability and reduced work support compared to the EHR they used before the new already implemented data system. The consequences of using the new data system have become salient only after go-live. As a result, the implementing organizations and their users have predominantly found themselves in a reactive mode of fending off problems rather than a proactive mode of realizing benefits.

This research's findings on dynamics in entry to and exit from the two nationwide services in Finland suggest that there exist a major administrative burden on public or private healthcare organizations as well as the Kela. For example from testing to production is a demanding phase since before starting production use, the information system provider must successfully complete joint testing and, possibly, deployment testing. In general, healthcare provider organizations are using a legally certified commercial information system that they already have implemented and adopted in the organization. In addition, both parties must accept and sign an agreement on issues of starting to use and actually using the appropriate nationwide Kanta Services and stating the responsibilities of the parties.

A major strength of the present study is access to comprehensive and detailed official national register data from public and private sector healthcare provider organizations. Due to this comprehensive data access, registered services' entry and exit dates are up-to-date in real time. The unique material in this research consisted of dates from the official registry in 2010–2023. To the author's knowledge, almost no previous studies exist on the implementation of two national HIS services conducted in a time-series fashion [34].

There are also limitations in the present study. The target registry – the official Social Welfare and Healthcare Organization Registry – contains information on organizations that use the nationwide Kanta Services, e.g. Prescription and Patient Data Repository Services, and their service entry and exit data. However, the registry data and information excludes private practitioners and individual professionals that contribute to information volume in the nationwide services. Information on professionals is confidential and is not directly accessible via internet. Furthermore, the registry does not include information on pharmacies whose information can be found in the official Pharmacy Register (*Fimea Apteekkirekisteri*) maintained by the Fimea.

The latest strategy for digitalization and information management in healthcare and social welfare in Finland vision is building a digital foundation for healthcare and social welfare [41]. Strategy timespan covers years 2024–2035. Citizens will be provided with better opportunities to independently take care of their wellbeing and health as individuals, service customers or as persons managing the affairs of their close family members. The flexibility and efficiency of healthcare and social welfare services will be enhanced through customer and service counselling and the introduction of advanced technology, while at the same time, the workload of the personnel will be reduced. Health and social services will be organized on the basis of effectiveness data and evidence (research findings or evaluated data) on higher quality basis and in a socially, economically and ecologically sustainable manner. A total of 13 sets of tasks are listed in the strategic roadmap.

In digitalization operating practices are developed and updated using information management as a basis [41]. It involves the changing of an organization's processes and electrification of services in line with the advances of information and communications technology (ICT). Planned digitalization measures can only be successfully implemented if the change is planned and coordinated by the key actor instead of allowing the change to be driven by ICT. Information management means the definition of the contents and uses of information as well as the collection, organization and storage of information in such a manner that the information can be retrieved and used appropriately and in a controlled manner. In information management, ICT solutions are combined with an organization's activities and the flow of information in the organization. Information management and ensuring interoperability are prerequisites for digitalization.

Acknowledgments. The contributions of the THL national Code Server process, the Kela (Kanta Services) and private and public healthcare organizations are acknowledged in preparing, development, specifications and maintenance of the official Social Welfare and Healthcare Organization Registry (*SOTE-organisaatiorekisteri*) in Finland.

Disclosure of Interests. The author has no competing interests to declare.

References

1. Aarts, J., Peel, V.: Using a descriptive model of change when implementing large scale clinical information systems to identify priorities for further research. Int. J. Med. Inform. **56**, 43–50 (1999). https://doi.org/10.1016/s1386-5056(99)00045-3
2. Glouberman, S., Mintzberg, H.: Managing the care of health and the cure of disease—Part I: differentiation. Health Care Manage. Rev. **26**, 58–71 (2001). https://doi.org/10.1097/000 04010-200101000-00006
3. Coiera, E.: Building a national health IT system from the Middle Out. J. Am. Med. Inform. Assoc. **16**, 271–273 (2009). https://doi.org/10.1197/jamia.M3183
4. Justinia, T.: Implementing large-scale healthcare information systems: the technological, managerial and behavioural issues. Saarbrücken (Germany): Scholars' Press, 2014. Dissertation approved by University of Wales Swansea (2009)
5. Bowden, T., Coiera, E.: Comparing New Zealand's 'middle out' health information technology strategy with other OECD nations. Int. J. Med. Inform. **82**, e87–e95 (2013). https://doi.org/10.1016/j.ijmedinf.2012.12.002
6. Couffinhal, A., Cylus, J., Elovainio, R., et al.: International expert panel prereview of health and social care reform in Finland. Reports and Memorandums of the Ministry of Social Affairs and Health 2016:66. Ministry of Social Affairs and Health, Helsinki (2016)
7. Ludwick, D.A., Doucette, J.: Adopting electronic medical records in primary care: lessons learned from health information systems implementation experience in seven countries. Int. J. Med. Inform. **78**, 22–31 (2009). https://doi.org/10.1016/j.ijmedinf.2008.06.005
8. Coiera, E., Aarts, J., Kulikowski, C.: The dangerous decade. J. Am. Med. Inform. Assoc. **19**, 2–5 (2012). https://doi.org/10.1136/amiajnl-2011-000674
9. Adler-Milstein, J., Ronchi, E., Cohen, G.R., et al.: Benchmarking health IT among OECD countries: better data for better policy. J. Am. Med. Inform. Assoc. **21**, 111–116 (2014). https://doi.org/10.1136/amiajnl-2013-001710
10. Esmaeilzadeh, P., Sambasivan, M.: Health information exchange (HIE): a literature review, assimilation pattern and a proposed classification for a new policy approach. J. Biomed. Inform. **64**, 74–86 (2016). https://doi.org/10.1016/j.jbi.2016.09.011

11. Sadoughi, F., Nasiri, S., Ahmadi, H.: The impact of health information exchange on healthcare quality and cost-effectiveness: a systematic literature review. Comput. Methods Programs Biomed. **161**, 209–232 (2018). https://doi.org/10.1016/j.cmpb.2018.04.023

12. Yusof, M.M., Stergioulas, L., Zugic, J.: Investigating evaluation frameworks for health information systems. Int. J. Med. Inf. **77**, 377–385 (2008). https://doi.org/10.1016/j.ijmedinf.2007.08.004

13. Coiera, E., Kocaballi, B., Halamka, J., et al.: L. The digital scribe. NPJ Digit. Med. **1**, 58 (2018). https://doi.org/10.1038/s41746-018-0066-9

14. Ammenwerth, E., Neyer, S., Hörbst, A., et al.: Adult patient access to electronic health records. Cochrane Database Syst. Rev. **2021**, CD012707 (2021). https://doi.org/10.1002/146 51858.CD012707.pub2

15. Fennelly, O., Cunningham, C., Grogan, L., et al.: Successfully implementing a national electronic health record: a rapid umbrella review. Int. J. Med. Inform. **144**, 104281 (2020). https:// doi.org/10.1016/j.ijmedinf.2020.104281

16. Oderkirk, J.: Readiness of electronic health record systems to contribute to national health information and research. OECD Health Working Papers No. 99. OECD Directorate for Employment, Labour and Social Affairs, Health Committee, Paris, pp. 1–78 (2017). https:// one.oecd.org/document/DELSA/HEA/WD/HWP(2021)4/En/pdf

17. Essén, A., Scandurra, I., Gerrits, R., et al.: Patient access to electronic health records: differences across ten countries. Health Policy Technol. **7**, 44–56 (2018). https://doi.org/10.1016/j.hlpt.2017.11.003

18. Ammenwerth, E., Duftschmid, G., Al-Hamdan, Z., et al.: International comparison of six basic eHealth indicators across 14 countries: an eHealth benchmarking study. Methods Inf. Med. **59**, e46–e63 (2020). https://doi.org/10.1055/s-0040-1715796

19. Houghom, J.L.: Implementation of an electronic health record. BMJ **343**, d5887 (2011). https://doi.org/10.1136/bmj.d5887

20. Flyvbjerg, B.: What you should know about mega-projects and why: an overview. Project Manage. J. **45**, 6–19 (2014). https://doi.org/10.1002/pmj.21409

21. Ellingsen, G., Hertzum, M., Melby, L.: The tension between national and local concerns in preparing for large-scale generic systems in healthcare. Comput. Supported Coop. Work (CSCW) **31**, 411–441 (2022). https://doi.org/10.1007/s10606-022-09424-9

22. Lehtonen, M.: Evaluating megaprojects: from the 'iron triangle' to network mapping. Evaluation **20**, 278–295 (2014). https://doi.org/10.1177/1356389014539868

23. Price, C., Green, W., Suhomlinova, O.: Twenty-five years of national health IT: exploring strategy, structure, and systems in the English NHS. J. Am. Med. Inform. Assoc. **26**, 188–197 (2019). https://doi.org/10.1093/jamia/ocy162

24. Reponen, J., Tervonen, O., Kiviniitty, K., et al.: Digitaalitekniikan aikakausi. Suom Lääkäril **50**, 3321–3323 (1995)

25. Harno, K., Paavola, T., Carlsson, C., et al.: Improvement of health care process between secondary and primary care with telemedicine: assessment of an intranet referral system on effectiveness and cost analysis. J. Telemed. Telecare **6**, 320–329 (2000). https://doi.org/10.1258/1357633001935996

26. Ohtonen, J. (ed.): Satakunnan Makropilotti: tulosten arviointi. FinOHTA raportti 21/2002. Stakes, Helsinki, 2002. (Abstract in English) (2002). https://www.julkari.fi/bitstream/handle/10024/76116/r021f.pdf?sequence=1

27. Winblad, I., Reponen, J., Hämäläinen, P., et al.: Informaatio- ja kommunikaatioteknologian käyttö Suomen terveydenhuollossa vuonna 2007: tilanne ja kehityssuunnat. Raportti 37/2008. Helsinki: Stakes; 2008. (Abstract in English) (2008). https://urn.fi/URN:NBN:fi-fe2012103 19557

28. Ahokas, S.: Sähköiset potilastietojärjestelmät, sähköinen resepti. In: Laitinen, L.A. (ed.) HUS siunatkoon: kommentteja terveydenhuollon johtamisesta. Kustannus Oy Duodecim, Helsinki, pp. 141–147 (2010)
29. Koponen-Piironen, H.-M., Kiiski, M.: Sähköistä reseptiä koskeva esiselvitys. STM työryhmämuistio 2001:27. Helsinki: Sosiaali- ja terveysministeriö (2001). http://urn.fi/URN:NBN: fi-fe201504226931
30. Varsi, C., Solberg Nes, L., Birna Kristjansdottir, O., et al.: Implementation strategies to enhance the implementation of eHealth programs for patients with chronic illnesses: realist systematic review. J. Med. Internet Res. **21**, e14255 (2019). https://doi.org/10.2196/14255
31. Fahy, N., Williams, G.A., et al.: Use of digital health tools in Europe before, during and after COVID-19. Policy Brief 42. Eur Observatory Health Systems Policies. WHO Regional Office for Europe, Copenhagen (2021). https://eurohealthobservatory.who.int/publications/i/use-of-digital-health-tools-in-europe-before-during-and-after-covid-19
32. WHO: Global strategy on digital health 2020–2025 (2021). https://www.who.int/docs/def ault-source/documents/gs4dhdaa2a9f352b0445bafbc79ca799dce4d.pdf
33. WHO: Classification of Digital Interventions, Services and Applications in Health. A Shared Language to Describe the Uses of Digital Technology for Health, 2nd edn. World Health Organization, Geneva (2023). https://www.who.int/publications/i/item/9789240081949
34. Jormanainen, V.: Large-scale implementation of the national Kanta Services in Finland 2010–2018 with special focus on electronic prescription. Dissertationes Scholae Doctorandis Ad Sanitatem Investigandem Universitatis Helsinkiensis 8/2023. University of Helsinki, Helsinki (2023). https://helda.helsinki.fi/items/4d4b1506-77e2-4f57-845e-98f4041c1388
35. Ministry of Social Affairs and Health. Wellbeing services counties will be responsible for organising health, social and rescue services. https://stm.fi/en/wellbeing-services-counties
36. Greenhalgh, T., Wherton, J., Papoutsi, C., et al.: Analysing the role of complexity in explaining the fortunes of technology programmes: empirical application of the NASSS framework. BMC Med. **16**, 66 (2018). https://doi.org/10.1186/s12916-018-1050-6
37. Melvin, K., Hunter, D., Bengoa, R.: Leading health system transformation to the next level. In: Expert Meeting 12–13 July 2017 in Durham (U.K.). WHO Regional Office for Europe, Copenhagen (Denmark), pp. 1–58 (2018)
38. Sligo, J., Roberts, V., Gauld, R., et al.: A checklist for healthcare organisations undergoing transformal change associated with large-scale health information systems implementation. Health Policy Technol. **8**, 237–247 (2019). https://doi.org/10.1016/j.hlpt.2019.08.001
39. Villumsen, S., Adler-Milstein, J., Nohr, C.: National monitoring and evaluation of eHealth: a scoping review. JAMIA Open **3**, 132–140 (2020). https://doi.org/10.1093/jamiaopen/ooz071
40. Hertzum, M., Ellingsen, G., Cajander, Å.: Implementing large-scale electronic health records: experiences from implementations of Epic in Denmark and Finland. Int. J. Med. Inform. **167**, 104868 (2022). https://doi.org/10.1016/j.ijmedinf.2022.104868
41. Ministry of Social Affairs and Health (MSAH): Strategy for digitalization and information management in healthcare and social welfare. MSAH Publications 2024:1. Ministry of Social Affairs and Health, Helsinki, pp. 1–36 (2024). http://urn.fi/URN:ISBN:978-952-00-5404-5. Accessed 24 Jan 2024

92   V. Jormanainen

Closing the Loop for Controlled Substances Surveillance: A Field Study of the Usability and User Experience of an Integrated Electronic Narcotic Consumption

Annika Häkkinen[1](✉) , Johanna Viitanen[3] , Kaisa Savolainen[3] ,
Ville-Matti Mäkinen[3] , Mia Siven[2,4] , Tinja Lääveri[3,5] ,
and Hanna M. Tolonen[1]

[1] HUS Pharmacy, HUS Helsinki University Hospital Helsinki, Helsinki, Finland
annika.hakkinen@hus.fi
[2] Faculty of Pharmacy, University of Helsinki, Helsinki, Finland
[3] Department of Computer Science, Aalto University, Espoo, Finland
[4] Helsinki Institute of Sustainability Science, HELSUS, Helsinki, Finland
[5] Inflammation Center, HUS Helsinki University Hospital and University of Helsinki, Helsinki, Finland

Abstract. The distribution and handling of controlled substances (CSs), i.e., narcotics, is strictly regulated to decrease the risk of abuse and drug diversion. In Finland, hospital pharmacies are mandated to keep records of CS distribution and consumption in healthcare through a labor-intensive paper-based process. After implementing a new electronic health record (EHR) system, a large university hospital started to streamline the process by transferring the CS documentation process from paper to digital format. Although the benefits of digital archiving, surveillance, and consumption monitoring are self-evident from the hospital pharmacy's perspective the advantages at wards remain less explored. Therefore, our goal was to explore the usability and user experience (UX) of the recently implemented electronic narcotic consumption card (eNCC) solution built into the EHR system, and the related workflows of nurses, pharmacists, and physicians. The field study consisted of two parts and was conducted using observation, interviews, and survey methods in two wards. Our findings suggest that the digitalized process enables reliable real-time documentation of CSs and improves process efficiency, particularly for oral tablets and capsules. Considering diverse end-users' perspectives is crucial when assessing the practical benefits of newly implemented digital solutions targeted at several healthcare professional groups. This approach enables a broader understanding of UX; supports development efforts, including usability improvements; and facilitates broader implementation. More research is needed to analyze the long-term impacts of the digital CSs' consumption documentation workflow and surveillance at different healthcare units.

Keywords: electronic narcotic consumption card · electronic health record · usability · user experience · nurse · pharmacist · physician · healthcare professional · controlled substance · narcotics

---

T. Lääveri and H. M. Tolonen—Equal contribution.

© The Author(s) 2024
M. Särestöniemi et al. (Eds.): NCDHWS 2024, CCIS 2083, pp. 93–109, 2024.
https://doi.org/10.1007/978-3-031-59080-1_7

Abbreviations

CS   controlled substance
EHR   electronic health record
eNCC   electronic narcotic consumption card
ERP   enterprise resource planning system
HCP   healthcare professional
pNCC   paper-based narcotic consumption card
UX   user experience

1 Introduction

Diversion of controlled substances (CSs) in healthcare poses a risk of harm for patients by exposing them to insufficient pain management, incorrect medications and their documentation, possible risk of infection from contaminated needles, and healthcare personnel incapacitated by narcotics misuse [1]. In the USA, it has been estimated that 1% of healthcare workers divert drugs [2], which underscores the necessity to strictly monitor and control the use of these substances.

In Finnish healthcare, the distribution and handling of CSs has been strictly regulated by national legislation since 1971. Both narcotics and psychotropic medicines are considered CSs; despite their therapeutic value for medical purposes, such as pain relief, they present a risk for drug abuse and diversion [3]. Hospital pharmacies are required to keep records of the distribution and consumption of CSs in hospital settings [4]. Traditionally, the CS documentation process has relied on paper-based practices. CSs are delivered with a package-specific consumption monitoring form from a hospital pharmacy to a healthcare unit [4]. When a CS package is empty, the filled consumption form (i.e., the consumption record), accompanied by the physician's verification signature, is returned to the hospital pharmacy for examination and approval. CS consumption records are required to be archived for at least six years after the end of the year in which the document was prepared [5].

Modern electronic health record (EHR) systems, however, allow the paper-based CS surveillance process to be digitalized. In Finland, HUS Helsinki University Hospital and four municipalities implemented a new EHR system between 2018 and 2021 [6]. The Epic-based Apotti system brought about closed-loop electronic medication management within the same EHR: ordering, pharmacy verification, reconstitution, patient identification, barcoded medication administration, and monitoring are executed electronically without manual copying [7]. It also enables automated data transfer between the EHR and smart infusion pumps or automated dispensing cabinets. All of these features decrease the need for error-prone manual work and reduce the risk of medication documentation errors [8–10]. These functionalities also enable automatic entries into an electronic narcotic consumption card (eNCC), which was built into the EHR and thereafter implemented gradually at HUS Helsinki University Hospital. The first pilot took place at three inpatient wards in November 2021 to examine whether the digitalized process is applicable for broader implementation. Thereafter, three implementations were completed successfully from 2022 to 2023. By the end of 2023, more than 80 units had begun using the eNCC.

There are many anticipated benefits of the eNCC for hospital pharmacies related to the distribution and handling of CSs. However, this implementation of new digital processes may create new challenges for the healthcare professionals (HCPs) using the EHR, including nurses, physicians, and clinical pharmacists. Research into the digital solutions related to NCC workflows and eNCC solutions remains scarce [11]. Putri et al. [12] evaluated the usability of the narcotics and psychotropic reporting system and found that pharmacies were quite satisfied with the system.

From end users' perspectives, the usability of the solution impacts work efficiency, error-free task completion, and user experience (UX) [13–15]. The objective of this study was to explore the usability and UX of the eNCC solution built into the EHR system, and the related end-user workflows of nurses, pharmacists, and physicians in the wards by comparing the new digitalized process to a conventional paper-based narcotic consumption card (pNCC). The research questions were as follows:

- How do the HCPs' workflows using eNCC differ from the conventional paper-based process?
- What kinds of experiences do HCPs have with the recently implemented eNCC?

2 Methods

A qualitative approach was used for this research because the eNCC was only in the pilot phase in spring 2022, and very few wards had begun using it. This field study was conducted using semi-structured interviews, observations with usability measurements, and surveys for HCPs. Semi-structured interviews were selected as the primary method to research workflows and UX, because interviews can be used to gather in-depth and detailed information while giving interviewees a chance to bring up themes absent from the interview script [16] Through observations, data can be collected that end-users may not be able to express verbally [17]. In field studies, observations can be conducted without interrupting the observed individuals [17, 18], which is particularly important in clinical environments. During observations, measurements related to tasks and usability can also be carried out, and information about the work environment can be gathered to support interviews [17]. The usability of interactive systems can be measured in terms of effectiveness, efficiency, and satisfaction [19]. Suitable metrics for measuring these variables include task completion time and error rates during task completion as well as standard usability questionnaires [19]. Finally, the study included a validated usability survey, System Usability Scale (SUS) [20], with complementing open-ended questions about development ideas related to the evaluated solution.

The research data were collected at a large university hospital (HUS Helsinki University Hospital) from the hospital pharmacy, one inpatient ward that used the eNCC, and one ward that used the pNCC in spring 2022. We selected these two wards because they were surgical units that cared for patients who frequently needed opioid-based postoperative analgesics. All the nurses and physicians working in these wards were invited to participate in the study, though the final participants for the study were selected through convenience sampling. The research data were collected during the daytime, which limited the potential participants. Moreover, the study was affected by labor actions, which affected the number of nurses available for the study. The number of personnel varies at the wards that involved in the study, but is typically 20–50 nurses and 10–20 physicians.

The study was conducted in two parts. The first part focused on the workflows related to the NCC (both paper-based and electronic). The aim was to describe and validate workflow descriptions. The initial versions of the descriptions were created before the interviews based on documentation available from the hospital pharmacy, the EHR system administrators, and discussions with domain experts. Two hospital pharmacists and a nurse participated in the interviews, which were conducted in their real working environments. The interviews included questions related to workflows, document handling, and the challenges and advantages of the eNCC. As part of the interviews, the participants were also asked to demonstrate the workflows in practice. Experiences from the first part were utilized when planning the data gathering and practical arrangements for the second part.

The second part focused on the usability and UX of the eNCC. The procedure included observations with discussion of the processes, observations with measurements, and a semi-structured interview, including a survey. All observations were conducted in medication rooms and focused on time measurements related to handling and documentation of CSs. The researcher utilized a predefined template to document observations and time measurements. Interview questions were designed based on the expertise of the research group. The data gathering was conducted in nine sessions, which lasted from three to four hours and included one to three participants. Each participant was interviewed and observed one at a time. The duration of an individual time measurement event was only a few minutes within the observation sessions. The interviews lasted about 15–30 min with each participant. After the interview the participants were asked to answer to the SUS questionnaire on a paper format. Field notes were written during the observations, and both interviews and observations were audio recorded.

In total, the second part included 13 participants: ten nurses, two pharmacists, and one physician. Table 1 provides the number of participants and their categorization between NCC types and professions. The physician participated only in an interview and survey; observations were not conducted due to the small sample size and the different work tasks.

The study had a research permit from HUS Helsinki University Hospital, and the participants signed a consent form before the interviews and observations. Audio recordings were used to ensure that no patient data would be unintentionally recorded, which might have occurred with photos or video recordings. The research data were pseudonymized for analysis. The study data consisted of participants' background information, audio recordings from the interviews and observations, measurements from the observations, and responses to the survey.

In the first part, the analysis was conducted forming process charts of the workflows with verbal descriptions. The audio recordings of the interviews and the participants' comments were transcribed and coded thematically by one researcher. The thematic coding [21] utilized predefined codes that are commonly used in usability and UX research (such as, problems, positive and negative experiences and technical challenges) and in addition to these new codes were added (such as, development suggestions). Affinity diagrams [22] were utilized in the analysis process. The affinity diagram of usability and UX findings consisted of approximately 350 observations that were grouped under 26 different thematic groups and further combined under three main themes and five sub-themes.

Table 1. Number of participants in the second part of the study and their categorization between the use of paper-based narcotic consumption card (pNCC) and electronic narcotic consumption card (eNCC).

Professional	Interview (n)	Observation (n)	SUS survey about eNCC (n)
Pharmacist			
eNCC	1	1	1
pNCC	1	1	-
Nurse			
eNCC	4	4	4
pNCC	6	6	-
Physician			
eNCC	1	-	1
pNCC	-	-	-
Wards total	13	12	6
eNCC	6	5	6
pNCC	7	7	-

SUS – System Usability Scale

From the observation data, we recorded elapsed time, usability findings, and irregular instances. From the elapsed time, the averages, standard deviations and interquartile ranges were calculated. Data from the observations were mostly analyzed with a qualitative approach. Responses to the SUS were analyzed with the standard analysis method [20], which results in a score between 0 and 100 points. The open-ended questions also were analyzed thematically and combined with the interview results.

3 Results

3.1 Workflows

At the hospital pharmacy, there were three differences in the workflows between the conventional paper-based pNCC process and the digitalized eNCC process. First, paper prints were handled in the conventional process. Second, the digitalized process required the use of 2D codes to create the eNCCs in the EHR. Third, eNCCs were created in the EHR system though all other pharmacy-related workflows were documented in the pharmacy enterprise resource planning (ERP) system. The process of CSs delivery at the hospital pharmacy is presented in Fig. 1.

CSs were ordered, and packages were identified similarly regardless of the NCC process. Each package was marked with a unique identification number label that connects the CS package and the NCC although the type of barcode varies depending on the process type. After the CS package was used, an empty package was discarded and the NCC with the physician verification signature (hand-written for pNCC and digital for eNCC) was returned to the pharmacy for examination, approval, and archiving (Fig. 2). The most remarkable change in pharmacy activities was to render manual paper archives unnecessary with eNCC. Digital archiving does not require a separate room, and the NCC records are accessible in the EHR system.

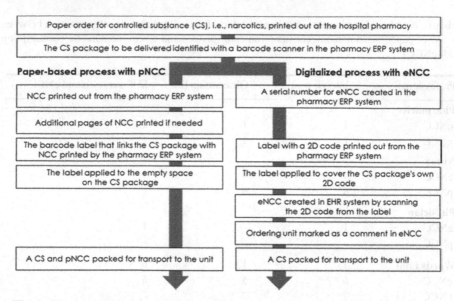

Fig. 1. The processes of paper-based and digitalized CS delivery at the hospital pharmacy

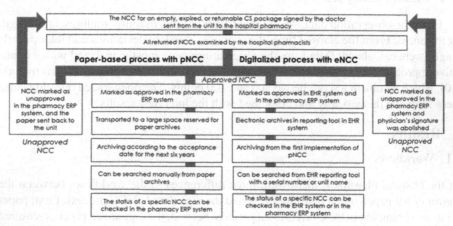

Fig. 2. The processes for paper-based and digitalized NCC examination, approval, and archiving at the hospital pharmacy

For administration, medications were prepared in the EHR system via two different workflows depending on the administration route or dosage form (Fig. 3). The barcodes or 2D codes of tablet and capsule packages were scanned in the medication room, and the CSs were placed in a container with the patient's identification label. Each injection required a printed label with specific patient information; then, the label and a package were scanned in the medication room, and the label was scanned again in the patient room. Workflows were the same regardless of the NCC process, except for the last step of the dispense preparation workflow. Double verification for the waste of partial injection vials by another HCP was not required in the pNCC process but was mandatory in the eNCC. In the eNCC, all unused CSs were considered waste requiring double verification. By contrast, separate documentation for medication administrations in the pNCC was omitted in the digitalized process with the eNCC.

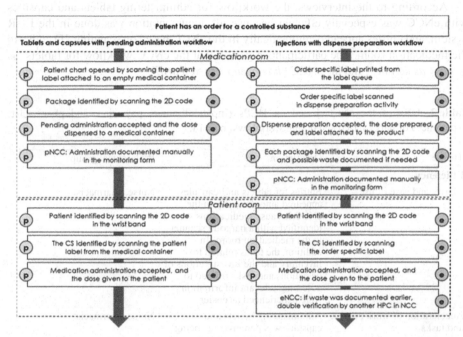

Fig. 3. Medication administration process for controlled substances (CSs) with paper-based (p) and electronic (e) narcotic consumption card (NCC) at hospital units in the EHR system

The medication administration process remained almost unchanged in the wards that had implemented the eNCC (Fig. 3). In the paper-based process, all required information had to be copied manually into the separate pNCC although most information was already recorded in the EHR system. By comparison, the eNCC automatically utilized all documented information and displayed it in the patients' charts. There were no more hand-written notes in the wards, which made reading the NCCs easier.

Barcode scanners were used in medication administrations regardless of the NCC process although scanning was a prerequisite for fluent documentation in the eNCC. If the scanning was skipped, automatic entries would not appear in the eNCC. Because hand-written entries in the pNCC were separate from the medication administration documentation in the EHR, skipped scanning did not influence entries in the pNCC.

Handling of the pNCC required physical access, whereas the eNCC could be accessed through the reporting tools in the EHR system. The consumption balances in the pNCC had to be counted manually in contrast to the eNCC where the balances were counted automatically in the EHR system based on earlier entries.

3.2　Usability and UX

Based on the interviews, user experiences of the digitalized process with eNCC were divided into three main themes (efficiency, reliability, and technical challenges) and six sub-themes (Table 2).

According to the interviews, the workflow for administering tablets and capsules with eNCC was especially efficient because all documentation was done in the EHR system, and entries appeared automatically in the eNCC based on scanning 2D codes in the medication room. The participants reported that the eNCC workflow for tablets "*is as easy as can be,*" and the eNCC "*has been easy to learn.*"

Table 2. UXs of the eNCC based on HCPs (inpatient nurse, physician, and pharmacist) experiences of paper-based and digital workflows, n = 14.

Theme	Description	Professional group
Efficiency		
Clarity and ease of use	Entries for tablets and capsules appeared automatically in the eNCC because medications were identified with a barcode scanner in the medication room. In addition, the tasks related to inventory and the investigations of deviations and tasks related to accessing relevant information were experienced as easier	Nurse, pharmacist
Acceleration of work process and tasks	Administering tablets and capsules was perceived as being faster because time was not consumed for written documentation. The total workflow was perceived as faster if there was no waste, and most information was already available and documented in the EHR system	Nurse, pharmacist
Reliability		
Reduced possibility of errors	Errors were perceived to occur less often if standardized workflows were followed, including barcode scanning. Tracing and correcting possible errors was usually possible because necessary information could be found in the EHR system	Nurse, pharmacist, physician
Increased reliability due to predefined workflows	Entries were perceived as easy to read, and there weren't problems with unclear handwriting. In particular, the workflow with tablets and capsules was considered unambiguous	Nurse, pharmacist

(*continued*)

Table 2. (*continued*)

Theme	Description	Professional group
Technical challenges		
Waste entries and double verification	In the EHR, injections were prepared using a different workflow than tablets and capsules. The workflow had multiple steps, most of which had to be done appropriately according to predefined procedure to produce automatic entries in the eNCC. Waste entries were considered laborious and hard to remember	Nurse, pharmacist
Reports of eNCC entries	Reporting tools in the EHR were considered to be challenging to use. Reports included eNCCs for several wards, and physicians had to filter the results in order to do the verification signatures for a specific ward	Physician

Interviews also indicated that eNCC has increased reliability for CS documentation. One participant commented that "[the documentation is] *faster and more reliable, and not many erroneous entries presumably.*" Another stated that "*everything is more visible, even though the right workflow wasn't followed.*" The eNCC was considered to be "*easy to read; everything seems to be unambiguous,*" and "*everything is visible because of the automatic workflow, and there is no unclear handwriting.*"

Most of the experienced challenges were related to injections. All unused amounts of CSs from injection vials had to be verified by another HCP's signature, which was quite easily forgotten if not done immediately after the administration. As one of the participants reported, "*There are multiple steps for injections; one must also remember to document an entry for the waste and ask for a double verification from a colleague, which is complicated.*"

When comparing the paper-based and digitalized workflows, the main advantages and challenges experienced were as follows:

- The digitalized process is easier and faster for tablets and capsules preparation, mainly because of the automatic workflow and the use of barcode scanners. With the digitalized process, possible errors in workflows are more visible; it is easier to find errors and make corrections.
- Perceived challenges are related to injections because they are prepared using a different workflow. Due to multiple steps, the process of injection preparation is prone to errors in the eNCC. In addition, injections usually require double verification for waste entries.

Based on the observations and measurements, the digitalized workflow appeared to be faster than the paper-based one (Table 3). For the paper-based process, the average time taken for pending administrations of tablets and capsules was 107 s, and for the digitalized process, it was 80 s. Some interruptions in the workflows were recorded that affected task completion times. Most exceptions were part of the normal workflow, such as a rush in a medication room, opening new CS packages, inventory of the tablets and capsules from used packages. If interruptions were irrelevant to the task, they were not included in the study measurements. Administration workflow in the patient room was identical irrespective of the NCC process, so no measurements were conducted related to this task.

Table 3. Time consumed for pending administrations of tablets or capsules in paper-based and digitalized NCC processes, in seconds (s)

	Paper-based NCC (n = 7), time (s)	Digitalized NCC (n = 5), time (s)	Difference, time (s)
Average	107	80	27
Median	102	75	27
SD	38	21	
IQR	30	31	

Inventory of CSs appeared faster with eNCC than pNCC at wards. Workflow was observed for both processes, but completion times were not comparable as only two cases were observed. However, the most remarkable differences in the inventory workflow were the use of the EHR system and handling of papers. The EHR system was required in eNCC, whereas all of the consumption information is found on paper in the pNCC.

As a part of the interviews, the participants responded to a SUS questionnaire. The questionnaire was completed by four nurses, one ward pharmacist, and one physician. The average score was 58 and the median was 65. One participant gave an extremely low score (8), which lowered the overall score. In the SUS scoring scale, the score 58 can be considered as marginal, between not acceptable and acceptable [23]. A SUS score below 50 is considered not acceptable, above 70 acceptable, and a good score is 73.

4 Discussion

The distribution and handling of CSs, such as narcotics, is strictly monitored in health-care. The full digital integration of CS surveillance and medication administration processes offered by the eNCC reduces the opportunities for drug diversion. HCPs often criticize EHRs for not supporting and facilitating routine tasks [24]. Therefore, while studying the usability and UX of a recently implemented eNCC in inpatient wards participating in the pilot, we wanted to ensure that the increased monitoring of quality and hospital pharmacy digital workflow efficiency would not negatively impact the HCPs' end-user experiences. To our knowledge, this was the first implementation of fully digital CS surveillance process in Finland..

The main result of our field study was that the digital process may even improve UX by reducing the need for manual steps. The end users believed that the eNCC enables faster and easier workflows for tablets and capsules, more reliable entries, and higher traceability for all CSs in comparison to the pNCC. In addition, the eNCC provided better opportunities to investigate and fix errors.

4.1   Comparisons of the Paper-Based and Digital Processes

From a CS surveillance perspective, the main difference between the paper-based and digital processes was that the entries from the EHR were automatically transferred to the eNCC. In practice, this automation may reduce the possibility of diversion, as entries to the eNCC could only be falsified by falsifying the medication administration documentation in the EHR. Indeed, most medication administration documentations in modern EHR systems are based on identifying the patient and the medication by barcode scanning [6]. Moreover, a physician's order in the EHR is technically required to document the administration of all medications, including CSs, which increases the reliability of documentation and may further reduce the risk of diversion [9]. In the paper-based process, systematic verification of all pNCC entries from the EHR would be practically impossible as it would require a laborious manual process. In addition, in the paper-based process, hand-written entries may result in interpretation errors; the digital process allows the hospital pharmacy personnel to concentrate on genuine discrepancies; in essence, the possibility of detecting actual diversion attempts is likely to be higher. Although interpretation errors are irrelevant in the eNCC, omitting steps in the medication administration process may cause new types of errors compared to the pNCC. Fully integrated eNCC in EHR provides easier and more frequent access to CS consumption records because a separate login is not required, as Witry et al. [25] suggested. Moreover, there is always a risk that pNCCs can disappear intentionally or accidentally.

4.2   Benefits of a Digital Process from the Hospital Pharmacy Perspective

In Finland, hospital pharmacies are mandated to keep records of CS consumption in hospital settings, which was already identified as an advantage of the digitalized NCC process before implementation of the eNCC. Archiving of the eNCCs can be done without extra effort, and all necessary information is found in the EHR system. Some problems related to drug diversion are completely precluded; for instance, it is impossible to steal eNCCs, and entries are hard to falsify due to automation. The generally identified [26] benefits of paperless processes could be seen with the digitalized eNCC process: 1) it can be remotely accessed; 2) it does not require archiving space; 3) it can be used simultaneously by several end users; and 4) it cannot be easily destroyed.

4.3   Perceived Benefits for Digitalized Processes from the HCP Perspective

The participants reported noticing a reduction in the potential for documentation errors for tablets and capsules. In general, the pharmacists' routine CS-related tasks at wards, such as local monitoring, inventory, and investigation of errors, were considered easier with the digitalized process. Because the pharmacists may work at several wards, the reporting tools in the EHR provide them with access to CSs' consumption data independently of their location, which was not possible with the pNCC. This benefit of remote access has been identified in other paperless processes [26].

In Finland, nurses primarily dispense and administer medications, including CSs. All interviewed nurses believed that the eNCC accelerated and eased NCC documentation for tablets and capsules. Indeed, the manual documentation phase in pNCC can be totally omitted with the eNCC by scanning the 2D code from the packages during the medication preparation and administration. If the predefined workflows were followed, all necessary information would be automatically documented in the eNCC. However, the preparation of injections was considered more time-consuming, complicated, and prone to errors. While the workflow for administering injections in the EHR did not change due to the implementation of the eNCC, it includes multiple steps, and skipping any of those steps was likely to cause errors in the eNCC. Injections are prepared differently in the EHR system than tablets and capsules because of a distinct workflow in the medication room. Tablets and capsules must be identified by scanning the package once in the medication room. By comparison, injections and other intravenous medications have to be identified twice; a label and components of the injection are scanned first in the medication room after which the label of the prepared injection is scanned in the patient room. The use of labels and barcode scanners can be considered as technology-based systemic defenses that are required for closed-loop electronic medication management to mitigate medication safety risks [27, 28]. Thus, workflows in the EHR aim for closed-loop medication administration for injection but require barcode scanning in multiple phases of the process. Although the EHR system requires end users to administer medications with medication safety, standardized workflows are partially based on instructions, and end users are not forced to use the standardized workflow for the specific dosage form by the EHR system.

We only interviewed one physician, who felt it was too complicated to use reports for signing the eNCCs. Moreover, the physician apparently had not recognized the benefit of the eNCC of not needing to manually copy from the EHR; this removes the possibility of human error, whether intentional or unintentional. To our knowledge, physicians hardly ever actually verify that the entries in the pNCC also appear in the EHR. Interviewed pharmacists also used reporting tools in the EHR, but they did not report the same usability problems. According to an earlier Finnish study related to the usability of EHR systems, physicians experienced the ease of use of their EHR systems worse than nurses, for instance [24]. After the pilot, more attention was given to training the physicians to use the reports. Additionally, after the interview, the usability of the physicians' reports was improved.

4.4   The eNCC Revealed Existing Workarounds in Medication Processes

Regardless of the different workflows for tablets and capsules or injections, our study identified that documentation- and workflow-related errors became more visible with the eNCC than with the pNCC. Most of the increased transparency was due to scanning and automatic entries. In fact, the documentation processes for the pNCC and eNCC were almost identical except for documenting waste for partly used ampoules with the eNCC. The introduction of the eNCC revealed that the end users had used workarounds instead of the correct and more medication safety-oriented workflows. The correct, predefined workflow required by the closed-loop electronic medication management process is suggested to increase safety [7, 9, 29] but is different from the workflows used before the implementation of the new EHR. Indeed, digitalization often reveals workarounds that may contribute to the dissatisfaction of end users and compromise patient safety [30]. HCPs may adopt workarounds to avoid new additional steps in workflows when transitioning from a paper-based systems to EHRs [31]. Barcoded medication administration systems are known to improve medication safety, but workarounds can nullify the effects of error prevention; for instance, documenting the medication administration in the EHR after giving the medication to the patient poses a risk to medication safety [32]. Although the new EHR system was implemented several years ago [6], the eNCC seemed to disclose some workarounds in the medication administration workflow.

4.5 Opportunities for Improved CS Surveillance

The closed-loop electronic medication management process has improved medication safety by ensuring that the right patient receives the right medication and dose at the right time with seamless information sharing and documentation [7]. However, the surveillance of CSs often includes manual steps leaving an opportunity for drug diversion [1, 9]. We implemented a digital eNCC process to close the surveillance loop from the hospital pharmacy to dispensing and administering the CSs at wards and back to the hospital pharmacy that utilizes the same entries as in the actual medication process. The digitalized eNCC process is also likely to prevent incorrect interpretation of narcotics consumption records because the eNCC is not based on handwriting like the pNCC. Compared to the pNCC, it is more difficult to falsify entries in the eNCC, mainly due to the automated process and the requirement of a physician's order. Although digitalizing the CS surveillance process is a great step forward in preventing drug diversion, it cannot be the only action to limit CS theft and illegal nonmedical use at healthcare organizations [1]. Other actions include, for instance, regular inventory of CSs, physical access controls for HCPs, and auditing.

Although the digitalized process relies on scanning workflow and automatic entries, waste entries always required double verification by another HCP regardless of the amount of waste. With the pNCC, double verification for the waste of partial injection vials was not needed. The tightened requirements related to double verification could improve CS surveillance, but the results also suggested that participants experienced double verification as hard to remember if not done immediately after administration.

4.6 Strengths and Limitations of the Study and Future Research

The process described in this paper was aimed at further reducing the risk of diversion of CSs and to streamline the legislation-driven process in hospital settings. However, a remarkable share of narcotics, especially weak opioids, are dispensed from community pharmacies [33] and, thus, eNCC is only one measure to manage and control the handling of CSs. Moreover, we have not deployed any automated algorithms to identify potential drug diversion situations; however, there is inconclusive evidence on the efficacy of these algorithms [34].

There are some other limitations that deserve to be discussed. As this study was related to the piloting of the eNCC, there were few HCPs at the hospital using the eNCC at the time of the study. The study focused on wards; therefore, the pharmacy side of the processes was not addressed. Consequently, the number of participants in the study was rather small.

In the study, we primarily applied a qualitative approach on researching user experiences, and the numeric usability results could not be analyzed quantitatively. The use of three complementary field research methods in the study can be seen as a clear strength. Even though the number of participants in the study was limited, the study managed to research the UX of three HCP groups with the eNCC. It is important to explore multiple perspectives of end-user groups instead of focusing on only one when the aim is to understand the practical benefits of recently implemented digital solutions and to provide information to support development work and wider implementation.

Our study provided initial results about usability measurements related to eNCC benefits. However, the small sample size needs to be considered. It was difficult to research and observe usability and user experiences related to unexpected events and exceptions because they occur rarely in workflows and would require extensive observation times over long periods in the wards. In the future, it would be beneficial to utilize log-data together with observations to gather rich data about errors and exceptions related to eNCC use and digitalized workflows. In addition, it should be noted that the practices and timing of medication distribution were not entirely consistent among the two wards in the study. Due to these differences, the measurement results should be considered very preliminary, and further research is needed to conduct additional measurements and strengthen the generalizability and validity of the findings. For future research, we are planning a larger-scale study once the eNCC is being used in more wards.

Digital medication processes are intended to improve medication safety and surveillance. However, after the first implementations of the new EHR system, ordering errors increased [6], and several usability problems were identified, particularly after the first go-live [35]. Therefore, we wanted to analyze possible usability problems before the large-scale implementation of the eNCC solution. Indeed, several usability problems were identified after the first pilot and this research project and fixed before the broader implementations. Moreover, as new workflows need to be followed, communication and trainings were improved for later phases of the implementation. Our findings underscore the importance of piloting new EHR features with a smaller group of end users whenever possible.

5   Conclusions

While the benefits of a digitalized process (i.e., the eNCC) were obvious from the hospital pharmacy point of view already before the implementation, changes in the workflows and usability from the clinicians' perspectives deserved deeper attention. Compared to paper-based practices and processes, the main advantages were related to improved efficiency and reliability. Based on HCPs' experiences, the eNCC enabled faster and easier workflows for tablets and capsules and higher traceability for documentation regardless of the workflow. Additionally, the eNCC with automated entries might reduce the number of errors in the documentation. However, a successful eNCC process requires following precise and predefined workflows, which emphasizes the role of training and communication before and during implementation.

Acknowledgments. We would like to thank all of the healthcare professionals who participated in this study.

Contributions. The empirical research was mostly carried out by VMM whose work was supervised by JV and KS. HMT participated in the study design. The main advisor regarding hospital practices and recruitment was AH, who wrote the first draft of the manuscript with JV and TL. All authors commented on and modified the draft and approved the final manuscript.

Disclosure of Interests. AH, JV, KS, MS, and HMT have no competing interests to declare that are relevant to the content of this article. TL is and VMM was employed by the software provider, Apotti, but the employer was not involved in the interpretation of data for this paper.

References

1. Clark, J., et al.: ASHP guidelines on preventing diversion of controlled substances. Am. J. Health-Syst. Pharm. **79**(24), 2279–306 (2022). https://doi.org/10.1093/ajhp/zxac246
2. Protenus: Diversion Digest 2023. https://www.protenus.com/diversion-digest. Accessed 14 Jan 2024
3. European Monitoring Centre for Drugs and Drugs Addiction: Classification of controlled drugs – topic overview. https://www.emcdda.europa.eu/publications/topic-overviews/classi fication-of-controlled-drugs/html_en. Accessed 14 Jan 2024
4. Finlex: Narcotics Act (548/2008). https://www.finlex.fi/fi/laki/ajantasa/2008/20080548. Accessed 23 Jan 2024
5. Finlex: Government Decree on Narcotics Control (373/2008). https://www.finlex.fi/fi/laki/aja ntasa/2008/20080373. Accessed 15 Jan 2024. Accessed 23 Jan 2024
6. Linden-Lahti, C., Kivivuori, S.M., Lehtonen, L., Schepel, L.: Implementing a new electronic health record system in a university hospital: the effect on reported medication errors. Healthcare **10**(6), 1020 (2022). https://doi.org/10.3390/healthcare10061020
7. Shermock, S.B., Shermock, K.M., Schepel, L.L.: Closed-loop medication management with an electronic health record system in U.S. and Finnish hospitals. Int. J. Environ. Res. Publ. Health **20**(17), 6680 (2023). https://doi.org/10.3390/ijerph20176680
8. Ciapponi, A., et al.: Reducing medication errors for adults in hospital settings. Cochrane Database System. Rev. **11**, CD009985 (2021). https://doi.org/10.1002/14651858.CD009985. pub2
9. Zheng, W.Y., Lichtner, V., Van Dort, B.A., Baysari, M.T.: The impact of introducing automated dispensing cabinets, barcode medication administration, and closed-loop electronic medication management systems on work processes and safety of controlled medications in hospitals: a systematic review. Res. Social Adm. Pharm. **17**(5), 832–841 (2021). https://doi. org/10.1016/j.sapharm.2020.08.001
10. Franklin, B.D., O'Grady, K., Donyai, P., Jacklin, A., Barber, N.: The impact of a closed-loop electronic prescribing and administration system on prescribing errors, administration errors and staff time: a before-and-after study. Qual. Saf. Health CareSaf. Health Care **16**(4), 279 (2007). https://doi.org/10.1136/qshc.2006.019497

11. Farzandipour, M., Meidani, Z., Riazi, H., Jabali, M.S.: Functional requirements of pharmacy's information system in hospitals. Front. Health Inform. **6**(1), 1–10 (2017). https://doi.org/10.24200/ijmi.v6i1.111

12. Putri, D.K., Pribadi, P., Setiawan, A.: The evaluation of narcotic and psychotropic reporting systems (SIPNAP). In: Advances in Social Science, Education and Humanities Research, pp. 1212–1216 (2020). https://doi.org/10.2991/assehr.k.200529.254

13. International Organization for Standardization: Ergonomic Requirements for Office Work with Visual Display Terminals, Part 11: Guidance on Usability, ISO 9241-11:1998

14. International Organization for Standardization: Human-centered design for interactive systems, ISO 9241-210:2019

15. Nielsen, J.: Usability Engineering. Morgan Kaufmann, San Francisco (1994)

16. Lazar, J., Feng, J.H., Hochheiser, H.: Interviews and focus groups. In: Research Methods in Human Computer Interaction, pp. 187–228. Elsevier (2017). https://doi.org/10.1016/B978-0-12-805390-4.00008-X

17. Hackos, J.T., Redish, J.C.: User and Task Analysis for Interface Design. Wiley, New York (1998)

18. McNaughton Nicholls, C., Mills, L., Kotecha, M.: Observation. In: Ritchie, J., Lewis, J., McNaughton Nicholls, C., Ormston, R. (eds.) Qualititative Research in Practice A Guide for Social Science Students and Researchers. Sage Publications, London (2013)

19. Hornbaek, K.: Current practice in measuring usability: challenges to usability studies and research. Int. J. Hum.-Comput. Stud. **64**, 79–102 (2006). https://doi.org/10.1016/j.ijhcs.2005.06.002

20. Brooke, J.: SUS: a quick and dirty usability scale. Usab. Eval Ind. **189** (1995)

21. Braun, V., Clarke, V.: Using thematic analysis in psychology. Qual. Res. Psychol. **3**(2), 77–101 (2006). https://doi.org/10.1191/1478088706qp063oa

22. Holtzblatt, K., Beyer, H.: The affinity diagram. In: Contextual Design, pp. 127–46, Morgan Kaufmann, Boston (2017)

23. Bangor, A., Kortum, P.T., Miller, J.T.: An empirical evaluation of the system usability scale. Int. J. Hum.-Comput. Interact. **24**(6), 574–594 (2008). https://doi.org/10.1080/10447310802205776

24. Kaipio, J., Kuusisto, A., Hyppönen, H., Heponiemi, T., Lääveri, T.: Physicians' and nurses' experiences on EHR usability: comparison between the professional groups by employment sector and system brand. Int. J. Med. Inform. **134**, 104018 (2019). https://doi.org/10.1016/j.ijmedinf.2019.104018

25. Witry, M., Marie, B.S., Reist, J.: Provider perspectives and experiences following the integration of the prescription drug monitoring program into the electronic health record. Health Inform. J. **28**(3) (2022). https://doi.org/10.1177/14604582221113435

26. Oliveira, J., Azevedo, A., Ferreira, J.J., Gomes, S., Lopes, J.M.: An insight on B2B firms in the age of digitalization and paperless processes. Sustainability **13**(21), 11565 (2021). https://doi.org/10.3390/su132111565

27. Kuitunen, S., Niittynen, I., Airaksinen, M., Holmström, A.R.: Systemic defenses to prevent intravenous medication errors in hospitals: a systematic review. J. Patient Saf.Saf. **8**, e1669 (2021). https://doi.org/10.1097/PTS.0000000000000688

28. Cho, J., Chung, H.S., Hong, S.H.: Improving the safety of continuously infused fluids in the emergency department. Int. J. Nurs. Pract.Nurs. Pract. **19**(1), 95–100 (2013). https://doi.org/10.1111/ijn.12022

29. Kinlay, M., et al.: Stakeholder perspectives of system-related errors: types, contributing factors, and consequences. Int. J. Med. Inform. **165**, 104821 (2022). https://doi.org/10.1016/j.ijmedinf.2022.104821

30. Awad, S., Amon, K., Baillie, A., Loveday, T., Baysari, M.T.: Human factors and safety analysis methods used in the design and redesign of electronic medication management systems: a systematic review. Int. J. Med. Inform. **172**, 105017 (2023). https://doi.org/10.1016/j.ijmedinf.2023.105017
31. Patterson, E.S.: Workarounds to intended use of health information technology: a narrative review of the human factors engineering literature. Hum. Factors **60**(3), 281–292 (2018). https://doi.org/10.1177/0018720818762546
32. Lichtner, V., Dowding, D.: Mindful workarounds in bar code medication administration. Stud. Health Technol. Inform. **294**, 740–744 (2022). https://doi.org/10.3233/SHTI220575
33. Finnish Medicines Agency Fimea, Social Insurance Institution: Finnish statistics on medicines 2021. https://urn.fi/URN:NBN:fi-fe2022121672024. Accessed 21 Jan 2024
34. Canan, C., Polinski, J.M., Alexander, G.C., Kowal, M.K., Brennan, T.A., Shrank, W.H.: Automatable algorithms to identify nonmedical opioid use using electronic data: a systematic review. J. Am. Med. Inform. Assoc. **24**(6), 1204–1210 (2017). https://doi.org/10.1093/jamia/ocx066
35. Palojoki, S., Saranto, K., Reponen, E., Skants, N., Vakkuri, A., Vuokko, R.: Classification of electronic health record-related patient safety incidents: development and validation study. JMIR Med. Inform. **9**(8), e30470 (2021). https://doi.org/10.2196/30470

A User-Centric Exploration of a Digital Health Experience

Milka Haanpää[✉] and Saila Saraniemi

Oulu Business School, Erkki-Koiso Kanttilan Katu 1, 90570 Oulu, Finland
{milka.haanpaa,study.business}@oulu.fi

Abstract. This paper explores digital health experience through focus on the experiences of diabetics who utilize digital health technology in their daily diabetes management. Theoretically, the paper draws from research on digital experience and from theoretical discussions concerned with digital health. Empirically, it analyzes three multimodal datasets using reflective thematic analysis. Three interlinked themes – always on, co-creation through interaction, and it makes things so much easier – are revealed. These themes reveal the key characteristics of users' digital health experiences and highlight how users shape their experiences in their daily lives. The study contributes theoretically to digital experience literature within which user-centric, longitudinal studies are scarce. Practically, it demonstrates to health professionals and developers how digital health technology becomes integrated into their users' lives.

Keywords: digital health · user experience · digital experience · diabetes · wearable technology

1 Introduction to the Study

In the contemporary consumption environment, characterized by constant interaction and information exchange between people, devices and other entities [1], consumers utilize digital technologies to track various aspects of their daily lives [2]. Since it has been argued that digital technologies have a tremendous potential to improve individuals' quality of life [3], it is only fitting that technological innovations, such as wearables, are increasingly adopted within the healthcare sector [4].

Earlier research demonstrates that healthcare professionals have adopted digital technology, for example, to promote weight control [5] and to assists in the care of health conditions such as cancer [6] and rheumatism [7]. Alongside this, connected mobile devices, such as wearables and sensors are progressively utilized to improve individuals' health and wellbeing [8]. Interestingly, while such technologies are adopted in an increasing rate, research that takes a user-centric approach into digital health experience is limited, and has, for the most part, focused on experiences with "wellbeing" technology, such as smart and -fitness watches [9]. Since it has been identified that the focus of the digital health market is progressively shifting towards developing technology for

© The Author(s) 2024
M. Särestöniemi et al. (Eds.): NCDHWS 2024, CCIS 2083, pp. 110–120, 2024.
https://doi.org/10.1007/978-3-031-59080-1_8

disease-specific uses and management of chronic conditions such as diabetes [8], more research is needed to understand user's daily experiences with such technology.

In line with that, this paper adopts a user-centric approach, i.e., an approach focused on the experiences of the users, into the exploration of digital health experience. Theoretically, this is done with reference to marketing literature focused on experience, and multidisciplinary research concerning the digital health domain. Empirically, this paper relies on three qualitative datasets concerned with the experiences of diabetics who utilize a wearable sensor to support their daily diabetes management. According to the World Health Organization [10], the prevalence of diabetes has been steadily increasing over the past decades, making it the 7th leading cause of death globally. Arguably, diabetes technology not only makes diabetes management easier, but also has the possibility to improve the health of people with diabetes [11]. Thus, by exploring user's day-to-day experiences with diabetes technology, this paper aims to identify characteristics of such experiences and provide insights into the ways in which users shape their digital health experiences in their daily lives to ease up their diabetes management and to improve their overall wellbeing.

This paper begins with an introduction, after which the theoretical concepts relevant for the study – experience and digital health – will be introduced. That will be followed by a chapter focused on the study's methodology and empirical data, after which the findings of the study will be presented. The paper concludes with a discussion of the study's contributions and suggestions for future research.

2 Literature Review

2.1 Defining Experience

Experience, "an all-embracing term which is often used to indicate some experience that a person has during everyday life" [12, p. 269] has captured the interest of researchers across disciplines for centuries. As research on experience has expanded throughout the years, nuances on how experience is understood have become prevalent. For example, while some regard experiences as something we passively go through, others regard them as being influenced by the actions individuals consciously take [12]. Overall, these different perspectives inevitably affect not only how experience is understood, but also how it is approached in research.

Across disciplines, interest in digital experiences has grown in recent years. Within the marketing research domain, it has been stipulated that as reliance on digital technologies has increased across sectors, consumption has started to progressively move from commercial settings, such as retail spaces, to non-commercial ones, such as consumers' homes [1, 13]. As a result, it is perceived that individuals can get access to a number of services through digital technologies wherever and whenever they so desire [14]. As reliance on networked devices increases, we become "tethered to technologies" in a way that makes us adapt our modes of interaction into something that accommodate the bounds of the digital solutions in use [15]. In light of these developments, there is an increasing demand for capturing a qualitative, in-depth understanding of the digital experience phenomenon [16] from a perspective which regards experience as something individuals can consciously shape to fit their preferences in their day-to-day lives.

2.2 Defining Digital Health

The digital health field, characterized by hybrid objects that can perform multiple activities [17], presents itself as a promising, relevant context wherein to study digital experiences. While digital health technologies and solutions, e.g., telemedicine, wearables and electronic health records are frequently used in clinical settings, namely hospitals, to enhance quality of care and cut costs [18], digital health solutions are increasingly relied on also by individuals to help in the management of health and wellbeing.

To make sense of the quickly evolving field of digital health solutions, three prominent, overlapping domains have been identified: 1) health in our hands (monitoring, tracking, and informing about health through technology), 2) interacting for health (relying on technology to communicate about health information, for instance, between professionals and patients), and 3) data enabling health (collecting, managing, and utilizing health data) [19]. This paper focuses principally on the domain of "health in our hands", as the focus is on users' experiences of utilizing a digital health solution to monitor, track, and inform about their health.

The "health in our hands" domain can arguably be divided into two categories – wellness management solutions and health condition management solution - in line with arguments presented by IQVIA, the Institute for Human Data Science [8]. While wellness management solutions, are designed for the monitoring of fitness and lifestyle factors, such as steps [20], diet [21], and sleep [22], health management solutions are used for the daily monitoring and treatment of specific illnesses and chronic conditions [23]), such as diabetes.

Previous studies have primarily explored the ephemeral nature of user experiences with digital health solutions utilized for wellness management, including fitness trackers [24] and happiness applications [25]. These studies demonstrate that experiences with digital health solutions can be fleeting as a result of eventual disuse, neglect, or inconsistent usage [26]. Although this body of work has shed some light into the transient nature of users' experiences, there is a growing demand for studies that explore the sustained use of digital health solutions over time [27]. A promising way to do this is to examine the experiences of individuals who utilize digital health solutions for the management of chronic conditions, such as diabetes, where continuous care is necessary. In these situations, it is challenging for users to simply abandon or overlook their interactions with digital health solutions, which makes it possible to access longitudinal insights about the user's digital experience.

3 Methodology and Data Analysis

By adopting a qualitative, exploratory research approach, this paper seeks an in-depth, user-centric understanding of digital health experiences. This approach facilitates the generation of novel ideas and theoretical insights from empirical observation [28, 29]. This paper employs a social constructionist perspective, which advocates for the comprehension and elucidation of social worlds and processes from the perspective of actors involved [30]. Coupled with "Thick Data", meaning data rich in context and authentic in details of individuals' emotions, narratives, and worldviews [31], the paper aims to uncover the nuances of users' digital health experiences within the context of their everyday lives.

The empirical material considered in this paper consists of three qualitative datasets collected by the first author between March 2020 and August 2021. Overall, the combination of the three datasets ensured access to a detailed, holistic understanding of the studied phenomenon. The first dataset, consisting of 15 in-depth open-ended interviews with diabetics assisted in producing a comprehensive understanding about the daily lives of diabetics and about the role of digital technology in diabetes management. Based on the initial analysis of the interviews, wherein it was stated by a number of interviewees that they utilize online platforms to share and discuss their experiences with other diabetics, a decision was made to acquire online data to expand on the insights gathered during the interview process.

The first online dataset was collected from a discussion forum web mastered by a Finnish diabetics' foundation. A total of 53 discussion threads with approximately 1000 messages were identified by using the brand name of a digital health solution named by the interviewees as the one they utilize in their daily diabetes management as a keyword. To ensure the identification of all relevant data, keyword combinations [brand name] + experience and experience of [brand name] were also used. After the initial analysis revealed the tendency of the discussants to share YouTube videos with each other on the forum, the same keywords were used on YouTube to identify relevant videos. A total of 142 videos were identified and collected from YouTube to form the study's second online dataset. Overall, the study's three datasets ensured data triangulation [32] and access to multiple perspectives of the same phenomenon. Details of the paper's three empirical datasets can be accessed from Table 1 below.

Table 1. Summary of the paper's three empirical datasets

Data type	In-depth open-ended interview	Discussion forum posts	YouTube videos
Data collection period	March-August 2020	August 2020 (posts shared 2014–2020)	June-August 2021 (videos released 2013–2021)
Details about the collected data	15 in-depth open-ended interviews with Finnish diabetics ranging in duration from 25 to 87 min (average 56 min) The interview participants ranged in age from 22 to 76	53 discussion forum threads with app. 1000 messages from a discussion forum for diabetics. The data was identified through the use of a brand name mentioned in the interviews as a keyword	142 videos identified using the same brand name as a keyword as within the discussion forum. The dataset influenced videos from individuals from multiple different countries

After the data collection was finalized, the paper's multimodal media data consisting of recollections of digital health user experiences presented both in oral and written form were "fused" [33] to gain rich insights of the studied phenomenon. In practice, this was done through the transcription of all non-textual data (i.e., audio recordings of the interviews and videos from YouTube) into textual Form. to analyze the empirical data, the paper relies on reflexive thematic analysis, which enables the identification and organization of qualitative data into patterns of meaning (themes) through the process of coding [34].

This paper's reflexive thematic analysis consisted of the six phases defined by Braun and Clarke [34]. In the first phase, *familiarization with the dataset*, the data transcripts were read through multiple times to ensure optimal level of immersion. Some initial notes were written down during this phase as a reference for the upcoming phases. In the second phase, *coding*, the three datasets were systematically explored to identify and code segments connected to the study's objectives. A new code was generated every time something new and interesting in relation to the studied phenomenon emerged from the data transcripts. Examples of codes established during the coding process included 'customization of the experience' and 'feeling like a robot'. When no new codes relevant for the studied phenomenon were identified, the coding process was finalized and the analysis moved to the third phase, *generation of initial themes*. During this third phase, the codes were clustered into categories that reflected key ideas relevant for the paper's aims. The initial theme development highlighted, for instance, users' active involvement in the construction of experiences, and the emerging sense of safety enhanced by the digital health solution. In the fourth phase, *development and review of themes*, the connections between initial themes were explored, resulting in the unification of some themes. Overall, this helped to clarify the process and set the stage for the fifth stage of *refining, defining and naming of themes*. During this penultimate stage of the reflexive thematic analysis process, three themes were refined and named as *always on, co-creation through interaction*, and *it makes things so much easier.* The final phase, *the writing up of the thematic analysis*, is presented in the following sections.

4   Findings of the Study

As the previous section indicates, the qualitative, thematic analysis of the empirical material regarding diabetics' experiences of digital health technology resulted in the identification of three themes: *always on, co-creation through interaction,* and *it makes things so much easier.* These themes, both separately and put together, aid in identifying characteristics of users' experience with a wearable sensor designed for the measurement of glucose levels from interstitial fluid, and shed light on the ways in which the users shape their experiences with the digital health solution in their daily lives.

4.1   Theme 1: Always on

The data indicates that though diabetes can be defined in simple terms as a chronic condition that affects how one's body processes blood sugar (glucose), the experience of living with diabetes is different for everyone. Since diabetes requires recurring care activities and careful monitoring, it can be regarded as something that is "completely part of one's life" (Interview 1) and thus "always on". As one of the interviewees indicated, "It's always part of my life. There's no break or vacation from diabetes" (Interview 3).

The empirical data demonstrates that in addition to the "always on" nature of diabetes, the digital health solution designed for its care is also regarded as something that is always present. The wearable sensor, which measures glucose levels from interstitial fluid, is inserted into one's skin for a 14-day period, after which it is replaced with a new sensor. Resulting from this, the sensor goes wherever its wearer goes, as is indicated in the data through recollections wherein the sensor is part of one's vacations, gym trips, dates, swimming hall visits, and so on. The always on nature of the wearable sensor comes with many benefits, demonstrated, for instance, through access to "trend arrows and graphs" (Discussion forum), and "information about blood glucose movements at all times (YouTube). Yet, acknowledgement is also made of the adverse consequences of the always on presence of the digital health solution and the data it supplies, such as unwanted attention, neuroticism about the data it provides, feelings of anxiety, and the sense that one is like a machine or a barcode that is "scanned repeatedly" (Discussion forum).

Overall, this complexity in perspectives points towards the subjective nature of the user's experience and the possibility to perceive the digital health experience as something that consists of both positive and negative aspects. It should be noted, though, that the majority consensus identified from the empirical material points towards a tendency to perceive and highlight the positive influence of the always on nature of the wearable sensor in diabetes management, as a result of which less attention is paid to the negative and/or aesthetic aspects of the experience.

4.2   Theme 2: Co-creation Through Interaction

To use the wearable sensor in its designed way and to its full benefit, users are expected to interact with it and the data it provides in a recurring manner. As a result of this, the experience with the digital health solution can be perceived as co-created through interaction that takes place between the user and the digital health solution. The data indicates that in the users' day-to-day lives, recurring interactions take the form of, for instance, checking the graphs displaying trends in blood glucose levels to get a "sense of direction for the day" (Interviewee 4) or utilizing the data to "know whether to have insulin, sugar, or just keep living life" (YouTube).

Thus, the co-creative nature of the user's digital health experience is reliant on the following facts: 1) the user must interact with the device in order to access data and 2) the data from the device is relevant only if the user reacts on it. While the interactions with the digital health solution make it possible for the device to produce, for instance, trend graphs, the data becomes relevant only if the user acts on it. Otherwise, it is just numbers and lines of a graph. At the time of the data collection, the interactions with the device involved scanning the sensor at least once every eight hours, either with a sensor reader or a mobile phone. While updates to the technology have made scanning unessential, interactions with the data are still required as the users are expected to use the data to modify their care actions, if necessary. In practice, this means that the digital health solution does not have the capability to take over the daily care activities associated with diabetes. Rather, it is designed to take on an assistive role, making the care of diabetes more convenient and balanced. Thus, "you're responsible for your own care" (Interview 7), which can be made "so much easier" (Interview 6) with the help of the digital health solution.

4.3 Theme 3: It Makes Things so Much Easier

Defined as "life changing" (YouTube), the data reveals that the digital health technology offers significant benefits for its users, including continuous access to data and the possibility "to stay fit for work for years, even decades longer than I would without it" (Discussion forum). Interestingly, the empirical material demonstrates that the digital health technology is often perceived as an educative tool that has the capacity to increase the user's awareness of their condition. This is demonstrated, for example, by the following: "While using the sensor, I noticed how the point where I inject insulin affects how long it takes to work. Now I use this information, for example, when I know that dinner will take longer and inject insulin in my thigh, as the effect will not be felt instantly. Conversely, if I eat fast food, I will inject insulin to my stomach because then the effect will be quicker" (Discussion forum). Overall, such improvements are seen not only to improve daily life and wellbeing by reducing the chance of complications and additional illnesses, but also to benefits to society as better balance of diabetes ensures "fewer additional costs" (Interview 3).

The analysis indicates that the capability to shape their experiences with the digital health solution further improves the potential of it in meeting subjective care needs. As was indicated previously, everyone's diabetes is different, which means that everyone's needs for care are different too. While the digital health device comes with some set parameters, perhaps most importantly the need to wear the sensor at all times for a period of 14-days at a time, the data shows that beyond this requirement, the experience is actually quite modifiable. The three most common ways of shaping the experience identified from the empirical material include 1) altering the placement site of the sensor from upper arm to other areas of the body, such as one's abdomen, 2) altering the appearance of the sensor, and 3) altering the technological aspects of the digital health solution.

The data demonstrates that altering the placement site of the wearable sensor is motivated by the desire to hide the sensor, to make its placement more convenient and secure when engaged in physical activity, and/or by the desire to experiment with the technology to test out the accuracy of glucose readings from different placement sites. Importantly, whatever the reason for alternative placement is, it is acknowledged in the data that such altering is done "at your own risk" (YouTube), as it goes against the instructions given by the digital health solution's manufacturer. Therefore, those shaping their experience through alterations of the placement site are willing to take the risk in order to modify the digital health experience into something that better serves their subjective needs.

Shaping the appearance of the sensor points towards practices that help to hide, secure and/or emphasize its appearance. While the desire to hide the sensor can also lead to trying out alternative placement sites, the data demonstrates that by utilizing tapes and stickers, users are able to diminish the appearance of the sensor. Interestingly, such hiding is associated in the empirical material with the wish to "avoid questions from strangers"

(YouTube) and to save oneself from awkward and even potentially hurtful interactions wherein one is expected to act like a "traveling dictionary who has to explain everything related to diabetes to people […] who just happen to spot the sensor" (Discussion forum). Yet, while some wish to diminish the appearance of the sensor, others are looking for ways to accessorize and personalize it, to "make it pretty" (YouTube) and turn it into something that people, including other diabetics, can easily spot. By making the sensor "cute" (YouTube), the user is able to turn the sensor into something that they carry similarly to a piece of jewelry or another wearable accessory.

Finally, the empirical material indicates that if the user so desires (and has the technological capability to do so), the technological aspects of the experience can be modified. In practice, this means, for instance, the insertion of a third-party Bluetooth transmitter on top of the sensor to make it possible to get alerts to one's smartwatch and to "see my blood glucose levels on my watch at the same time as I check the time" (Discussion forum). Overall, the empirical material shows that such shaping practices are less common as they tend to require a certain level of technological expertise and financial input.

4.4 Summary of the Findings

Altogether, the findings of the study demonstrate that the digital health solution utilized for diabetes management becomes integrated into its user's daily life and through that has the potential to improve not only the users' management of diabetes, but also their overall wellbeing, both in the short and long term. By having the capability to shape their interactions with the technology that is "always on", the user is able to modify the experience into something that best serves their subjective needs and wants, both in relation to diabetes management and to their wishes regarding the visibility of their diabetes for others.

5 Contributions and Future Research Suggestions

The seeking out of an understanding of digital health experience from a user-centric perspective offers various contributions to existing literature. Firstly, while research on digital experience has increased in recent years [14], in the digital health context studies which adopt a user-centric approach have been limited [35]. Secondly, by focusing on experiences of those who utilize digital health technology for health condition management, the paper answers to recent calls for research regarding users' longitudinal experiences with digital health technology [27] and the influence of digital health technology in shaping users' daily lives [26]. Thirdly, in particular for marketing researchers, this paper offers fresh insights into the understanding of user, or customer experience in the contemporary consumption environment, and especially within a domain, which has not been studied extensively in the marketing context despite the digital health market's immerse growth [8].

Since users are increasingly looking for digital solutions that can effectively and fluidly serve their subjective needs [36], this paper highlights the importance for health professionals and health technology developers to understand how digital solutions become integrated into users' lives. Importantly, the paper indicates that allowing users to modify their experiences with digital health technology, at least to some degree, is likely to positively affect the formation of an ongoing relationship between the user and the digital health solution.

It is also important to note that as the digital health market becomes more and more saturated with solutions possessing similar technological functionalities, companies developing digital health solutions must find ways to differentiate themselves on the market. Thus, an understanding of the user perspective will undoubtedly become even more relevant in the future, as it offers digital health companies the possibility to communicate on their promises and values more efficiently for existing and potential users. In practice, a user-centric exploration into digital health experience, such as the one presented in this paper, can be used by digital health companies, for example, to generate brand promises, i.e. assurances of what the digital health brand will and will not deliver to its users [37].

To expand the user-centric understanding of digital health experience beyond this paper, future research should concern itself not only with how experiences are reflected on, either in speech or writing, but also on depicting how the experiences actually look like. Such research could adopt an ethnographic approach through which the daily life of the user and the role digital health technology plays in it could be observed in more detail. Alternatively, research could rely on a combination of videography [38] and diary method [39] to capture both how the experiences look like and how, for example, the role of contextual factors, such as users' education, economic status, and technological know-how potentially influence digital health experience. In order to expand the understanding of digital experiences of users (or customers), marketing researchers in particular should pay more attention to the co-creative nature of the interactions that take place between users and digital health devices, and conduct, for instance, studies focused on users' motivations to engage in recurring interactions with digital health solutions. Though earlier research has indicated the necessity of considering negative user/customer experiences, for the most part focus has been on experience as a positive phenomenon [40]. Thus, future research could expand on this by more carefully considering the factors that have the possibility to contribute negatively to digital health experiences.

Disclosure of Interests. The authors have no competing interests to declare that are relevant to the content of this article.

References

1. Swaminathan, V., Sorescu, A., Steenkamp, J.-B.E.M., O'Guinn, T.C.G., Schmitt, B.: Branding in a hyperconnected world: refocusing theories and rethinking boundaries. J. Mark. **82**(2), 24–46 (2020)
2. Wieczorek, M., O'Brolchain, F., Saghai, Y., Gordjin, B.: The ethics of self-tracking: a comprehensive review of the literature. Ethics Behav. **33**(4), 239–271 (2023)
3. Vial, G.: Understanding digital transformation: a review and a research agenda. J. Strat. Inf. Syst. **28**(2), 118–144 (2019)

4. Frennert, S., et al.: Materiality and the mediating roles of eHealth: a qualitative study and comparison of three cases. Digit. Health **8**, 1–14 (2022)
5. Thomas, J.G., Bond, D.S.: Review of innovations in digital health technology to promote weight control. Curr. Diab. Rep. **14**, 485 (2014)
6. Kemp, E., et al.: Health literary, digital health literary and the implementation of digital health technologies in cancer cure: the need for a strategic approach. Health Promot. J. Austr. **32**(1), 104–114 (2020)
7. Solomon, D.H., Rubin, R.S.: Digital health technologies: opportunities and challenges in rheumatology. Nat. Rev. Rheumatol. **16**, 525–535 (2020)
8. IQVIA Institute for Human Data Sciences. Digital Health Trends 2021: Innovation, evidence, regulation, and adoption. IQVIA Institute, Parsippany (2021)
9. Väinämö, M.: It Makes Things So Much Easier: Exploring Brand Experience in a Digital Health Context. Acta Universitatis Ouluensis, Oulu (2023)
10. World Health Organization homepage. https://who.int. Accessed 19 Jan 2024
11. Elsayed, N.E., et al.: Diabetes technology: standards of care in diabetes – 2023. Am. Diab. Assoc. **46**(1), 111–127 (2023)
12. Carú, A., Cova, B.: Revisiting consumption experience: a more humble but complete view of the concept. Mark. Theory **3**(2), 267–286 (2003)
13. Lipkin, M.: Customer experience formation in today's service landscape. J. Serv. Manag. **27**(5), 678–703 (2016)
14. Gummerus, J., Liljander, V., Weman, E., Pihlström, M.: Customer engagement in a Facebook brand community. Manag. Res. Rev. **35**(9), 857–877 (2019)
15. Markham, A.: The dramaturgy of digital experience. In: Edgley, C. (ed.) The Drama of Social Life, pp. 279–294. Routledge, London (2016)
16. Kawaf, F.: Capturing digital experience: the method of screencast videography. Int. J. Res. Mark. **36**, 169–184 (2019)
17. Ferreira, J.J., Fernandes, C.I., Rammal, H.G., Veiga, P.M.: Wearable technology and consumer interaction: a systematic review and research agenda. Comput. Hum. Behav. **118** (2021)
18. Gleiss, A., Lewandowski, S.: Removing barriers for digital health throughout organizing ambidexterity in hospitals. J. Publ. Health **30**, 21–35 (2022)
19. Shaw, T., McGregor, D., Brunner, M., Keep, M., Janssen, A., Barnet, S.: What is eHealth? Development of a conceptual model for eHealth: qualitative study with key informants. J. Med. Internet Res. **19**(10), e324 (2017)
20. Jin, D., Halvari, H., Maehle, N., Olafsen, A.H.: Self-tracking behaviour in physical activity: a systematic review of drivers and outcomes of fitness tracking. Behav. Inf. Technol. **41**(2), 242–261 (2022)
21. Abril, E.P.: Tracking myself: assessing the contribution of mobile technologies for self-trackers of weight, diet, or exercise. J. Health Commun. **21**(6), 638–646 (2016)
22. Kim, J.: Analysis of health consumers' behavior using self-tracker for activity, sleep, and diet. Telemed. eHealth **20**(6), 552–558 (2014)
23. Seixas, A.A., Olaye, I.M., Wall, S.P., Dunn, P.: Optimizing healthcare through digital health and wellness solutions to meet the needs of patients with chronic disease during the Covid-19 era. Front. Publ. Health **9**, 667654 (2021)
24. Pinto, M.B., Yagnik, A.: Fit for life: a content analysis of fitness tracker brands use of Facebook in social media marketing. J. Brand Manag. **24**, 49–67 (2016)
25. Belli, J.: Unhappy? There's an app for that – tracking well-being through the quantified self. Digit. Cult. Soc. **2**(1), 89–104 (2016)
26. Kristensen, D.B., Ruckenstein, M.: Co-evolving with self-tracking technologies. New Media Soc. **20**(10), 3624–3640 (2018)
27. Pantzar, M., Ruckenstein, M.: The heart of everyday analytics: emotional, material and practical extensions in self-tracking market. Consum. Mark. Cult. **18**(1), 92–109 (2015)

28. Corbin, J., Strauss, B.: Basics of Qualitative Research: Techniques and Procedures for Developing Grounded Theory. Sage, London (2015)
29. Swedberg, R.: Exploratory research. In: Elman, C., Gerring, J., Mahoney, J. (eds.) The Production of Knowledge: Enhancing Progress in Social Science, pp. 17–43. Cambridge University Press, Cambridge (2020)
30. Burrell, G., Morgan, G.: Sociological Paradigms and Organizational Analysis. Heinemann Educational Books, Portsmouth (1979)
31. Moisander, J., Närvänen, E., Valtonen, E.: Interpretative marketing research: using ethnography in strategic management development. In: Visconti, M., Penaloza, L., Tolouse, N. (eds.) Marketing Management: A Cultural Perspective, 2nd edn. Routledge, London (2020)
32. Lincoln, Y., Guba, E.G.: Handbook of Qualitative Research. Sage, London (2000)
33. Boughanmi, K., Ansari, A.: Dynamics of musical success: a machine learning approach for multimedia data fusion. J. Mark. Res. **58**(3), 1034–1057 (2021)
34. Braun, V., Clarke, V.: Thematic Analysis: A Practical Guide. Sage, London (2022)
35. Kolasa, K., Kozinski, G.: How to value digital health interventions? A systematic literature review. Int. J. Environ. Res. Publ. Health **17**(6), 2119 (2020)
36. Ramasundaram, A., Pandey, N., Shukla, Y., Alavi, S., Wirtz, J.: Fluidity and the customer experience in digital platform ecosystems. Int. J. Inf. Manag. **39**, 102599 (2023)
37. Anker, T.B., Kappel, K., Eadie, D., Sandøe, P.: Fuzzy promises: explicative definitions of brand promise delivery. Mark. Theory **12**(3), 267–287 (2012)
38. Belk, R.W., et al.: Envisioning consumers: how videography can contribute to marketing knowledge. J. Mark. Manag. **34**, 432–458 (2018)
39. Komulainen, H., Saraniemi, S.: Customer centricity in mobile banking: a customer experience perspective. Int. J. Bank Mark. **37**(5), 1082–1102 (2019)
40. Barari, M., Ross, M., Surachartkumtonkun, J.: Negative and positive customer shopping experience in an online context. J. Retail. Consum. Serv. **53**, 101985 (2020)

Fatigue Assessment with Visualizations of Patient-Generated Data: An Evaluation with Informatics-Savvy Healthcare Professionals

Sharon Guardado[1]([✉]) [iD], Terhi Holappa[2] [iD], and Minna Isomursu[1] [iD]

[1] University of Oulu, Oulu, Finland
sharon.guardadomedina@oulu.fi
[2] Lapland University of Applied Sciences, Rovaniemi, Finland

Abstract. Severe and chronic fatigue is a prevalent symptom in multiple chronic conditions. Its complexity, its multifaceted nature and its varied manifestations across different conditions require a nuanced approach for accurate assessment by healthcare professionals. In our research, informatics-savvy public health nurses from a Digital Health Services and Health Promotion Master's program evaluated various visualizations of patient-generated health data which could potentially be collected through a mobile app designed for people with Multiple Sclerosis. The data visualization prototypes could be a tool to support fatigue assessment and effective communication during consultations and their design was based on prior suggestions from healthcare professionals with experience in fatigue assessment. The patient-generated health data represented in the prototypes comprised a combination of fatigue-related factors and physical activity tracked by Google Fit. This study presents the recommendations of the participants regarding various aspects linked to the visualizations of patient-generated health data, including their utility in the clinical setting, the most suitable types of data summaries, usability aspects and the possibility of meaningful interrelations between distinct types of data. The results of our study emphasize the importance of well-designed data visualizations to support healthcare professionals in decision-making and to improve patient participation in the chronic care process. The iterative design process of the prototypes ensures that the final visualizations have proper usability and the potential to become clinically relevant, and instrumental in the effective assessment of fatigue in chronic management.

Keywords: Data Visualization · Patient-generated health data · mHealth · Fatigue Assessment

1 Introduction

Severe and chronic fatigue is a prevalent symptom observed in a variety of chronic conditions e.g. chronic obstructive pulmonary disease, type I diabetes mellitus, asthma, and multiple sclerosis. Its assessment can vary depending on the context, the underlying condition, and the patient's overall health [1]. Due to its multifactorial causes, accurate

© The Author(s) 2024
M. Särestöniemi et al. (Eds.): NCDHWS 2024, CCIS 2083, pp. 121–130, 2024.
https://doi.org/10.1007/978-3-031-59080-1_9

assessment of fatigue demands a blended approach which combines multiple methods such as patient-reported outcome measures, clinical interviews, physical examination, and review of symptoms and medical history.

The increased acceptance of mobile health (mHealth) apps and tracking devices among individuals with chronic conditions presents a unique opportunity to integrate these innovative tools into the healthcare processes. The data produced through wearable devices and mobile health applications can be utilized both to empower people to monitor their health and to enhance the healthcare process [2]. Patient-generated health data (PGHD) can be a way to understand patients' environments and self-perceived states of health. Now, patients can record data and report health outcomes whenever and wherever they happen. However, this ubiquitous data collection increases the complexity of data security and data analysis and visualization. A major challenge in dealing with such a large volume of complex data is interpreting and extracting useful knowledge about users' health [3] and research about effective methods to represent PGHD to cater for the diverse needs of users is still in the early stage of design [4].

Understanding the status of a person's health and the underlying factors behind the data produced by mHealth solutions is not a simple task [5]. In the case of fatigue, measurement and impact on patients' lives still pose a challenge. Fatigue represents a widespread symptom reported by 90% of people with Multiple Sclerosis (PwMS), making it one of the most frequent and disabling symptoms of that condition. Assessing the impact fatigue has on patients' lives can support healthcare professionals (HCPs) in their efforts to personalise care to the specific needs of each patient. The most typical goal for the visualization of symptoms data is understanding the relationships of symptoms to disease processes and their symptoms or treatments [6]. Previous studies have shown that patients find visual representations of their health data beneficial because they allow them to better recall past symptoms and relayed clinically relevant patterns that might be difficult to describe, especially when the current health status is not representative of the patient's experiences over previous weeks or months [7].

Investigating how individuals interpret their self-generated data is important [4], especially if this data could potentially aid in improving care. Although previous research has explored efficient and effective ways to present data visualizations for lay audiences, similar research on PGHD from mobile technologies for the clinical context is limited [4]. In general, data visualizations play a significant role in helping different users comprehend data, facilitate communication, and support decision-making processes. Visualizations are also known to lower the cognitive load, enabling users to quickly understand the data [4]. In the clinical setting, effective data visualizations could assist HCPs in chronic care management, enhancing communication and decision-making, while facilitating data analysis, thereby benefiting the patient.

The primary objective of this study is to evaluate the efficacy of various data visualization prototypes designed to present patient-reported data on fatigue in a manner that is clear, concise, and actionable for HCPs. This paper seeks to identify the specific insights and requirements of experiences and informatics-savvy HCPs in assessing patient fatigue, to improve the development of visual representations of fatigue-related factors based on those needs, and to empirically validate the utility of these visualizations in the clinical setting.

2 Methods

To achieve our objective, we employed the focus group methodology with a group of HCPs, who at the time of the study were enrolled in a Digital Health Services and Health Promotion Master's program. A previously defined guide led the execution of the focus group. The design of the evaluated prototypes utilized findings from previous participatory research. In a prior study, HCPs experienced with fatigue assessment created paper prototypes of PGHD that they considered could be useful in the clinical setting[8]. The visualization prototypes were based on the data generated by the "More Stamina" mobile app, which is a self-management solution designed for efficient energy management [9]. The solution was designed to support PwMS in self-management, leveraging wearable sensors and PGHD to provide personalized recommendations and, through anonymized data collection, aids in identifying patterns in living with fatigue [10].

2.1 Development of the Visualization Prototypes

Teams of experienced HCPs, specialized in the care of PwMS, collaborated to develop paper prototypes for the visualization of PGHD collected through the More Stamina app. The prototypes aimed to leverage the use of PGHD during regular consultations, to enhance patient-clinician communication and monitoring in a concise format, adhering to a review time of five minutes or less. The details of the initial prototyping process have been documented in a previous publication [8]. Basic design principles were later used to improve the data visualization prototypes. The type and objectives for the different data visualization prototypes are explained in Table 1.

Utility of PGHD on Energy Expenditure
The use of mHealth solutions for the self-management of patients with chronic disease has been explored and positive results have been found, including the improvement of symptoms in conditions such as asthma, chronic pulmonary diseases, diabetes, and hypertension [2] and the improvement of pain and fatigue outcomes in cancer survivors [11], yet the potential of using the data generated by these solutions in the clinical context remain vastly underexploited. To evaluate the efficacy of patient-reported energy levels and how they are related to fatigue, we designed various data visualisations of energy expenditure by tasks and periods. A sample prototype is shown in Fig. 1.

Periodicity of Visual Data Summaries
In a prior study, we identified that HCPs felt summaries related to physical activity and changes in energy levels during specific periods could give them a better understanding of factors affecting their patients in between appointments[12]. Considering the scarce time availability HCPs have during appointments, it was pertinent to evaluate whether summaries would be more effective on a daily, weekly, or monthly basis, or since the last appointment had occurred. To explore potential differences, we designed variations of data visualisations of energy expenditure of different periods.

Usability of Data Visualizations and Combination of Types of Data
Usability evaluations are of utmost importance to ensure efficient use of, suitable workload, and acceptance of healthcare technologies in the clinical context, [13]. Prior

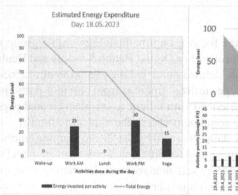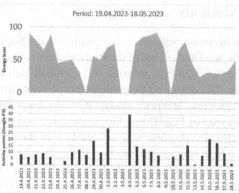

Fig. 1. Sample visualizations of energy expenditure by day and month.

Table 1. Types of visualizations assessed.

Type of Visualization	Explanation	The objective of the Evaluation
Daily energy expenditure	Representation of the energy different activities consume and how they affect the daily energy level	To validate if a patient's daily energy expenditure would be an understandable measure for HCPs
Daily and Monthly energy trends with Google Fit data	Representation of patient-reported energy level against activity tracked in Google Fit	To validate if the combination of patient-reported data with the passively tracked on a longer period would be useful for HCPs
Summaries of energy expenditure by activities	Various representations of patient-reported energy usage by type of activity and period (day, week, and month)	To validate in which periods summaries of patient-reported energy expenditure would be more meaningful for HCPs
Monthly activity level tracked by Google Fit	Various visual representations of activity tracked by Google Fit in a month	To validate if specific colour schemes and designs would facilitate the identification of high and low activity levels

research supports the validity of the Google Fit smartphone application in estimating the stepping activity of individuals with chronic stroke suggesting it is a cost-effective alternative which could be suitable for the clinical context [14]. We designed data visualizations to evaluate if representing patient-reported data generated in combination with the passively tracked data from Google Fit would be useful for HCPs in fatigue assessment.

2.2 Implementation of the Focus Group Methodology

The focus group was conducted during an Innovation Workshop organized by Lapland University of Applied Sciences, which has recently intensified its cooperation with companies related to well-being, health technology and digital solutions in the social and healthcare sectors. Due to its densely sparse distances, Lapland offers an interesting value-adding environment for piloting digital solutions related to well-being and health.

During the workshop, the participants were first introduced to the distinctive features of the More Stamina app by the first author. Afterwards, the focus group was facilitated by the first and second authors, who guided the participants through the different visualization prototypes and related discussions. After participants had the opportunity to write down their observations on each prototype, discussion allowed for further understanding of the participants' perceptions on each topic At the end, participants completed an exit questionnaire about their current utilization of mobile technologies and perception of PGHD. This focus group provided a good opportunity to understand the experience of first-time potential users, who were able to analyse each prototype and provide feedback as experts in the healthcare context.

No personal data was collected throughout the study and before the evaluation was conducted, all participants provided informed consent for their participation in the session and potential utilization of the results for research purposes.

3   Results

3.1   Descriptive Statistics

The participants of our study were nine public health nurses, students in a Master´s program in Digital Health Services and Health Promotion. All of them were female and the average years of working experience was 10.3 (SD = 6.24). Ownership of activity trackers was 85.7% and 100% for mobile phones.

3.2   Perception of Data Visualizations Prototypes

The participants found the visualization prototypes were clear and comprehensible, particularly for HCPs familiar with the topic. The visualizations were effective in representing energy expenditure. However, participants suggested that additional context would be helpful for HCPs less familiar with the specific data. This could be particularly beneficial for public health nurses who collaborate with a diverse patient base and require more detailed background information to interpret the visualizations accurately.

Utility of PGHD on Energy Expenditure
HCPs recognised the value of these data visualizations in understanding the relationship between patient activity levels and energy expenditure. Participants proposed that such a tool could be used to evaluate the effects of medications on patients' fatigue levels, and potentially aid in treatment adjustments or preparation of rehabilitation plans.

Moreover, long-term data summaries were perceived as beneficial for setting realistic patient goals and customizing care plans, identifying energy expenditure patterns related to various activities.

Periodicity of Visual Data Summaries
Although HCPs deemed detailed be essential for initial patient assessments and establishing patterns, in the long term, their preference leaned towards summarized data due to its clarity and practicality. Summarized data, whether weekly or monthly, seemed more practical for monitoring and providing meaningful insights without the intensity of daily analysis. Monthly summaries, or a summary since the last check-up were more suitable for ongoing patient evaluations and routine assessments. HCPs indicated this preference may vary depending on the clinical role or the specific needs of the patient; However, 22% of our participants noted that daily summaries could be useful for HCPs at certain points in the care process.

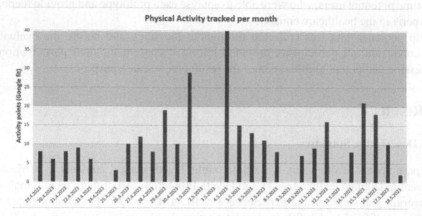

Fig. 2. Sample summarization of activity points tracked with Google Fit in a month.

Usability of Data Visualization and Combination of Types of Data
HCPs reviewed various visualizations which integrated data from the Google Fit application, each with distinct design elements and colour schemes. A unanimous preference emerged for a specific prototype, which was deemed the most effective in illustrating patient activity levels. Participants felt this design intuitively facilitated the identification of varying activity intensities (see Fig. 2).

3.3 Support in Understanding Patients

From the responses to the exit questionnaire, we identified all participants agreed on the value of PGHD from health apps and activity trackers in comprehending patient conditions. Despite over half (55%) of them not having previously recommended mHealth apps to patients, they acknowledged the potential of integrating PGHD with conventional clinical data for a comprehensive understanding of patient health particularly when patients are discharged from the hospital, to understand how they continue at home by themselves. Additionally, almost half of the participants (44%) reported an increase in patient inter-actions which involved patients wanting to share data from mHealth solutions, reflecting a growing trend in patient-driven health data sharing.

4 Discussion

Our study revealed a notable trend: patients are increasingly using mHealth solutions and are willing to share their health data with HCPs to support treatment effectiveness. This can be related to prior studies where participants reported using visualizations from their self-tracking apps to foster higher-quality dialogue with their care team [7].

Effective visualization of PGHD requires a thorough design that aligns with specific data types and the intended functions of the data visualization [4]. Our approach to developing the visualization prototypes was iterative, initially led by HCPs skilled in fatigue assessment with PwMS. The initial designs were refined using basic design principles, resulting in prototypes that were well-received by our participants. However, the feedback obtained during the focus group highlighted the need to include more descriptive elements to enhance the usability of the visualizations to understand PGHD effectively.

In designing PGHD visualizations for HCPs it is crucial to recognize that patients, as the primary users of self-management mHealth solutions, are willing to spend time reviewing their health data. Conversely HCPs, as secondary users, may benefit from PGHD to support their work but do not require the same level of detail as patients, since they already utilize various clinical methods for fatigue assessment. Simple and efficient visualizations significantly enhance HCPs' ability to access and comprehend data[15] allowing for increased patient involvement. HCPs highlighted the importance of clarity and intuitive design for those familiar and unfamiliar with the. This underscores the need for accompanying explanations or legends that can provide the necessary background to understand the visualized data. This is pivotal in clinical settings, where time constraints demand clear, concise information that can critically influence patient care and decision-making.

The participants agreed on the potential for PGHD visualizations to enhance various aspects of patient care, from preventive health to treatment evaluation. The visualizations were viewed as tools to gain a more nuanced understanding of the patient's condition, which can lead to more informed decision-making and personalized care strategies. HCPs indicated that summarized data, whether weekly or monthly, seemed more practical for monitoring, yet they remarked on the need for adaptability in the frequency and depth of data summaries, striking a balance between detail and usability to effectively represent the patient's overall health status.

5 Limitations

The present study, while comprehensive in its approach to evaluating data visualiza-tion prototypes of PGHD for HCPs, has limitations that should be acknowledged. First, the study focused on patient-reported fatigue data generated by a mHealth solution for

PwMS. Fatigue, while a common symptom across various chronic conditions, can manifest differently in different conditions and patients, requiring different approaches for accurate assessment. Therefore, further research would be required to validate whether patient-reported fatigue data generated by people with other conditions would be as meaningful when visualized in a similar way.

Furthermore, the study does not extensively address potential data privacy concerns or the regulatory implications related to utilizing PGHD in clinical decision-making. The integration of PGHD into the healthcare process must be conducted with consideration for patients' data security and compliance with the corresponding regulations. However, the study's main objective is to evaluate the potential of PGHD visualizations as a supplementary tool for clinical practice. The use of this type of tool would imply the active participation and collaboration of patients. Potential data privacy concerns and regulatory matters need to be addressed in more detail in future studies.

In addition, while the study provides insights into the perceived utility of the proposed data visualizations, the long-term benefits, and potential risks or drawbacks of using these tools in chronic care management could not have been explored extensively using our study design and context. Future research would be required to assess the long-term impact and potential challenges of implementing these tools in clinical practice.

6   Conclusions

The utilisation of mHealth apps like "More Stamina" and the integration of patient-reported fatigue with passively collected data from tools such as Google Fit highlight the potential of PGHD for improving the assessment of severe and chronic fatigue.

Our research has shown that HCPs can leverage data visualizations of PGHD to gain a more nuanced appreciation of patients' energy levels and activity patterns. This could inform more personalized and effective treatment plans, medication management, and rehabilitation programs. The feedback on our data visualization prototypes was positive, suggesting that the data representations were understandable and potentially effective for HCPs; however, further research in varied clinical settings would be necessary to validate these results and assess their utility in the treatment of other health conditions.

The iterative design and evaluation process for the data visualization prototypes is a step in the right direction, as it aligns the development of mHealth solutions that can cater for the needs and preferences of different users. As healthcare systems continue to evolve with technological innovations, integrating mHealth solutions into the clinical practice holds significant promise for improving patient outcomes and healthcare experiences by leveraging the use of PGHD.

Acknowledgments. The authors would like to thank Milla Immonen, Anu Kinnunen, Guido Giunti, Vasiliki Mylonopoulou and Octavio Rivera Romero. Without your contributions, this study would not have been possible.

Disclosure of Interests.   The authors have no competing interests to declare, that are relevant to the content of this article.

References

1. Goërtz, Y.M.J., et al.: Fatigue in patients with chronic disease: results from the population-based lifelines Cohort study. Sci. Rep. **11**(1), 1–12 (2021). https://doi.org/10.1038/s41598-021-00337-z

2. Marcolino, M.S., Oliveira, J.A.Q., D'Agostino, M., Ribeiro, A.L., Alkmim, M.B.M., Novillo-Ortiz, D.: The impact of mHealth interventions: systematic review of systematic reviews. JMIR Mhealth Uhealth **6**(1), e8873 (2018). https://doi.org/10.2196/mhealth.8873

3. Alrehiely, M., Eslambolchilar, P., Borgo, R.: Evaluating different visualization designs for personal health data. In: Proceedings of the 32nd International BCS Human Computer Interaction Conference, vol. 32, pp. 1–6 (2018). https://doi.org/10.14236/ewic/hci2018.205

4. Kim, S.H.: A systematic review on visualizations for self-generated health data for daily activities. Int. J. Environ. Res. Publ. Health **19**(18) (2022). https://doi.org/10.3390/ijerph191811166

5. Ledesma, A., Nieminen, H., Valve, P., Ermes, M., Jimison, H., Pavel, M.: The shape of health: a comparison of five alternative ways of visualizing personal health and wellbeing. In: Proceedings of the Annual International Conference of the IEEE Engineering in Medicine and Biology Society, EMBS, pp. 7638–7641. IEEE (2015). https://doi.org/10.1109/EMBC.2015.7320161

6. Lor, M., Koleck, T.A., Bakken, S.: Information visualizations of symptom information for patients and providers: a systematic review. J. Am. Med. Inform. Assoc. **26**(2), 162–171 (2019). https://doi.org/10.1093/jamia/ocy152

7. Polhemus, A., et al.: Data visualization for chronic neurological and mental health condition self-management: systematic review of user perspectives. JMIR Ment. Health **9**(4), e25249 (2022). https://doi.org/10.2196/25249

8. Guardado, S., Mylonopoulou, V., Rivera-Romero, O., Patt, N., Bansi, J., Giunti, G.: An exploratory study on the utility of patient-generated health data as a tool for health care professionals in multiple sclerosis care. Methods Inf. Med. **62**(05/06), 165–173 (2023). https://doi.org/10.1055/s-0043-1775718

9. Giunti, G., Mylonopoulou, V., Romero, O.R.: More stamina, a gamified mHealth solution for persons with multiple sclerosis: research through design. JMIR Mhealth Uhealth **6**(3), e9437 (2018). https://doi.org/10.2196/mhealth.9437

10. Giunti, G., et al.: Evaluation of more stamina, a mobile app for fatigue management in persons with multiple sclerosis: protocol for a feasibility, acceptability, and usability study. JMIR Res Protoc **9**(8), e18196 (2020). https://doi.org/10.2196/18196

11. Hernandez Silva, E., Lawler, S., Langbecker, D.: The effectiveness of mHealth for self-management in improving pain, psychological distress, fatigue, and sleep in cancer survivors: a systematic review. J. Cancer Survivorsh. **13**(1), 97–107 (2019). https://doi.org/10.1007/s11764-018-0730-8

12. Guardado, S., Isomursu, M., Giunti, G.: Health care professionals' perspectives on the uses of patient-generated health data. In: Challenges of Trustable AI and Added-Value on Health, vol. 294, pp. 750–754 (2022). https://doi.org/10.3233/SHTI220577

13. Scherf, J., Mentler, T., Herczeg, M.: Healthcare and usability professionals' performance in reflecting on visualized patient-reported outcomes. In: 2020 IEEE International Conference on Healthcare Informatics, ICHI 2020, pp. 20–22 (2020). https://doi.org/10.1109/ICHI48887.2020.9374392

130 S. Guardado et al.

14. Polese, J.C., et al.: Google Fit smartphone application or Gt3X Actigraph: which is better for detecting the stepping activity of individuals with stroke? A validity study. J. Bodyw. Mov. Ther. **23**(3), 461–465 (2019). https://doi.org/10.1016/j.jbmt.2019.01.011
15. Gustafson, W., Holt, C., Gustafson, J.W., Jones, C.H., Pape-haugaard, L.: Designing a dashboard to visualize patient information designing a dashboard to visualize patient information. In: 16th Scandinavian Conference on Health Informatics, Linköping University Electronic Press, pp. 23–29 (2018)

Older Adults´ Emotional User Experiences with Digital Health Services

Paula Valkonen(✉) ⓘ and Sari Kujala ⓘ

School of Science, Department of Computer Science, Aalto University, P.O. Box 11000, 00076 Aalto, Finland
paula.valkonen@aalto.fi

Abstract. Older adults are at risk of being excluded from digital society. They do not always find digital health services appealing, or they may have challenges with them. We investigated older adults´ emotional user experiences with digital health services and aimed to give designers tools to make digital health services more appealing for older adults. We interviewed 16 older adults about their experiences with digital health services. The use of digital health services brought joy and increased self-confidence. On the other hand, older adults had many negative emotional user experiences, including fear of pressing buttons and embarrassment of incompetence. In the future, designers should actively look for solutions that alleviate older adults´ fears and further encourage them to use digital health services. To enable that, proposals are made for designing digital health services.

Keywords: Older Adults · Emotional User Experiences · Positive Design · Positive Computing

1 Introduction

Older adults are at a great risk of being excluded from digital society [1–3]. As we age, the risk of chronic disease and multimorbidity and the need for health care increase [4, 5]. Moreover, in this digital age, healthcare is evolving and relying more on digital health services [2, 6]. This can lead to inequalities between different citizen groups [7]: those who need healthcare services most often have challenges using new digital health services. In addition, they face challenges in accessing digital services and available knowledge, and they might sometimes experience being socially excluded [1, 5, 8]. Older adults may experience that they do not have enough knowledge, self-efficacy or support with digital health services, and the benefits of digital health services are not clear them [5].

The exclusion of older adults from digital health services points to technology-driven development processes, where end-users are not involved in design processes [1]. Designers should give attention to the needs of older adults, otherwise the situation will never change [1, 8]. For example, designers should consider older adults´ cognitive capabilities and cognitive changes, such as reduced working memory in their design decisions [9]. At the same time, healthcare providers should take their needs and abilities

© The Author(s) 2024
M. Särestöniemi et al. (Eds.): NCDHWS 2024, CCIS 2083, pp. 131–146, 2024.
https://doi.org/10.1007/978-3-031-59080-1_10

into account and offer digital health services that are easy to use and motivate older adults to use them [2, 5].

Emotions are central to user experience [10–12]. Emotional user experiences are an important part of being human, and in human-computer-interaction, emotional user experiences play a significant role [12, 13]. Emotional user experiences and digital services´ usability become entangled and affect each other [12, 14]. Emotional user experiences together with memories are central when individuals evaluate product success [14], but older adults´ emotional user experiences are especially important to investigate and consider when making design decisions because older adults´ first experiences with new digital services count the most [15]. At the same time, older adults may feel that learning something new, like using digital services, is a labor-intensive process, which challenges the engagement of older adults with digital services [15]. The successful use of technology supports self-efficacy and positive emotions when unsuccessful use of technology may cause even rejection of use [16]. Therefore, we believe that if the emotional user experiences of using digital health services are negative, older adults will reject new services, and their risk of inequal digital health service access will increase.

In this study, we collect emotional user experiences of older adults using digital health services, focusing on citizen´s digitally offered health services (e.g., nationwide patient portals), municipal or private service providers' digital healthcare services (e.g., digital appointment booking to health centers), and digitally offered social services. We will refer to these various services as "digital health services." We also give designers and developers tools (as a mode of design proposals) to take older adults experiences into account in design and development decisions, to lower the existing barriers to the use of digital health services and reduce older adults´ fears.

This research is guided by two questions: 1) What emotional user experiences do older adults have with digital health services? and 2) How can older adults be considered when designing digital health services?

2   Related Work

2.1   Older Adults´ Emotional User Experiences with Digital Services

Among all age groups, digital services cause experiences with full of emotions. At least 1) frustration 2) feeling of competent 3) pleasantness, 4) anxiety, 5) confusion, 6) desperation, 7) pride, 8) determination, 9) annoyance, 10) excitedness, 11) feeling of success, 12) feeling of self-efficacy, 13) vigilance, 14) fear, 15) trust, 16) sorrow, 17) pleasantness, 18) unpleasantness, and 19) confidence of digital services use have been recognized [13, 16, 17].

When older adults´ experiences using computers and search engines were investigated it was found, for example, that content with unfamiliar language was problematic: too-difficult terminology in the user interface caused confusion and emotional user experience of helplessness [18].

The negative emotional user experiences, like fear, frustration, or worries, arise when older adults try to cope with the challenges of technology [19]. Challenges again rise, for example, when training materials are poor, support is not available, the user interfaces change too quickly, or older adults face physical limitations, such as hand tremors [15, 19]. The importance of support and the availability of manuals are emphasized [15].

2.2 Older Adults' Emotional User Experiences with Health Technology

Older adults' needs for health technology is increasing. When the older adults' emotional user experiences with health technology, including the internet, computers, and healthcare applications were studied, both love and hate were identified, as well as concerns, confusion, and frustration, but emotional user experiences of being safe and getting help were also present [9, 20]. For example, older adults with health problems such as diabetes found that health technology benefited them, but the user interface and the use process bought challenges. In the interview study for older adults (n = 50) in Hong Kong was recognized that they had a fear of making mistakes with the devices and user interfaces [9]. Some of them did not want to use health technology at all, and behind the frustration was suspected to be a lack of skills and overly complex devices [9, 20]. The health technology should empower older adults; instead of increasing worries, it should offer experiences of self-confidence and improve older adults' self-esteem [9].

Ware et al. [21] concentrated especially on barriers to older adults using digital health services, such as health portals or mobile apps related to health. Their interviewees reported frustration when trying to find relevant information about their health on the internet and trying to recognize the reliability of the information available. Respondents felt that they did not have good enough access to their health information. For example, medical records were kept in multiple places, which challenged access to information. From the other perspective, digital health services offer the possibility of peer support and communication, especially with other people in the same health situation; however, potential privacy issues worried older adults [21].

Privacy concerns [5, 22] are also reported with older adults, and challenges related to the use of language in patient portals, especially medical terminology, or Latin phrases that healthcare professionals use, were common among the participants. The lack of information available in time or errors with the information in the patient portal brought frustration to older adults [22].

2.3 Designing for Older Adults

With the careful design decisions, it's possible to influence the emotions caused by digital services. Although older adults is a heterogeneous group with varying user needs [15, 23], the design proposals for older adults often differ based only on their age [23].

A positive design approach underlines the maximization of positive emotional user experiences and the minimization of negative ones [24, 25]. With the positive design approach, it is possible to increase older adults' overall well-being and help them flourish [24, 25]. Moreover, negative emotional user experiences can be alleviated through design, supporting the experience of autonomy instead of forcing older adults to comply and offering value instead of frustration.

Positive computing shares the positive design philosophy's targets in many ways. In positive computing, the information technology concentrates improving a human's wellbeing focusing originally especially on psychological wellbeing, but also seen health and wellbeing in a larger context [26–28]. The information technology should support, help, and strengthen end-users´ capabilities [26, 27].

The health conditions of older adults should be considered during design. When older adults might have many chronic diseases at the same time, and the need for assisting digital health services is high, the digital health services should adapt in changing health conditions to support older adults´ health self-management [29].

Seeing the benefits of digital services strongly motivates older adults [5, 15]. Therefore, it is important to understand older adults´ needs for digital health services as a part of the design process [15], as well as communicate the potential benefits to older adults [5]. In addition, with the careful user interface design decisions (e.g., restricting the number of available options, hierarchy, and process steps, and offering enough time to operate) it is possible to do help older adults to use digital services [15].

3 Study Design and Methods

3.1 Participant Recruitment

The material for this research was collected as part of a larger study [3], in which the focus was to recognize them, who are potentially in vulnerable positions, and their challenges with digital health services. The data of the larger study was analyzed and coded anew by PV using this study´s focus. In this study, 16 older adults between the ages of 67 and 90 (mean = 75.4 years) from different parts of Finland were interviewed. The interviews were conducted from 11/2020 to 01/2021, while the COVID-19 pandemic was in its second wave in Finland. Since the availability of physical services varies based on an individual's distance from a city, participants both from cities and the countryside were included in the sample. Participants had different life situations and technological skills, and they were fairly well educated (the average of the years of education 12.5 years, range 7–20 years). The sample of the study did not include the most vulnerable older adults. All participants lived at home and were active. 13 participants were recruited using purposive sampling via two older adults´ affairs promotion associations. Three participants were found using snowball sampling.

3.2 Interview Design

The main interview structure was planned together with a group of 10 researchers, but the questions were modified by this study´s researchers (PV and SK) to be easier to understand by those older adults who may not have many information technology skills. The edits were, for example, the addition of examples to explain the interview questions. The interview questions of the emotional user experiences were add-ons to the larger study´s interview structure this study´s researchers (PV and SK). A pilot interview with an older adult was organized, and some minor changes were made to the interview questions. The data of the pilot interview were included in the data set with the permission of the interviewee. Due to the COVID-19 situation, the interviews were conducted remotely. The interviews were recorded with Audacity® (Version 3.2.5).

3.3 Data Analysis

The data were transcripted, pseudonymized and classified into themes, which were decided together with other researchers of the main study [3]. Next to the collaborative data analysis of the main study in Microsoft Excel (Version 2208 (Build 15601.20680) ("Excel"), data were collected (PV) under two extra themes as well: interviewees' ideas about how older adults could participate in digital society better in the future and older adults´ experiences among healthcare, which were raised during the interviews on an ad hoc basis. Therefore, next to the collaborative analysis of the main study [3], the data were further analyzed and re-grouped in detail (PV) in ATLAS.ti (Version 8.4.26.0) and Excel.

In this further analysis, the data were reviewed again following the grounded theory´s code recognition practices [30, 31], and to identify emotions based on the literature [13, 16, 17]. For example, some new, lower-level codes were created, and the digital health services that older adults use in their everyday lives were identified. At this stage of the analysis, situations with some emotional user experiences were also picked, and coded to understand the background, possible values, expectations, and life situations behind the emotions. The recognized emotional experiences (emotions) were grouped again under the emotion categories from the literature [13, 16, 17]: 1) frustration 2) feeling of competent 3) pleasantness, 4) anxiety, 5) confusion, 6) desperation, 7) pride, 8) determination, 9) annoyance, 10) excitedness, 11) feeling of success, 12) feeling of self-efficacy, 13) vigilance, 14) fear, 15) trust, 16) sorrow, 17) pleasantness, and 18) un-pleasantness, and 19) confidence [13, 16, 17]. Finally, it was calculated how many different emotional experiences belonged to each category. This further review of the data focused on content related to digital health services (including social services).

4 Results

The data of this study consisted of a total of 931 min of recording (average length 58 min, range 46–72 min), which was transcribed into 225 pages (Verdana 11, line spacing 1). The codes for emotional user experiences that were highlighted in the analysis relating to this study are presented in Fig. 1.

Most of the emotion categories (A-E, G) were opened based on the emotions recognized [13, 16, 17]. In addition to that, the emotion categories F, H-K (Disgust, Rebellion, Experience of being forced, Embarrassment, and Stress) were formed via identifying new codes. The most frequently mentioned emotional user experience was joy and contentment (Category A.) with digital health services use. Participants liked the ease of accessing services digitally. They were also proud that they could use digital health services, which seemed to bring self-confidence (Categories G, H). From another perspective, digital health services brought a lot of negative emotional user experiences, such as anger, irritation, worries, and even fear to participants (Categories B-F, I-K). Often, those older adults in our study who could use digital health services were very worried about those who cannot use digital health services because they do not have enough guidance and support to use digital health services or do not have well-functioning devices.

Next, we specify with examples the emotional user experiences that caused the emotions presented in Fig. 1. We concentrate on joys first and continue to frustration. Finally,

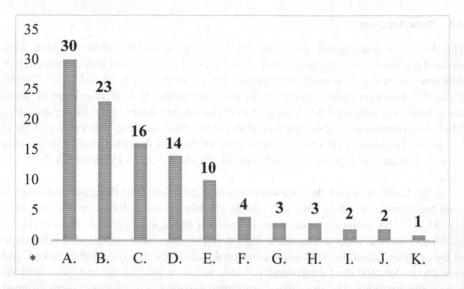

*A) Pleasantness, feeling of success, trust. B) Frustration, annoyance. C) Fear. D) Anxiety, confusion. E) Sorrow. F) Disgust (not in the literature). G) Experience of being competent, feeling of self-efficacy, pride, trust, confidence, determination. H) Rebellion. I) Experience of being forced. J) Embarrassment. K) Stress.

Fig. 1. Emotional user experiences and the number of the mentions per each emotion category.

we suggest some design aspects to consider when designing digital health services based on the existing literature and the findings of our study.

4.1 Joys

Delight with the Ease that Digital Health Services Bring to Everyday Life. Making appointments remotely delighted older adults. Using digital devices and services was a joy for those who knew how to take advantage of them. Digital health services brought ease to their everyday lives.

> *For example, a blood test time can be booked in advance digitally. No need to sit there on the spot for long periods queuing. What a great relief! (Male, 75)*

> *Once the devices work and you know how to use them, [using digital health services] is great. When you can do with them what you need. (Female, 69)*

> *Well, in general, appointments booking digitally [with digital health services] goes well. I'm alive. I have not had any problems with them. (Male, 79)*

> *Before, I always walked there [to the healthcare service provider] and made an appointment from there. Now I book appointments through the internet. (Female, 69)*

The Joy of Learning Something New. The digital health services can bring joy to older adults. Learning to use digital health services and devices can activate and motivate older adults.

> *Someone should just tell the older adults that feel free to get to know digital devices and digital health services through their grandchildren or a friend first.--- You will learn to use them! Luckily, I have my family who always want to inspire me to get involved. So, I have that good side in my life. And besides, I'm brave and accept* [digital health services], *that's it. There's nothing stopping me, like thinking that I can't or don't want to. But rather, I think that I want to, and I learn! (Female, 90)*

> *It's a pleasure to know for sure that especially that button should be pressed* [in the user interface]. *(Female, 70)*

> *Digital health services have become pretty well more, and I think they work well. They are easy to use once you get used to them. (Male, 71)*

Increasing Self-confidence with the Success of Using Digital Health Services. The success of using digital health services improves older adults´ self-confidence. They rejoice in being able to manage their affairs digitally and independently, although the use of digital health services is not always without problems.

> *I feel that I will succeed* [using digital health services] *if I just focus properly. In a way, digital technology has told me that yes this is taken care of, and this is for your benefit. I have accepted the use* [of digital health services] *step by step. --- So, this doesn't evoke any such wow-effect, but the emotional user experience that I will probably succeed the next time* [using digital health services] *as well. That emotional user experience is neutral. I kind of forget the emotional user experience until the next time comes* [using digital health services]. *(Female, 69)*

> *However, I am quite pleased I can handle those most important things online. That is, banks, My Kanta pages* [national patient portal] *and emails. (Female, 78)*

> *--- I can use some* [digital health services] *myself. All alone, even if I don't support, and I'll get along pretty well. --- I am glad that I know this much, and that I have the devices* [and digital health services]. *(Female, 70)*

> *--- Then my husband and I took care of things together* [via digital health services]. *I didn't have to take responsibility for it alone* [using digital health services], *and it seemed to work quite easily. (Female, 69).*

4.2   Frustrations

Anger About Poorly Designed Digital Health Services. Older adults demand better-designed services. They understand that their use problems with digital health services are not just due to their limitations but also to poor design. Older adults feel that digital health services are too confusing and complex and that they change too much with development. Poorly designed services annoy older adults.

I think digital health services are in the worst condition of all. They are so confusing! The only thing that works in digital health services is an appointment booking. Elsewhere, digital health services are developed in a haphazard way. (Male, 71)

Fear of Using Devices for Digital Health Services. Pressing the function keys on the user interface is scary. Older adults know that pressing a button starts a process that is important for their everyday life or well-being. The fear of pressing a button includes the concern that the process will go wrong, that the wrong process will start, or that the process cannot be canceled. Fear of a disaster includes fear of breaking either the device or the digital health service and is also related to older adults´ concerns about the lack of help available. If one is not used to dealing with digital health services, it takes a lot of courage to try again when the first try has failed. Overly complicated digital health services confuse older adults and complicate the situation.

If I must take care of something through the internet, I stop when I can't and don't know how to act, and I'll start to be afraid of where I'll click. Then I quit very suddenly and make a phone call to my eldest son for help. (Female, 69)

Many are afraid to press a button: what happens then and so on. I don't know how that fear could then be dispelled. (Female, 67)

If you haven't normally been using them [referring to the devices], *many are afraid of doing something like that... So, I always say that don't be afraid; that it's a device* [tablet, computer, or mobile phone], *and it won't break down now or go out of order, and if you click something a little wrong, it doesn't break. It will not be a disaster. (Male, 75)*

Concerns About Competence. Even for them from older adults who know how to take advantage of the basic functions of digital health services, problem situations cause a lot of headaches. They have uncertainty about whether their skills are sufficient to solve potential computer problems.

While I may be able to look for the bugs or problems that now always arise when working on a computer, and even if I can navigate in the right files, I don't have enough know-how to solve the problems. (Male, 78)

When you don't know how to use them perfectly, yes, it keeps you watching out about what you do there [in digital health services]. *(Male, 79)*

Worry of Lack of Support in Crisis. Older adults need support both in the use of digital health services and in the crisis of digital health service use. If help is not available when needed, digital health services may not be fully utilized, and stress may increase.

I am not at all surprised that my peers and even older than me are without data connections and a computer. It's hard to learn something new, pile yourself up, and focus on sitting still all day and searching for something specific from the Internet. (Female, 78)

I get frustrated when there is always a problem with my computer, which I then try to solve with the little digital know-how I have. That's when I always hope to have a friend to ask for help. How should I solve the problem, what should I do, and what is wrong here? At some point, I have a lot of stress. (Male, 78)

I don't have any young or older people I could ask for help if needed. I am now content with what I have. I think that this is just the situation now. I rub along somehow. I would like to be able to do a little more with the computer as it would make communication easier, and I could send those messages. --- I miss out a lot. (Male, 88)

Worry About not Understanding the Contents of the Digital Health Services (e.g., Language, Names of the Functions). Older adults become worried about digital health services when they can´t understand the content of the services, or the content is offered in another language that they do not understand. For example, overly challenging terminology in digital health services, such as specific medical terminology that healthcare professionals use, brings challenges to older adults when using digital health services.

So at least I think of that computer, that I kind of respect it because of that, because I don't understand what it means with the things what it tells me to do. (Female, 78)

I tried to search the internet for an appointment at an office. --- I didn't understand those texts (in the user interface of the digital health service). (Female, 69)

Embarrassment About Incompetence. Sometimes not being able to use digital health services embarrasses older adults. This embarrassment about incompetence is mixed with the worry that other people might find them stupid or simple or express pity that digital skills have not been learned in their time.

This digital world is not problem-free. Millions of Finnish adults do not use or do not know how to use this nonsense [referring to the digital health services]. Then the others [referring them who can use digital health services or developers] think that how stupid those millions are and turn their noses up at them. (Male, 72)

It's annoying that I have all that kind of digital, like computers, left out. --- It's a little hard to admit, but I feel stupid when everyone's talking about the internet and digital things. I feel like an outsider. (Male, 88)

4.3 Design Proposals

The aim of these design proposals (Table 1) is to reduce negative emotional user experiences, such as fear, and help older adults flourish when using digital health services in the spirit of the positive design approach and positive computing [24–26, 32]. Although these design proposals are aimed at older adults, they would probably benefit everyone [19]. The design proposals have been formed by combining the interview results and ensuring their relevance from the background literature. Both researchers participated in the design proposal creation. The targets of the design proposals are done in the light of positive design and positive computing [24–26, 32]. The design proposals 1, 3, 4, 5, and 8 target to increasing the older adults´ self-confidence with the success of using digital health services. The design proposals 3, 4, 5, 6, 8, and 9 target to bringing the delight with the ease that digital health services bring to everyday life. The design proposals 3, 7, and 8 target to offering the joy of learning something new. The design proposals 1, 2, and 8 target to lowering the worry of lack of support in crisis. The design proposal 2 targets to lowering the worry about not understanding the contents of the digital health services and the fear of using devices for digital health services. The design proposals 2, 7, 8, and 9 target to lowering and the concerns about competence. The design proposals 4, 5, 6 and, 8 target to lowering the anger about poorly designed digital health services. Finally, the design proposals 8, and 9 target to lowering the embarrassment about incompetence.

Table 1. Design proposals and the literature for ensuring the relevance.

Design Proposal	Background Literature
1. Contact information for support should be easily visible and use instructions should be available. We suggest offering manuals and guidance. An easy access to support should be offered in several channels next to digital health service	[3, 5, 15, 19]
2. Face-to-face guidance for use should be offered to those who need it. It still should be possible to meet service providers face-to-face alongside the remote services	[2, 3, 33]
3. Different user groups should be identified, and in the best case, the content of a digital health service and the support available should be adjusted based on the needs of the user group. The health and wellbeing of older adults is a diverse phenomenon, and older adults´ individual differences should be taken account in user experience design	[5, 8, 15, 17, 21, 23, 34–36]
4. The usability of a digital health service should often be tested as development progresses and participants should include older adults with different skill levels and in different health and life situations. The focus should be on consistency, simplicity, and minimizing the number of procedure steps and potential errors	[5, 15, 35–37]
5. Overly complex structures in menus and hierarchies should be avoided	[15, 18, 34, 37–39]
6. To older adults who like to make appointments online, easy appointment booking in digital health services should be supported	[33]
7. It is challenging for older adults to learn new habits. Therefore, minimal updates and other changes to the interface as development progresses could help older adults with their use challenges	[5, 15]
8. Building the trust between older adults and digital health services should be emphasized by: 1) Simple interface language, 2) A clear feedback on successful performance, 3) Openly informing about potential security issues and how to avoid them, and 4) Providing help for important maintenance procedures, like security updates	[3, 5, 18, 21, 22, 34, 37, 40, 41]
9. Clarify the older adults´ real values: do they need a new digital channel for their health issues, or does some other channel fit to their real needs better. Take account also the older adults´ changing health situations	[3–5, 8, 11, 15, 16, 29, 35, 42]

5 Discussion

In this interview study, emotional user experiences of older adults regarding to their digital health service use were gathered. In addition, this study presented design proposals for digital health services which take the older adults account, based on the quantitative and qualitative research.

The interviews showed that the older adults experienced strong emotions about digital health services. This came out even when the emotions were just a side plot in the interview structure. They also describe their experiences in a rich way. In the spirit of Kujala and Miron-Shatz [14], many of the older adults we interview have emotional user experiences that affect their behavior, for example, their choice to use or not to use digital health services. Based on the interviews, positive experiences encouraged the use of the digital health services, while negative experiences could even cause the digital health services not to be used. For example, a successful digital health service's first use motivates one to use it again. On the other hand, due to negative testing experiences, the use of the services has been completely abandoned.

We identified many positive emotions in the use of digital health services by older adults. Interestingly, the most often mentioned emotional user experience in our study was joy. The joy came out for example in situations, where the digital health service functioned well or supported the older adults´ lives especially well. Learning new digital health self-management ways motivated older adults in the study. Other literature has also observed positive effects by older adults of using digital health services [e.g., [3, 5]. These can be supported for example with the positive design approach and positive computing [24–28, 32]. If the use of digital health services produces mostly negative emotional user experiences, a negative cycle is possible, the ageing population´s self-confidence decreases, and using the services starts to make older adults anxious or can even cause them stress [16]. Therefore, it is not enough to concentrate in helping older adults to get practices to use digital health services. It is also important to build older adults´ self-confidence with digital health services. Our results show that not only the capability to use digital health services counts; the experiences of success are at least as important.

To gain the feeling of success was not obvious in this study either. Older adults had emotional user experiences, such as many fears, anger, and embarrassment, when they failed to use digital health services. For example, fear arose when an older adult did not know how to use devices or user interfaces and thus rejected digital health services. On the other hand, anger or frustration arose when the benefits of digital health services were not understood, and the interest in using them was lacking. The result of this study shows that self-confidence and self-efficacy are one of the main factors to older adults related to their willingness to use digital health services, which is in line with Wilson et al. [5]. If they don´t have self-confidence and self-efficacy with digital health services, the use of digital health services brings negative emotional user experiences, such as anger, embarrassment, or experience of being outsider of the community. This is somewhat in line with Saariluoma and Jokinen [13], where was found that the smooth technology use follows the experience of competence and presented even in more detail: poor usability in digital services activates negative emotional experiences. Also, other studies emphasize the importance of emotions and experiences to been investigated and taken account in human–technology interaction design and remark the connection between the end-users' feelings of their competence levels and the possible frustration with technology use [16, 17]. However, our research did not deep dive in that correlation but recognized older adults´ emotional experiences when using digital health services.

Our study shows that older adults have a fear of using digital health services, and they are unsure of the consequences of continuous updates and other maintenance work on devices. This may come from the fact that they can be from different generations of technology than the user interfaces have been designed for [43], and older adults´ mental models do not always match the performance of younger adults' mental models [44]. In addition, maintenance procedures for devices, such as security updates, can feel terrifying to older adults due to, for example, fear of changes in the user interface's layout after the update [40]. This fear was mentioned in the interviews.

Therefore, it´s also important to help older adults to strengthen their knowledge and capability to 1) use digital health services, but also 2) maintenance their devices for example with security updates themselves. This might empower older adults and to calm them down with possible security issues and reduce their concerns about competence. On the other hand, like mentioned in the interviews, older adults get the joy of learning something new as well.

When designing digital health services, it is important to listen to the concerns of older adults and remember that some of them think that digital health services are frightening [3]. In many cases open communication of the benefits of digital health services might help to reduce older adults´ barriers to use digital health services [5].

Supporting successful use of digital health services enables older adults to independently live for as long as possible and provides them with the joy of success, as it was expressed in the interviews. Many are upset about being excluded from these digital services [1, 3]. Designers should therefore look for solutions that can reduce the fear of using digital health services. Older adults should be encouraged to overcome their concerns and to try to use digital health services more boldly.

5.1 Limitations and Future Research

This study investigated what older adults experience with digital health services. To refine and complement the design proposals presented in this article in line with positive design and positive computing, the lives of older adults in terms of health and well-being should be examined in more detail. The user needs of older adults for digital health services should be further explored. In addition to that, the testing, and prioritizing the design proposals will be necessary. The design proposals in this study were created to help strengthen positive experiences and reduce negative ones. Therefore, they were quite general and should not be viewed as user interface guidelines.

The study was conducted remotely during the COVID-19 pandemic. In Finland, older adults had been ordered to stay at home for safety reasons. At the same time, many health services were offered, mostly digitally for safety reasons. These circumstances may have influenced to the emotional user experiences in this study.

In the analysis phase, the emotional experiences were not comprehensively compared to the findings in other studies. Therefore, it´s not possible to distinguish whether the experiences were the same as in other studies. The study neither attempted this comparison. However, we got an idea of what kind of emotional experiences older adults have of digital health service use.

6 Conclusions

In this study, we collected older adults´ emotional user experiences of using digital health services. We found that the use of digital health services caused emotional user experiences on both ends of the spectrum, from frustration to joy. The experiences of joy showed the empowerment of older adults, and experiences of success using digital health services made their daily lives easier. Designers have both an excellent opportunity and a great responsibility to influence the experiences of older adults regarding digital health services in the future. Based on existing literature and our findings of emotional user experiences of older adults when using digital health services, we created design proposals to reduce the negative emotional user experiences and to highlight positive ones.

Acknowledgments. The work was supported by the Strategic Research Council at the Academy of Finland (grants 352501 and 352503), and NordForsk (project 100477). The study protocol was reviewed and approved by the Ethical Review Board of Aalto University. We would like to thank co-researchers from the DigiIN, DigiCOVID, and NORDeHEALTH projects for their help with research arrangements.

Disclosure of Interests. None.

References

1. Coleman, G.W., Gibson, L., Hanson, V.L., Bobrowicz, A., McKay, A.: Engaging the disengaged: How do we design technology for digitally excluded older adults? 2010, pp. 175–178. https://doi.org/10.1145/1858171.1858202
2. Heponiemi, T., Kaihlanen, A.-M., Kouvonen, A., Leemann, L., Taipale, S., Gluschkoff, K.: The role of age and digital competence on the use of online health and social care services: a cross-sectional population-based survey. Digital Health Sage Publications Ltd; 2022 Jan 1;8:20552076221074484 (2022). https://doi.org/10.1177/20552076221074485
3. Kaihlanen, A.-M., et al.: Towards digital health equity - a qualitative study of the challenges experienced by vulnerable groups in using digital health services in the COVID-19 era. BMC Health Serv. Res. **22**(1), 188 (2022). https://doi.org/10.1186/s12913-022-07584-4
4. Atella, V., Belotti, F., Kim, D., Goldman, D., Gracner, T., Piano Mortari, A., Tysinger, B.: The future of the elderly population health status: Filling a knowledge gap. Health Economics 2021 Mar 26; hec.4258 (2021). https://doi.org/10.1002/hec.4258
5. Wilson, J., Heinsch, M., Betts, D., Booth, D., Kay-Lambkin, F.: Barriers and facilitators to the use of e-health by older adults: a scoping review. BMC Public Health **21**(1), 1556 (2021). https://doi.org/10.1186/s12889-021-11623-w

6. Meier, C.A., Fitzgerald, M.C., Smith, J.M.: EHealth: extending, enhancing, and evolving health care. Annu. Rev. Biomed. Eng. **15**(1), 359–382 (2013). https://doi.org/10.1146/ann urev-bioeng-071812-152350

7. Heponiemi, T., Gluschkoff, K., Leemann, L., Manderbacka, K., Aalto, A.-M., Hyppönen, H.: Digital inequality in Finland: Access, skills and attitudes as social impact mediators. New Media & Society SAGE Publications; Jul 28;14614448211023008 (2021). https://doi.org/10. 1177/14614448211023007

8. Hanson, V.L.: Influencing technology adoption by older adults. Interact Comput Oxford University Press Oxford, UK **22**(6), 502–509 (2010). https://doi.org/10.1016/j.intcom.2010. 09.001

9. Chen, K.: Assistive technology and emotions of older people – adopting a positive and integrated design approach. In: Zhou, J., Salvendy, G, editors. Human Aspects of IT for the Aged Population Acceptance, Communication and Participation Cham: Springer International Publishing, pp. 21–29 (2018). https://doi.org/10.1007/978-3-319-92034-4_2

10. Hassenzahl, M.: Experience design: technology for all the right reasons. Synthesis Lectures Human-Centered Inform. **3**(1), 1–95 (2010). https://doi.org/10.2200/S00261ED1V01Y20100 3HCI008

11. Partala, T., Saari, T.: Understanding the most influential user experiences in successful and unsuccessful technology adoptions. Comput. Hum. Behav. **1**(53), 381–395 (2015). https:// doi.org/10.1016/j.chb.2015.07.012

12. Agarwal, A., Meyer, A.: Beyond usability: evaluating emotional response as an integral part of the user experience. In: CHI '09 Extended Abstracts on Human Factors in Computing Systems, pp. 2919–2930. ACM, Boston (2009). https://doi.org/10.1145/1520340.1520420

13. Saariluoma, P., Jokinen, J.P.P.: Emotional dimensions of user experience: a user psychological analysis. Int. J. Hum.–Comput. Interact. **30**(4), 303–320 (2014). https://doi.org/10.1080/104 47318.2013.858460

14. Kujala, S., Miron-Shatz, T.: Emotions, experiences and usability in real-life mobile phone use. In: Proceedings of the SIGCHI Conference on Human Factors in Computing Systems, pp. 1061–1070. Association for Computing Machinery, New York (2013). https://doi.org/10. 1145/2470654.2466135

15. Czaja, S.J., Boot, W.R., Charness, N., Rogers, W.A.: Designing for Older Adults: Principles and Creative Human Factors Approaches, 3rd edn. CRC Press (2019). ISBN:978-1-351-68225-1

16. Saariluoma, P.: User psychology of emotional interaction—usability, user experience and technology ethics. In: Rousi, R., Leikas, J., Saariluoma, P., (eds.) Emotions in Technology Design: From Experience to Ethics, pp. 15–26. Springer, Cham (2020). https://doi.org/10. 1007/978-3-030-53483-7_2

17. Jokinen, J.P.P.: Emotional user experience: Traits, events, and states☆. Int. J. Hum. Comput. Stud.Comput. Stud. **1**(76), 67–77 (2015). https://doi.org/10.1016/j.ijhcs.2014.12.006

18. Aula, A.: User study on older adults' use of the Web and search engines. Univ. Access Inf. Soc. **4**(1), 67–81 (2005). https://doi.org/10.1007/s10209-004-0097-7

19. Bhattacharjee, P., Baker, S., Waycott, J.: Older adults and their acquisition of digital skills: a review of current research evidence. In: 32nd Australian Conference on Human-Computer Interaction, pp. 437–443. Association for Computing Machinery, New York (2020). https:// doi.org/10.1145/3441000.3441053

20. Chen, K.: Why do older people love and hate assistive technology? – an emotional experience perspective. Ergonomics **63**(12), 1463–1474 (2020). PMID:32780683 https://doi.org/ 10.1080/00140139.2020.1808714

21. Ware, P., Bartlett, S.J., Paré, G., Symeonidis, I., Tannenbaum, C., Bartlett, G., Poissant, L., Ahmed, S.: Using eHealth technologies: interests, preferences, and concerns of older adults. Interactive J. Med. Res. **6**(1), e3 (2017). https://doi.org/10.2196/ijmr.4447

22. Eriksson-Backa, K., Hirvonen, N., Enwald, H., Huvila, I.: Enablers for and barriers to using My Kanta – A focus group study of older adults' perceptions of the National Electronic Health Record in Finland. Inform. Health Soc. Care **31**, 1–13 (2021). https://doi.org/10.1080/17538157.2021.1902331

23. Bobeth, J., Deutsch, S., Schmehl, S., Tscheligi, M.: Facing the user heterogeneity when designing touch interfaces for older adults: a representative personas approach. In: NordiCHI 2012 Proceedings. 14, pp. 1–4, October 2012

24. Desmet, P.M.A., Pohlmeyer, A.E.: An introduction to design for subjective well-being. Int. J. Des. **7**(3), 15 (2013)

25. Peters, D., Calvo, R.A., Ryan, R.M.: Designing for motivation, engagement and wellbeing in digital experience. Front. Psychol. (2018). https://doi.org/10.3389/fpsyg.2018.00797

26. Calvo, R.A., Peters, D.: Positive Computing: Technology for Wellbeing and Human Potential. MIT Press (2014). ISBN:978-0-262-32569-1

27. Calvo, R.A., Peters, D.: Positive computing: technology for a wiser world. Interactions **19**(4), 28–31 (2012). https://doi.org/10.1145/2212877.2212886

28. Peters, D., Ahmadpour, N., Calvo, R.A.: Tools for wellbeing-supportive design: features, characteristics, and prototypes. MTI **4**(3), 40 (2020). https://doi.org/10.3390/mti4030040

29. Doyle, J., Murphy, E., Kuiper, J., Smith, S., Hannigan, C., Jacobs, A., Dinsmore, J.: Managing Multimorbidity: Identifying Design Requirements for a Digital Self-Management Tool to Support Older Adults with Multiple Chronic Conditions, pp. 1–14 (2019). https://doi.org/10.1145/3290605.3300629

30. Corbin, J., Strauss, A.: Basics of Qualitative Research: Techniques and Procedures for Developing Grounded Theory. SAGE Publications (2014). ISBN:978-1-4833-1568-3

31. Boyatzis, R.E.: Transforming Qualitative Information: Thematic Analysis and Code Development. SAGE (1998). ISBN:978-0-7619-0961-3

32. Calvo, R.A., Vella-Brodrick, D., Desmet, P., M. Ryan R.: Editorial for "Positive Computing: A New Partnership Between Psychology, Social Sciences and Technologists." Psychol. Well-Being **6**(1), 10 (2016). https://doi.org/10.1186/s13612-016-0047-1

33. Valkonen, P., Kujala, S., Hörhammer, I., Savolainen, K., Helminen, R.-R., Vartia, I.: Health self-management of older employees: identifying critical peak experiences of a patient portal. FinJeHeW **15**(2) (2023). https://doi.org/10.23996/fjhw.126837

34. Nielsen, J.: Usability Engineering. Elsevier (1993). https://doi.org/10.1016/C2009-0-215 12-1. ISBN: 978-0-12-518406-9

35. Van Velsen, L., Wentzel, J., Van Gemert-Pijnen, J.E.: Designing eHealth that matters via a multidisciplinary requirements development approach. JMIR Res. Protoc. **2**(1), e2547 (2013). https://doi.org/10.2196/resprot.2547

36. Ekstedt, M., Kirsebom, M., Lindqvist, G., Kneck, Å., Frykholm, O., Flink, M., Wannheden, C.: Design and development of an ehealth service for collaborative self-management among older adults with chronic diseases: a theory-driven user-centered approach. Int. J. Environ. Res. Public Health Multidisciplinary Digital Publishing Institute **19**(1), 391 (2022). https://doi.org/10.3390/ijerph19010391

37. Nielsen, J.: Designing Web usability. Indianapolis, Ind: New Riders (2000). ISBN:978-1-56205-810-4

38. Zaphiris, P., Kurniawan, S.H., Ellis, R.D.: Age related differences and the depth vs. breadth tradeoff in hierarchical online information systems. In: Carbonell, N., Stephanidis, C., (eds.) Universal Access Theoretical Perspectives, Practice, and Experience, pp. 23–42. Springer, Heidelberg (2003). https://doi.org/10.1007/3-540-36572-9_2

39. Chun, Y.J., Patterson, P.E.: A usability gap between older adults and younger adults on interface design of an Internet-based telemedicine system. Work IOS Press; **41**(Suppl. 1), 349–352 (2012). https://doi.org/10.3233/WOR-2012-0180-349

40. Morrison, B., Coventry, L., Briggs, P.: How do older adults feel about engaging with cyber-security? Hum. Behav. Emerg. Technol. **3**(5), 1033–1049 (2021). https://doi.org/10.1002/hbe2.291
41. Scheerens, C., et al.: Developing eHealth tools for diverse older adults: lessons learned from the PREPARE for Your Care Program. J. Am. Geriatr. Soc.Geriatr. Soc. **69**(10), 2939–2949 (2021). https://doi.org/10.1111/jgs.17284
42. Hechinger, M., Hentschel, D., Aumer, C., Rester, C.: A conceptual model of experiences with digital technologies in aging in place: qualitative systematic review and meta-synthesis. JMIR Aging **5**(3), e34872 (2022). https://doi.org/10.2196/34872
43. Cutler, S.J.: Ageism and technology. Generations: J. Am. Soc. Aging **29**(3), 67–72 (2005)
44. Xie, B., Zhou, J.: The influence of mental model similarity on user performance: comparing older and younger adults. In: Zhou, J., Salvendy, G. (eds.) Human Aspects of IT for the Aged Population Applications, Services and Contexts, pp. 569–579. Springer, Cham (2017). https://doi.org/10.1007/978-3-319-58536-9_45

The Adoption of MyData-Based Health Applications Among Elderly Citizens in Nordic Countries and the UK

Chathurangani Jayathilake[1]([⊠]) [iD], Pantea Keikhosrokiani[2,3] [iD],
and Minna Isomursu[2,3] [iD]

[1] Martti Ahtisaari Institute, Oulu Business School, University of Oulu, Oulu, Finland
`chathurangani.weerasekaramudiyanselage@oulu.fi`
[2] Faculty of Information Technology and Electrical Engineering, University of Oulu, Oulu, Finland
[3] Faculty of Medicine, University of Oulu, Oulu, Finland

Abstract. This study addresses a crucial gap in current literature by examining the use of MyData-based health apps among individuals aged 50 and above in the UK and Nordic nations. With the advancement of personalized health technologies, understanding the factors influencing adoption among the elderly is essential. The research provides insights tailored to this demographic within the broader framework of digital health adoption. The primary scientific objective was to identify technological and health-related factors influencing the willingness of senior adults (50 and above) to use MyData-based preventive healthcare applications. The conditions for adoption, technological considerations, health-related variables, willingness to share MyData, and demographic variations were explored. Grounded in the Universal Theory of Acceptance and Use of Technology (UTAUT2) and Health Protection Motivation components, the research employed a quantitative approach, integrating a new concept called sharing personal data into the framework. Data collection occurred through an online survey in the UK and the Nordic region, yielding 374 responses from the Nordic sample and 1165 from the UK sample, resulting in a cleaned dataset of 1016. Findings revealed the significance of willingness to share MyData for both the UK and Nordic regions, with performance expectancy emerging as an outstanding technological factor for the Nordic population, but not for the UK. Across nations and genders, self-efficacy is portrayed as a strong driver in health-related aspects. These contribute to academic knowledge and have societal value by guiding the development of digital health solutions for the elderly, ultimately improving their quality of life and health outcomes.

Keywords: Mydata · Health Protection Motivation · UTAUT2

M. Särestöniemi et al. (Eds.): NCDHWS 2024, CCIS 2083, pp. 147–165, 2024.
https://doi.org/10.1007/978-3-031-59080-1_11

1 Introduction

1.1 Overview

The pervasive integration of technology in our daily lives has transformed healthcare solutions, drawing significant attention to medical issues. The If Nordic Health Report 2023 [28] highlights prevalent health concerns, yet a considerable percentage (26%) of those experiencing health issues do not seek help. Confidence in the public healthcare system is relatively low, with only 45% expressing trust. The State of Health and Care of Older People, 2023 (abridged) [29] reveals high rates of long-term health conditions among individuals over 85 in England, demanding a revival of healthcare systems due to these failures.

The adoption of technology in healthcare, particularly mobile health apps, has expanded the reach of patient treatment beyond traditional one-on-one interactions. However, the aging population and healthcare capacity constraints underscore the need for preventive health applications. These apps collect personal data of individuals. The MyData approach suggests a human-centric personal data model, empowering individuals with their data, transitioning from mere protection to enabling individuals to utilize their data for their benefit [19]. Additionally, it calls for open ecosystems, challenging the dominance of large platforms and promoting individual control over data flow [27]. The MyData principles include human-centric control, individual integration, empowerment, portability, transparency, and interoperability [27]. The study innovatively incorporates the willingness to share personal data, identified as a significant factor to represent MyData approach, into traditional UTAUT2 constructs, adding a novel dimension. Additionally, the study addresses gaps by exploring the role of MyData in preventive healthcare, an aspect often overlooked in previous studies.

Prior research has primarily focused on specific geographic regions, prompting this study to conduct a comparative analysis between two areas. Notably, there is a scarcity of studies targeting the elderly population, with fewer quantitative studies exploring the consumer perspective.

While existing studies on MyData-based healthcare services predominantly originate from China and the USA, emphasizing a government-centered data policy, European countries follow the GDPR, making the MyData concept more applicable. Despite a limited number of studies on consumer adoption in EU countries, this study contributes valuable insights to the literature from a European perspective.

1.2 Related Work

Following thorough literature research, eight key ideas explaining the adoption of a technology were found. These are: Technology acceptance model (TAM), Theory of reasoned action (TRA), Theory of planned behavior (TPB), Motivational model, Combined TAM and TPB, Model of personal computer use, Diffusion of innovations theory and Social cognitive theory [26]. Every theory has a distinct origin and diverse variables that measure in different contexts.

Recently, all eight of the aforementioned theories were combined to create the Universal Theory of Acceptance and Use of Technology (UTAUT), which was established by [24]. They discovered that the UTAUT performed better than the eight separate models, and it is thought to be the most comprehensive acceptance model.

Nevertheless, diverse frameworks have been employed in numerous studies examining the acceptance of healthcare technology applications by consumers. Specifically, [17] and [4] exclusively delve into MyData-based healthcare applications, employing the UTAUT2 model due to its contemporary and superior performance in technology adoption studies. However, [17], in addition to UTAUT2, incorporates three constructs from health behavior theories, rendering it more specialized and tailored to the consumer perspective within the healthcare services sector. Consequently, this research draws substantial inspiration from [17], as it seamlessly integrates both technical and healthcare domains.

1.3 Theoretical Framework

The conceptual framework for this study is a modification of Koivumäki et al. [17] which integrates UTAUT2 and health protection motivation constructs. Figure 1 shows the proposed conceptual framework for this study.

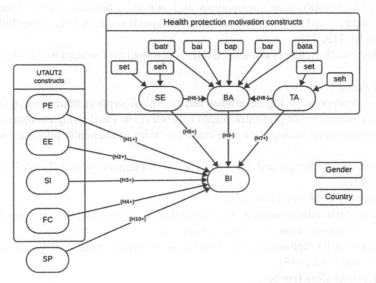

Fig. 1. The Proposed Conceptual Framework for this Study.

Utaut2

The traditional constructs of Performance Expectancy (PE), Effort Expectancy (EE), Social Influence (SI), Facilitating Conditions (FC) of UTAUT2, along new construct, willingness to share personal data has been introduced based on findings of [25].

Performance Expectancy (PE).

Anticipated benefits of using technology in preventive eHealth services play a crucial role in influencing behavioral intention, as individuals expect assistance in avoiding illnesses through technological applications [11]. Numerous studies focusing on the acceptance of information technology and preventive eHealth have consistently identified performance expectancy as the most influential factor influencing behavioral intention [24].

• Hypothesis 1: Behavioral Intention (BI) is positively influenced by Performance Expectancy (PE).

Effort Expectancy (EE).

The perceived ease of usage, known as effort expectancy, significantly influences the acceptance of preventive eHealth services, particularly among older consumers [22]. Individuals are more likely to embrace a new system if its adoption is perceived as straightforward [23]. Difficulties encountered in utilizing preventive eHealth technology are frequently associated with users' lack of familiarity with the internet in a broader context [13, 14]. The perception of a technology's ease of use is positively correlated with the intention to use that particular technology [24].

•Hypothesis 2: Behavioral intention (BI) is positively influenced by Effort expectancy (EE).

Social Influence (SI)

Various social circles, including friends, family, and healthcare professionals, significantly shape individuals' perceptions and attitudes. Social influence, manifested through guidance and motivation, is identified as a positive factor influencing Behavioral Intention (BI) [18, 24].

•Hypothesis 3: Behavioral intention (BI) is positively influenced by Social influence (SI).

Facilitating Conditions

Users' perception of organizational and technical support structures significantly impacts the utilization of preventive healthcare services. Facilitating conditions impact both the intention to use and the actual usage behavior of the health information system [1, 24].

•Hypothesis 4: Behavioral intention (BI) is influenced positively by Facilitating Conditions (FC).

Willingness to Share Personal Data

Upon understanding potential benefits and risks, many users express readiness to share data, with or without de-identification [25].

•Hypothesis 10: Behavioral intention (BI) is positively influenced by willingness to sharing Personal data (SP).

Health Related Constructs

The study incorporates three theories—Health Belief Model (HBM), Protection Motivation Theory (PMT), and Social Cognitive Theory (SCT) —to explore preventive eHealth.

The HBM looks at what makes people decide to do or not do health-related activities, emphasizing the idea that doing these activities can stop diseases. Perceived barriers, perceived benefits, severity, and vulnerability, with an added self-efficacy component from SCT forms the HBM. PMT was formulated to understand the impact of fears about health affect thoughts and actions, proposing that thinking about dangers and how well someone can handle them leads to the decision to adopt healthy behaviors. PMT considers factors like severity, vulnerability, response cost, response efficacy, and self-efficacy. SCT examines the intention to engage in health-protective activities, emphasizing self-efficacy and providing guidance for behavioral change [17].

Self-efficacy

Self-efficacy is the belief in effectively achieving positive outcomes which aligns with the Theory of Planned Behavior. It encourages ambitious goals, fosters learning, and positively influences the acceptance of preventive eHealth services. In adopting healthier habits through eHealth services, self-efficacy plays a crucial role, increasing the likelihood of success and the belief in improved health outcomes [21].

•Hypothesis 5: Behavioral intention (BI) is positively influenced by Self-efficacy (SE).

High self-efficacy plays a crucial role in overcoming cognitive barriers, as confident individuals see challenges as manageable and persist in pursuing goals [2]. In the context of protection motivation theory, individuals' choices for preventive health actions are influenced by evaluating benefits and threats, with high self-efficacy reducing perceived barriers and increasing commitment to goals [8].

•Hypothesis 6: Perceived barriers (BA) are negatively influenced by Self-efficacy (SE).

Threat appraisals

Individuals who perceive a higher threat are more motivated to adopt healthy behaviors, expecting stronger intentions to engage in preventive health actions and encountering fewer obstacles in using eHealth services [12]. This holds true even for those with higher healthcare needs, although they may pay less attention to risks. Furthermore, individuals with heightened threat perceptions find preventive eHealth services more useful, particularly if they perceive high health threats [15].

•Hypothesis 7: Behavioral intention (BI) is positively influenced by Threat appraisals (TA).

•Hypothesis 8: Perceived barriers (BA) is negatively influenced by Threat appraisals (TA).

Perceived Barriers

Concerns regarding information and technology risks, lifestyle changes, and technological anxiety among elderly users contribute to cognitive barriers against adopting preventive eHealth services [9]. These barriers include fears of information misuse, invasion of privacy, equipment imprecision, and high costs [6, 12, 22]. According to the Health Belief Model, perceived barriers strongly affect the intention to adopt health-protective actions. Consequently, individuals facing obstacles in using preventive eHealth technologies, including MyData-based services, are likely to have minimal intention to engage in health behavior.

•Hypothesis 9: Behavioral intention (BI) is negatively influenced by Perceived barriers (BA).

2   Methods

2.1   Research Approach

The study aimed to understand the factors influencing elderly citizens (aged 50 and above) in adopting MyData-based preventive health applications. Data was collected through a quantitative, web-based survey accessible via mobile devices, following similar approaches used in previous studies [16, 17]. Quantitative research, known for its numerical data and statistical analysis, was chosen as it addresses questions about who, what, when, where, and how many elements are being examined [7]. This method, favored by businesses for decision-making, aligns with the study's focus on the customer perspective.

The survey underwent verification and refinement with collaboration from Professor Timo Koivumäki from Oulu Business School and Aki Kuivalainen from Predicell. Initially prepared in English, it was later translated into Finnish and Swedish. Google Forms facilitated data collection due to its accessibility and user-friendly nature. Purposive sampling targeted citizens aged 50 and above in specific Nordic and UK regions. Various channels, including LinkedIn, Facebook, Twitter, and university of Oulu staff emails, were utilized for distribution. Motivational incentives included Amazon gift cards for raffle winners. Privacy measures ensured complete anonymity, explaining the purpose of data collection and obtaining consent from participants, separate collection of email addresses for the raffle, storing data for a maximum of a year and compliance with GDPR. The survey covered three sections: demographic information with age gender and level of education, a five-point Likert scale questions section with 1 for Strongly disagree and 5 for Strongly agree, and a conclusion with the raffle draw link. The UK demographic section differed slightly, collecting only age and gender.

2.2 Data Collection and Analysis

The UK survey received 1165 responses over one week, with the first 352 lacking demographic details initially. The Nordic survey spanned four months, accumulating 374 responses—330 English, 40 Finnish, and 4 Swedish. After closing the surveys, data was downloaded and underwent initial cleaning in Excel, including dropping unnecessary columns and renaming headers. Further preprocessing in Python involved filtering out respondents below 50, discarding entries lacking age and gender in the UK dataset, converting gender and country columns to numeric format, and merging the datasets into one with 1016 records. The highest number of responses for the Nordic survey was collected from e-mail followed by Twitter, Facebook and LinkedIn. In the UK survey, Facebook and Reddit were the primary sources of responses.

Initially, a sample analysis was conducted to identify the gender distribution in each market and overall. Subsequently, the distribution of responses by country was examined. Structural Equation Modeling (SEM), based on maximum likelihood estimation, was applied to analyze the conceptual framework of the research, following the approach of [17] and [4] using SPSS AMOS 28. While the overall SEM for the conceptual framework exhibited a good fit, none of the latent variables showed a significant relationship with the dependent variable 'behavioral intention.' Consequently, separate SEM analyses were conducted for UTAUT2, and health behavior constructs to explore their impact on behavioral intention. Multi-group analysis was performed to assess the influence of country and gender on behavioral intention.

The data analysis involved three steps:

1. Assessment of model fit:
   • Root Mean Square Error of Approximation (RMSEA): A low RMSEA value indicates a good fit, with a value below 0.8 considered reasonable [3].

- Tucker-Lewis Index (TLI) and Comparative Fit Index (CFI): Values close to 0.95 for both TLI and CFI are indicative of a good fit [10].

2. Confirmatory Factor Analysis:

This step examined the association of factors with latent variables, considering a confidence interval of 95%. P values below 0.05 were identified as significant, and insignificant relationships were omitted, repeating the analysis until all second-order constructs were significant.

3. Hypothesis Validation using SEM:

SEM was conducted, and correlations between latent variables with behavioral intention were accepted if the p value was less than 0.05, considering a 95% confidence interval and a significance level of 0.05.

3   Results

3.1   Sample Characteristics

Figure 2 displays the breakdown of responses from the UK and Nordic countries. The majority of the data, constituting 72.5%, has been gathered from the UK, while the remaining 27.5% represents data collected from the Nordic population. Figure 3 illustrates the percentage distribution of gender in the overall dataset. The sample is predominantly composed of males (61.4%), followed by females (38.4%), with the remaining 0.2% representing others or individuals who chose not to specify their gender.

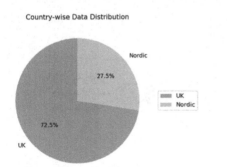
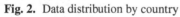
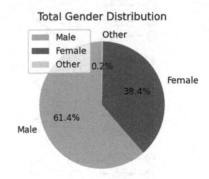

Fig. 2. Data distribution by country   **Fig. 3.** Data distribution by gender

Figure 4 displays the gender breakdown in the UK, with the majority consisting of 60.2% males, 39.6% females, and 0.1% falling into the other/not disclosed category. This distribution mirrors that of the total dataset and the Nordic populations. Figure 5 illustrates the gender distribution in the Nordic population, highlighting male dominance at 64.5%, females constituting 35.1%, and the others/not disclosed category making up 0.4%.

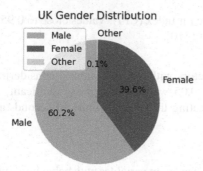

Fig. 4. Data distribution by gender in UK sample

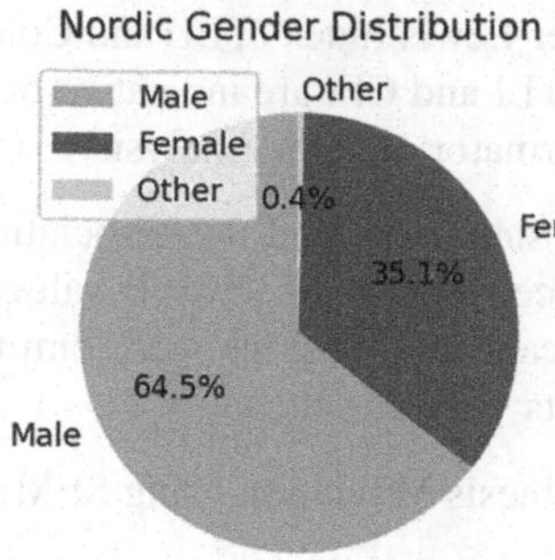

Fig. 5. Data distribution by gender in Nordic sample

3.2 Data Analysis Using SEM

Figure 6 presents the path diagram illustrating the UTAUT2 constructs drawn using SPSS AMOS 28. The latent variables include Performance Expectancy (PE), Effort Expectancy (EE), Social Influence (SI), Facilitating Conditions (FC) from UTAUT2, and sharing personal data (SP). Each latent variable consists of second-order factors, such as PE1, PE2, PE3, and PE4 for performance expectancy, and so forth. The Behavioral Intention (BI) serves as the dependent variable and has three second-order factors. The curved double-headed arrows indicate the correlations between the latent variables.

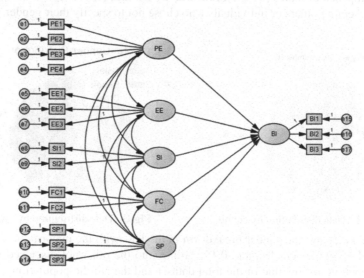

Fig. 6. Path diagram for UTAUT2

SEM was conducted for the path diagram of health protection motivation constructs through a multi-group analysis for the UK group and Nordic group, considering both males and females. The model fit indices are detailed in Table 1. According to Table 6, the UTAUT2 model demonstrates a good fit for the UK sample, meeting the baseline comparison values, including an RMSEA below 0.8, a TLI nearly equal to 0.95, and a CFI equal to 0.95. In all the scenarios when applying UTAUT2 irrespective of country and gender, the second order factors showed significant positive relationship to the corresponding latent variable further validating the model.

Table 1. UTAUT2 model fit indices

Fit Index	Value	Baseline comparison
RMSEA	0.029	< 0.8
TLI	0.936	$\cong 0.95$
CFI	0.95	$= 0.95$

The regression table (Table 2) for the UK group, utilizing maximum likelihood (ML) estimation, highlights the strength of the relationship, sign indicates the direction, Standard Error (S.E.), Critical Ratio (C.R.), and p-value of relationships between latent variables (PE, EE, SI, FC, and SP). Except SP other latent variables (PE, EE, SI, and FC) do not significantly impact behavioral intention.

Table 2. ML estimations for UK group using UTAUT2

Hypothesis	Estimate	S.E	C.R	P
BI <--- PE	0.797	0.51	1.562	0.118
BI <--- EE	-1.227	1.35	-0.909	0.363
BI <--- SI	-0.031	1.018	-0.031	0.976
BI <--- FC	-0.343	0.965	-0.355	0.722
BI <--- SP	1.708	0.756	2.26	0.024

Table 3 demonstrates significant positive associations among latent variables (PE, EE, SI, FC, and SP), indicating a robust interplay between these constructs.

Contrastingly, in the Nordic population (Table 4), performance expectancy (PE), willingness to share personal data (SP), and effort expectancy (EE) significantly influence behavioral intention. However, effort expectancy is negatively correlated with behavioral intention.

Table 5 confirms that all latent variables positively and significantly impact each other, emphasizing strong interrelations among the model's constructs.

For the entire male population (Table 6), the latent variables do not significantly influence behavioral intention.

Covariances in Table 7 reveal significant correlations among latent variables associated with PE, EE, SI, FC, and SP, indicating positive relationships.

Table 3. Covariances for UK group using UTAUT2

	Estimate	S.E	C.R	P
PE <-- > EE	0.414	0.033	12.354	***
PE <-- > FC	0.357	0.03	11.804	***
PE <-- > SP	0.347	0.03	11.373	***
PE <-- > SI	0.39	0.032	12.117	***
EE <-- > FC	0.356	0.031	11.656	***
EE <-- > SP	0.333	0.03	11.102	***
EE <-- > SI	0.364	0.031	11.61	***
FC <-- > SP	0.318	0.029	11.033	***
FC <-- > SI	0.352	0.03	11.65	***
SP <-- > SI	0.322	0.029	10.94	***

Table 4. ML estimations for Nordic group using UTAUT2

	Estimate	S.E	C.R	P
BI <--- PE	1.514	0.449	3.374	***
BI <--- EE	-1.591	0.46	-3.456	***
BI <--- SI	0.032	0.34	0.093	0.926
BI <--- FC	0.104	0.166	0.627	0.53
BI <--- SP	0.734	0.28	2.622	0.009
BI2 <--- BI	0.834	0.075	11.056	***

Table 8 illustrates that among females, latent variables PE, EE, SI, and FC do not significantly impact behavioral intention. Still, SP is significant. Table 9 highlights positive associations between latent constructs, with statistically significant estimates, suggesting robust relationships among these constructs.

Figure 7 depicts the path diagram for the health protection motivation constructs model, featuring latent variables like Self-Efficacy (SE), Threat Appraisals (TA), and Perceived Barriers (BA), each with its set of second-order factors. Behavioral Intention (BI) serves as the dependent variable, connected to three second-order factors. Curved double-headed arrows denote correlations between the latent variables.

Structural Equation Modeling (SEM) was employed for the health protection motivation constructs path diagram using multi-group analysis, considering the UK group, Nordic group, males, and females. The model fit indices in Table 10 indicate a well-aligned health model with the UK sample, meeting baseline comparison values with RMSEA below 0.8, TLI nearly equal to 0.95, and CFI nearly equal to 0.95. Except for the Nordic group, in all other groups, all second-order factors (set, seh, tav, tas, bai, bap,

Table 5. Covariances for Nordic using UTAUT2

	Estimate	S.E	C.R	P
PE <--> EE	0.462	0.054	8.476	***
PE <--> FC	0.315	0.046	6.902	***
PE <--> SP	0.462	0.058	8.02	***
PE <--> SI	0.382	0.054	7.099	***
EE <--> FC	0.312	0.046	6.837	***
EE <--> SP	0.448	0.058	7.76	***
EE <--> SI	0.332	0.05	6.619	***
FC <--> SP	0.336	0.052	6.486	***
FC <--> SI	0.23	0.043	5.377	***
SP <--> SI	0.297	0.051	5.784	***

Table 6. ML estimation for males using UTAUT2

	Estimate	S.E	C.R	P
BI <--- PE	-4.609	9.258	-0.498	0.619
BI <--- EE	-0.461	2.104	-0.219	0.827
BI <--- SI	7.847	14.089	0.557	0.578
BI <--- FC	-7.26	13.416	-0.541	0.588
BI <--- SP	5.669	8.217	0.69	0.49

bar, bata, batr) had a significant positive effect on their respective latent variables SE, TA, and BA.

In the UK population, Table 11 indicates that self-efficacy significantly influences behavioral intention, while threat appraisals and perceived barriers do not. Table 12 reports the covariances for UK using health model. For the Nordic group, an initial insignificant p-value for seh3 led to its removal, and in subsequent iterations, seh1 was also eliminated. The revised SEM analysis in Table 13 reveals that only self-efficacy significantly affects behavioral intention. TA and BA are not significant, with all second-order factors (post removal of seh3 and seh2) significantly influencing latent variables.

Table 14 highlights that threat appraisals significantly influence perceived barriers, while self-efficacy does not significantly impact threat appraisals or perceived barriers. In the male population (Table 15), all latent variables significantly impact behavioral intention, contrary to country-wise analyses. Notably, threat appraisals negatively affect behavioral intention. Table 16 indicates that perceived barriers significantly affect threat appraisals, while self-efficacy has no significant influence on either threat appraisals or perceived barriers. For females (Table 17), self-efficacy significantly affects behavioral intention, while TA and BA do not.

Table 7. Covariances table for males using UTAUT2

	Estimate	S.E	C.R	P
PE <--> EE	0.468	0.038	12.429	***
PE <--> FC	0.357	0.033	10.976	***
PE <--> SP	0.403	0.035	11.521	***
PE <--> SI	0.44	0.037	11.951	***
EE <--> FC	0.338	0.032	10.539	***
EE <--> SP	0.371	0.034	10.902	***
EE <--> SI	0.387	0.035	11.053	***
FC <--> SP	0.307	0.03	10.088	***
FC <--> SI	0.326	0.031	10.367	***
SP <--> SI	0.31	0.031	9.905	***

Table 8. ML estimations for females using UTAUT2

	Estimate	S.E	C.R	P
BI <--- PE	0.081	0.407	0.199	0.842
BI <--- EE	0.467	0.539	0.865	0.387
BI <--- SI	0.245	0.351	0.699	0.484
BI <--- FC	-0.472	0.32	-1.478	0.14
BI <--- SP	0.614	0.243	2.521	0.012

Table 18 confirms significant positive associations among all latent variables in the female population, with a negative association between SE and TA and also SE and BA.

3.3 Summary of Findings

The summary of the hypothesis validation under each group analysis is shown in Table 19. The Nordic population significantly embraces MyData-based healthcare applications when they perceive performance expectancy benefits in preventing illnesses, supporting the acceptance of H1. This contradicts [17], where performance expectancy was deemed non-significant, but aligns with [4], emphasizing its significance. Effort expectancy negatively affects behavioral intention in the Nordic population, implying an increased intention to use the application with higher perceived effort, though this seems logically implausible. This discrepancy leads to the rejection of H2, contrary to [17]. Social influence does not significantly impact behavioral intention in the Nordic population, contradicting H3 and aligning with [4] and [20]. Facilitating Conditions do not significantly influence behavioral intention in the Nordic population, leading to the rejection of H4, consistent with [17]. Self-efficacy positively influences behavioral intention in the overall UK population, Nordic population, and across genders, supporting H5. This

Table 9. Covariances table for females using UTAUT2

	Estimate	S.E	C.R	P
PE <--> EE	0.399	0.047	8.568	***
PE <--> FC	0.31	0.04	7.799	***
PE <--> SP	0.354	0.045	7.943	***
PE <--> SI	0.313	0.041	7.628	***
EE <--> FC	0.356	0.043	8.309	***
EE <--> SP	0.357	0.045	7.893	***
EE <--> SI	0.324	0.042	7.661	***
FC <--> SP	0.331	0.043	7.7	***
FC <--> SI	0.297	0.04	7.411	***
SP <--> SI	0.337	0.045	7.563	***

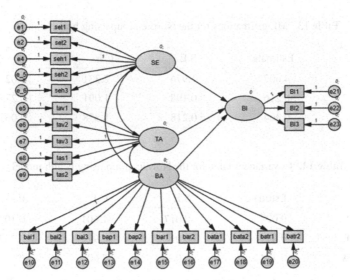

Fig. 7. Health model path diagram

Table 10. Health model fit indices

Fit Index	Value	Baseline comparison
RMSEA	0.039	< 0.8
TLI	0.823	≅ 0.95
CFI	0.841	≅ 0.95

Table 11. ML estimations for UK using health model

	Estimate	S.E	C.R	P
BI <--- SE	1.545	0.178	8.666	***
BI <--- TA	-0.074	0.085	-0.864	0.387
BI <--- BA	0.102	0.077	1.332	0.183

Table 12. Covariances table for UK using health model

	Estimate	S.E	C.R	P
SE < -- > TA	-0.04	0.012	-3.232	0.001
BA < -- > SE	-0.027	0.012	-2.346	0.019
BA < -- > TA	0.373	0.034	11.095	***

Table 13. ML estimations for the Nordic group using health model

	Estimate	S.E	C.R	P
BI <--- SE	4.607	1.976	2.331	0.02
BI <--- TA	-0.216	0.198	-1.091	0.275
BI <--- BA	0.404	0.218	1.858	0.063

Table 14. Covariances table for the Nordic group using health model

	Estimate	S.E	C.R	P
SE <--> TA	0.028	0.017	1.601	0.109
BA <--> SE	0.012	0.012	0.97	0.332
BA <--> TA	0.474	0.062	7.609	***

Table 15. ML estimations for males using health model

	Estimate	S.E	C.R	P
BI <--- SE	2.585	0.47	5.504	***
BI <--- TA	-0.285	0.112	-2.551	0.011
BI <--- BA	0.373	0.102	3.655	***

Table 16. Covariances table for males using health model

	Estimate	S.E	C.R	P
SE <--> TA	0.011	0.008	1.253	0.21
BA <--> SE	0.003	0.008	0.321	0.748
BA <--> TA	0.345	0.033	10.42	***

Table 17. ML estimations for females using health model

	Estimate	S.E	C.R	P
BI <--- SE	1.369	0.191	7.188	***
BI <--- TA	0.064	0.133	0.478	0.633
BI <--- BA	0.037	0.139	0.269	0.788

Table 18. Covariance table for females using health model

	Estimate	S.E	C.R	P
SE <--> TA	−0.093	0.029	−3.235	0.001
BA <--> SE	−0.092	0.026	−3.489	***
BA <--> TA	0.539	0.061	8.784	***

concurs with [17] and [16]. Self-efficacy negatively influences perceived barriers among females and in the UK, corroborating H6 and aligning with [17]. In the male population, threat appraisals negatively impact behavioral intention, contrary to H7 and differing from [17].

Across all groups, threat appraisals positively influence perceived barriers, rejecting H8 and aligning with [17], suggesting that higher perceived threat correlates with more perceived barriers. Perceived barriers positively influence behavioral intention in the male population, rejecting H9 and presenting a contradictory outcome to [17]. The newly introduced construct, willingness to share personal data, significantly influences behavioral intention in the UK, Nordic, and female groups, supporting H10. However, it does not significantly influence behavioral intention in males.

4   Discussion

4.1   Managerial Implications

Given that performance expectancy lacks significance in the UK, marketing efforts should shift focus towards other aspects, particularly highlighting the privacy and security features of MyData applications. Healthcare providers should underscore the personal health outcomes of MyData applications rather than focusing on general illness

Table 19. Hypothesis testing results

Hypothesis	Group Name			
	UK	Nordic	Male	Female
H1: BI is positively influenced by PE	Rejected	Accepted	Rejected	Rejected
H2: BI is positively influenced by EE	Rejected	Rejected	Rejected	Rejected
H3: BI is positively influenced by SI	Rejected	Rejected	Rejected	Rejected
H4: BI is positively influenced by FC	Rejected	Rejected	Rejected	Rejected
H5: BI is positively influenced by SE	Accepted	Accepted	Accepted	Accepted
H6: BA is negatively influenced by SE	Accepted	Rejected	Rejected	Accepted
H7: BI is positively influenced by TA	Rejected	Rejected	Rejected	Rejected
H8: BA is negatively influenced by TA	Rejected	Rejected	Rejected	Rejected
H9: BI is negatively influenced by BA	Rejected	Rejected	Rejected	Rejected
H10: BI is positively influenced by SP	Accepted	Accepted	Rejected	Accepted

prevention. The data privacy concerns in the UK should be acknowledged, necessitating the development of transparent policies and communication strategies to address these concerns. Service providers must emphasize the benefits and protective measures in place for personal data security.

The acknowledgment of performance expectancy influencing customer intention in the Nordic population underscores the importance of highlighting the advantages of eHealth services. Managers should continue promoting these perceived benefits to encourage adoption. Boosting the perceived benefits of the health application can increase the likelihood of user adoption. Strategies should concentrate on effectively communicating the advantages of the service to positively influence users' intention to use it. Additionally, service providers must leverage the willingness to share personal data in the Nordic population, developing strategies that highlight the advantages of data sharing for personalized healthcare services. Privacy policies and security measures must be clearly communicated.

The acceptance of self-efficacy across genders in both countries suggests a consistent positive influence. Managers should reinforce users' confidence in their ability to use eHealth services, with an emphasis on training or user-friendly interfaces. Sufficient training, guidance, and support are necessary to improve users' self-efficacy and boost their confidence in utilizing the application.

For females, the significant role of self-efficacy in overcoming perceived barriers implies the need for tailored interventions and support systems to boost confidence among female users. The negative influence of self-efficacy on perceived barriers among females suggests that efforts to enhance women's confidence in using the application can help reduce perceived obstacles. Managers should focus on providing support, training, and resources to boost self-efficacy among female users, ultimately contributing to a more positive perception and lower perceived barriers, promoting greater acceptance and use of the application.

Development of user-friendly interfaces and educational materials addressing the specific needs and concerns of the elderly is crucial. Investments in technology enhancing the perceived advantages of MyData applications and providing clear benefits to users could be considered. Regular assessments and updates based on evolving user perceptions and preferences must be conducted. Prioritizing user education and awareness campaigns is essential. A user-centric approach that actively seeks feedback and incorporates user insights into the development and marketing processes should be adopted.

4.2 Theoretical Implications

The study investigated the viability of incorporating the UTAUT2 model with health protection motivation constructs to evaluate consumer behavior intention in both Nordic and UK samples. The results suggest that, specifically within these demographics, the UTAUT2 model exhibits superior performance compared to health constructs when augmented with the new component of willingness to share data. Also, the majority of the latent variables had a significant impact on each other proving their interdependency and also the concreteness of the model. A noteworthy contribution is the customization of the UTAUT2 model, involving the exclusion of habit and hedonic motivation while incorporating willingness to share data. Unlike previous studies on MyData-related applications, where UTAUT2 included habit and hedonic motivation without addressing data sharing (as seen in [17]) or traditional UTAUT2 constructs (as in [4]), this research adopts a novel consumer-centric approach. This emphasis is significant considering the prevalent focus on medical journals in eHealth services research, highlighting the importance of interdisciplinary teams to support healthcare professionals, as highlighted by [5].

This theoretical foundation not only serves as a base of research for the healthcare service providers to tailor their MyData based preventive services according to the customer aspirations, but also could be customized by various stakeholders in the MyData based healthcare ecosystem such as physicians, investors, regulatory bodies and so on, according to their needs.

4.3 Limitations

While the study benefits from a substantial dataset of 1016 responses, providing reliable results, it is essential to acknowledge several limitations associated with the research. Firstly, participants were introduced to a hypothetical application, introducing a potential source of ambiguity in their responses as they did not have actual experience with the application. The study primarily focuses on behavioral intention, and the findings may not necessarily correspond to real-world application usage. Additionally, the majority of the total sample comprises respondents from the UK, posing a potential bias in the results. The Nordic sample is limited to Finland and Sweden only, lacking a comprehensive representation of all nations in the region. Furthermore, the respondent distribution is imbalanced, with a majority being Finnish, and there is an overall dominance of males in both regions. Achieving a more balanced gender distribution would have enhanced the study's generalizability.

4.4 Recommendations for Future Work

In future research endeavors, there is an opportunity to expand the model by examining participants' actual usage behavior through experimental studies. The scope of the sample selection could be widened to encompass representation from additional Nordic countries, promoting a more equitable distribution of responses. Investigating the impact of other moderating variables, such as the participants' level of education, on behavioral intention could offer valuable insights. Additionally, delving into variations in both actual behavior and behavioral intention among each Nordic country may uncover intriguing findings for further exploration. Moreover, future research efforts may benefit from exploring alternative methods for gathering data or integrating qualitative methodologies to gain deeper insights into participants' viewpoints and experiences.

References

1. Aggelidis, V.P., Chatzoglou, P.: Using a modified technology acceptance model in hospitals. Int. J. Medical Informatics. **78**, 2 (2009). https://doi.org/10.1016/j.ijmedinf.2008.06.006
2. Bandura, A.: Health promotion by social cognitive means. Health Educ. Behav.Behav. **31**(2), 143–164 (2004). https://doi.org/10.1177/1090198104263660
3. Browne, M.W., Cudeck, R.: Alternative ways of assessing model fit. Sociological Methods Res. **21**(2), 230–258 (1993). https://doi.org/10.1177/0049124192021002005
4. Choi, W., et al.: Study of the factors influencing the use of MyData platform based on personal health record data sharing system. BMC Med. Inform. Decis. Mak.Decis. Mak. **22**(1), 1–13 (2022). https://doi.org/10.1186/s12911-022-01929-z
5. Cobelli, N., Blasioli, E.: To be or not to be digital? a bibliometric analysis of adoption of eHealth services. The Tqm J. **35**(9), 299–331 (2023). https://doi.org/10.1108/tqm-02-2023-0065
6. Deng, Z.: Understanding public users' adoption of mobile health service. Int. J. Mob. Commun. **11**, 4, 351 (2013). https://doi.org/10.1504/ijmc.2013.055748
7. Ephraim Matanda: Research Methods and Statistics for Cross-Cutting Research. African Books Collective (2022)
8. Floyd, D.L., et al.: A meta-analysis of research on protection motivation theory. J. Appl. Soc. Psychol. **30**, 2, 407–429 (2000). https://doi.org/10.1111/j.1559-1816.2000.tb02323.x
9. Guo, X., et al.: Investigating m-health acceptance from a protection motivation theory perspective: gender and age differences. Telemed. e-Health. **21**(8), 661–669 (2015). https://doi.org/10.1089/tmj.2014.0166
10. Hu, L., Bentler, P.M.: Cutoff criteria for fit indexes in covariance structure analysis: conventional criteria versus new alternatives. Struct. Equ. ModelingEqu. Modeling **6**(1), 1–55 (1999). https://doi.org/10.1080/10705519909540118
11. Hung, M.-C., Jen, W.-Y.: The adoption of mobile health management services: an empirical study. J. Med. Syst. **36**(3), 1381–1388 (2010). https://doi.org/10.1007/s10916-010-9600-2
12. Janz, N.K., Becker, M.H.: The health belief model: a decade later. Health Educ. Q. **11**(1), 1–47 (1984). https://doi.org/10.1177/109019818401100101
13. Jung, M.-L., Berthon, P.: Fulfilling the promise: a model for delivering successful online health care. J. Med. Mark. **9**(3), 243–254 (2009). https://doi.org/10.1057/jmm.2009.26
14. Jung, M.-L., Loria, K.: Acceptance of Swedish e-health services. J. Multidiscip. Healthc.Multidiscip. Healthc. **3**, 55 (2010). https://doi.org/10.2147/jmdh.s9159

15. Kim, J., Park, H.-A.: Development of a health information technology acceptance model using consumers' health behavior intention. J. Med. Internet Res. **14**(5), e133 (2012). https://doi.org/10.2196/jmir.2143
16. Klossner, S.: AI powered m-health apps empowering smart city citizens to live a healthier life –The role of trust and privacy concerns. aaltodoc.aalto.fi. (2022)
17. Koivumäki, T., et al.: Consumer adoption of future mydata-based preventive ehealth services: an acceptance model and survey study. J. Med. Internet Res. **19**(12), e429 (2017). https://doi.org/10.2196/jmir.7821
18. Lin, S.P.: Determinants of adoption of Mobile Healthcare Service. Int. J. Mob. Commun. **9**(3), 298 (2011). https://doi.org/10.1504/ijmc.2011.040608
19. Poikola, A., et al.: MyData – an introduction to human-centric use of personal data (2020)
20. Sampa, M.B., et al.: Influence of factors on the adoption and use of ICT-based eHealth technology by urban corporate people. J. Serv. Sci. Manag.Manag. **13**(01), 1–19 (2020). https://doi.org/10.4236/jssm.2020.131001
21. Sun, Y., et al.: Understanding the acceptance of mobile health services: a comparison and integration of alternative models. J. Electron. Commer. Res.Commer. Res. **14**, 2 (2013)
22. Tang, P.C., et al.: Personal health records: definitions, benefits, and strategies for overcoming barriers to adoption. J. Am. Med. Inform. Assoc. **13**(2), 121–126 (2006). https://doi.org/10.1197/jamia.m2025
23. Tarhini, A., et al.: Extending the UTAUT model to understand the customers' acceptance and use of internet banking in Lebanon. Inf. Technol. People **29**(4), 830–849 (2016). https://doi.org/10.1108/itp-02-2014-0034
24. Venkatesh, V., et al.: User acceptance of information technology: toward a unified view. MIS Q. **27**(3), 425–478 (2003). https://doi.org/10.2307/30036540
25. Weng, C., et al.: A two-site survey of medical center personnel's willingness to share clinical data for research: implications for reproducible health NLP research. BMC Med. Inform. Decis. Mak.Decis. Mak. **19**, S3 (2019). https://doi.org/10.1186/s12911-019-0778-z
26. Zhang, Y., et al.: Factors influencing patients' intentions to use diabetes management apps based on an extended unified theory of acceptance and use of technology model: web-based survey. J. Med. Internet Res. **21**(8), e15023 (2019). https://doi.org/10.2196/15023
27. Declaration. https://mydata.org/participate/declaration/. Accessed 27 Feb 2024
28. The Nordic Health Survey 2023. https://www.if-insurance.com/large-enterprises/insight/the-nordic-health-survey-2023. Accessed 16 Nov 2023
29. The State of Health and Care of Older People, 2023 (abridged)

Digitalization in Health Education

Initial Experiences of Electronic Medical Record Simulation Environment in eHealth Education Course for Medical Students in Finland

Petra Kuikka[1]([⊠]) [iD], Paula Veikkolainen[1] [iD], Tiina Salmijärvi[2] [iD],
Timo Tuovinen[1,3] [iD], Petri Kulmala[2,3] [iD], and Jarmo Reponen[1,3] [iD]

[1] FinnTelemedicum, Research Unit of Health Sciences and Technology, University of Oulu, Oulu, Finland
petra.kuikka@oulu.fi
[2] Faculty of Medicine, University of Oulu, Oulu, Finland
[3] Medical Research Center Oulu, Oulu University Hospital, Oulu, Finland

Abstract. Different electronic medical record systems (EMR) have established themselves as part of the Finnish health care service provision. There is a need to ensure health care professionals' competence and training for such systems. The MEDigi project, aimed to modernize and harmonize the Finnish basic medical education, recognized EMR systems as a key competence area for medical professionals in eHealth topics. The project also led to the development of a new eHealth course and an EMR simulation environment targeted for medical students based on the Esko EMR system already in production use.

A new simulation environment was developed in cooperation with the Faculty of Medicine at University of Oulu and Esko Systems Ltd. The simulation environment was implemented as an optional exercise in a cross-institutional web-based course teaching eHealth topics to medical students in the spring 2023. Students' experiences with the simulation environment and associated exercise were collected with a feedback survey using 5- and 10-point Likert scales.

An EMR simulation environment "TrainingEsko" was successfully implemented into the "Basics in eHealth for Medical Students" course. Up to 11 medical students took part in the exercise, of which two participated in the associated feedback survey. They expressed satisfaction with the performance of the simulation environment and the associated exercise.

Our initial experiences with the EMR simulation environment give support for the further use of the EMR simulation environment in future course implementations. According to the feedback the students found the environment effective and the exercises beneficial for learning about EMR systems.

Keywords: Telemedicine · Medical Informatics · Professional Competence · Medical Education · Medical Students · Digitalization · EMR Simulation

M. Särestöniemi et al. (Eds.): NCDHWS 2024, CCIS 2083, pp. 169–180, 2024.
https://doi.org/10.1007/978-3-031-59080-1_12

1   Introduction

Reflecting the increasing digitalization of societies and health care, the International Medical Informatics Association (IMIA) published the second revision of the Recommendations on Biomedical and Health Informatics (BMHI) Education in 2023, suggesting the introduction of BMHI core principles, and fundamentals of other BMHI knowledge domains, in all health care profession curriculums, as a separate or integrated subject [1].

In Finland, efforts have been made to modernize basic medical education. One notable initiative was the national MEDigi project (2018–2021), funded by the Finnish Ministry of Education and Culture [2]. The project aimed to modernize and digitize the teaching of medicine and dentistry in Finland as well as to ensure that students possess a high-level competence in using electronic health care tools. This was achieved by establishing nationwide eHealth key competence themes. These areas of competence included topics such as electronic medical record systems (EMR), electronic databases, and clinical decision support systems [3].

Additionally, the MEDigi project aimed to promote flexible studying, cross-institutional learning, and other forms of educational cooperation [2]. During the project, a new course titled "Basics in eHealth for Medical Students" was introduced in spring 2021 [4]. The course provides students with an overview of the position of eHealth and telemedicine solutions within the Finnish health care information system. It also familiarizes them with the terminology of information and communication technology (ICT) in health care and offers insights into future health ICT trends. The course, offered to medical students at all Finnish medical campuses, was the first nationwide cross-institutional medical course in Finland. The implementation of the course has been continued even after the end of the project, and on average, 15 students from different universities have completed the course as part of their optional studies yearly.

1.1   Electronic Medical Records and Education

The terms electronic patient record (EPR), electronic medical record (EMR), and electronic health record (EHR) are often used interchangeably. However, some definitions restrict EPR and EMR to a single health care organization, while EHR is more comprehensive, extending across organizational borders [5]. All these terms describe the collection of medical and health-related data on an individual, generated and managed primarily by health care professionals.

Finland has been among the leading countries in electronic medical data management. EMRs had been implemented in all Finnish public health care provider organizations by 2007 [6], and another milestone was reached by 2015, with widespread integration of Kanta services into the public health care sector's record systems [7]. The Kanta services introduced the national e-prescription service, which became mandatory for all public health care provider organizations since 2017, the Patient Data Repository for central archiving and sharing of patient data between health care organizations, and the citizen health portal "My Kanta", which provides citizens with secure access to their own health data and the option to control the sharing of their health data between different organizations [8].

With the introduction of Kanta services in Finland, distinguishing between EMRs and EHRs has become more challenging. In this paper, we use the terms electronic medical record (EMR), and EMR systems to denote the primary systems within a single health care organization to store and manage patient data, regardless of Patient Data Repository integration.

Despite the widespread implementation of digital tools in clinical practice, 57% of Finnish medical doctors, who graduated between 2007 and 2016, felt that their training in these tools during basic medical education was inadequate [9]. Studies have indicated that longer extracurricular EHR experience correlates with higher confidence levels in using EHRs among the students [10]. A scoping review found that simulation training positively impacted the skills, attitudes, knowledge, and satisfaction of health profession students [11]. Moreover, simulated training in using EHRs can enhance medical students' knowledge and awareness of the limitations of these systems [12]. A review of current literature on EMR training among health professionals and health profession students highlighted Academic Electronic Medical Records (AEMRs) and EMR simulation as the most prevalent methods in EMR education [13].

Given the importance of EMR systems as a key competence area for medical professionals in eHealth topics, we set out to pilot an electronic medical record simulation environment in the "Basics in eHealth for Medical Students" course during its third iteration in 2023.

1.2   Objectives

Our objectives were:

1. To develop and implement an EMR simulation environment called "TrainingEsko", and the associated Moodle exercise targeted at training medical students in the principals and use of EMR systems, and
2. To gain initial user feedback about the environment and exercise for further development and improvement.

2   Materials and Methods

2.1   Electronic Medical Record System Esko

The "Esko" medical record system, developed by Esko Systems Ltd, is a browser-based modular system comprising of the core system with individual proprietary modules (e.g. Medication and Unit Situation Picture) and external integrations, such as LIS (laboratory information system) and RIS (radiology information system). First introduced in the Oulu University Hospital in 1996, the system has since been in use in specialized health care in four hospital districts. Esko has been among the highest rated systems in national usability studies both among physicians and registered nurses, especially for its ease of use and the technical functionality and stability [14, 15]. The system's logical, easy to use interface and browser-based accessibility commended its use as the basis for a simulation environment in basic medical education.

2.2 Development and Piloting of the EMR Simulation Environment

The TrainingEsko simulation environment was developed in cooperation with the Faculty of Medicine at University of Oulu and the system producer Esko Systems Ltd, during the MEDigi project. After the end of the MEDigi project, the development was continued by the Medical Faculty and the system provider, and the system was introduced to students through a remote connection with the help of the ICT specialists from the Oulu University Hospital, their service supplier Istekki Ltd, and University of Oulu. The simulation environment and associated exercise were implemented in a web-based course aimed at teaching eHealth topics to medical students, titled "Basics in eHealth for Medical Students", during the spring semester in 2023. The course was held in English and hosted on the Moodle learning platform. It was offered to all Finnish medical students as an optional course. As the simulation environment and exercises were in a pilot phase, they were an optional part of the course. Despite the course been held in English, the EMR simulation exercise was in Finnish due to the language restrictions of the system. Medical students were invited to participate in the pilot and associated feedback survey in a Moodle platform. The survey was conducted via Webropol survey tool to collect preliminary user experiences about the system and its implementation anonymously.

Student experiences with the exercise were surveyed using 5- and 10-point Likert scales in the survey. Students assessed their self-perceived competence on the subject themes on a scale from 0 (No competence) to 10 (Excellent competence) both before and after the exercise. The usefulness of the EMR simulation environment for independent learning was evaluated on a scale from 0 (Not useful) to 10 (Extremely useful), and students' readiness and eagerness to use the system in other courses were measured on a scale from 0 (None) to 10 (As much as possible). The construction and implementation of the exercise and its components were assessed using positive statements about each part of the exercise, and a 5-point Likert scale ranging from 1 (Strongly disagree) to 5 (Strongly agree). The perceived level of difficulty of each part of the exercise was rated on a scale from 1 (Too easy) to 5 (Too difficult). In addition, students' years of study as well as previous EMR experience were collected using a multi-choice question format.

We report the results of the feedback, and our experiences with the development of an EMR simulation environment and its implementation in an optional course as part of basic medical education.

2.3 Ethical Statement

The survey was conducted in accordance with the instructions of the Finnish Advisory Board on Research Integrity, and in compliance with EU data protection regulations as well as the established research practices of the University of Oulu and the Faculty of Medicine. Thus, no approval from the ethics committee was required. Full consideration was given to matters related to data protection in accordance with the ethical principles applicable to research subjects. The participation in the exercise and the feedback survey was voluntary and students were asked for their consent to collect and use data for the purpose of an academic paper. The students were informed of the purpose of the survey, their right to withdraw from it and prohibit the use of their data at any time. No incentives were offered for participation.

3   Results

3.1   Design and Implementation of the Electronic Medical Record Simulation Environment TrainingEsko

The Esko simulation environment "TrainingEsko" is a separate instance of the core Esko medical record system. Intended for educational and training purposes, the TrainingEsko includes functionalities such as medical history, progression and discharge notes, medication, and key certificate forms. Importantly, as an independent system, Training-Esko is not connected to the production version of Esko and does not contain any real patient data; instead, it features entirely fictional patient profiles. The simulation environment is hosted on secure servers, and students can access the simulation environment in a browser on their own computers, using personal Oulu University login ID to open a secure connection. Access to the system is granted only to the students enrolled in the course and only for the duration of the course. Login to the simulated EMR system itself uses login information intended for this purpose only. Personal login information to the production system is never used with the simulation system.

As a pilot feature, the simulation environment was introduced as an optional additional exercise designed to teach the anatomy and use of EMR systems. The exercise comprised of Moodle H5P-activity with branching scenarios and practical tasks performed in the EMR simulation environment. The H5P-activity in Moodle, with slide shows and interactive imagery, provided students with written instructions for navigating the exercise and managing the simulation environment. It presented activating questions from various viewpoints on the subjects for student contemplation. Screenshots of the training environment, equipped with interactive "hotspots" that opened additional information in floating windows, offered a practical method for presenting visual and dynamic instructions on the structure and use of the simulation environment. For this exercise, we created an imaginary patient case in the simulation environment, featuring a senior patient with a history of hypertension, heart infarction, and atrial fibrillation, along with appropriate medications.

The related learning exercise was divided into three parts, which students could perform separately and in the order of their choosing, although the numbered order was encouraged (see Fig. 1). Part 1, titled "Relevance and anatomy of EMRs", focused on the general structure and functions of EMRs using TrainingEsko as an example. It covered what information EMRs contain, and how this information is stored and organized. Students were instructed to navigate in the system and familiarize themselves with the general structures of EMRs by searching and opening the medical record of the fictional patient using a personal identity code (see Fig. 2–3).

Part 2, "Patient record and note entering", dealt with the medical record of an individual, exploring the differences between structured and unstructured medical data, as well as aspects of data security. As practical tasks, students reviewed the patient history and practiced note entering in the simulation environment (see Fig. 4). Part 3, "EMR and tools of care: medications", focused on the management of medication data. This section discussed the benefits and risks associated with electronic medication lists, and

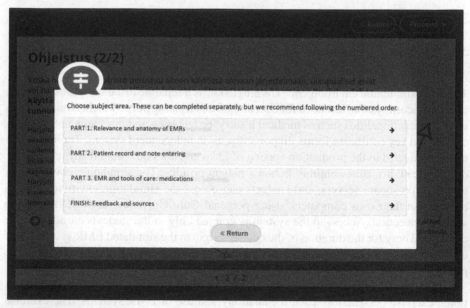

Fig. 1. Screenshot of student's view in the Moodle activity with branching scenarios. First three options direct to parts 1–3 of the exercise, and the last option to the feedback survey and used sources. English translations by authors.

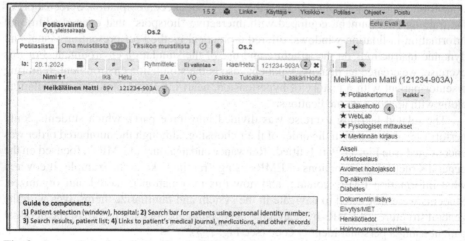

Fig. 2. Screenshot of student's view in TrainingEsko, as they search for the fictional patient's records. System language Finnish, English translations provided by authors.

relevant clinical decision support tools, such as drug interaction warning systems. Students engaged in different types of medication orders, which also demonstrated various levels of drug interaction warnings (see Fig. 5).

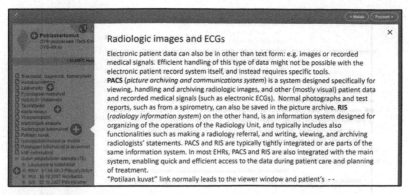

Fig. 3. Screenshot of the Moodle activity from part 1 of the exercise. After instructing the students to practice navigating the system themselves, screenshots of the respective views of the system with interactive hotspots (green plus signs) were used to educate students on different aspects of the system. English translation by authors.

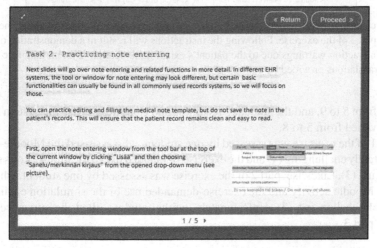

Fig. 4. Screenshot from Moodle for the part 2 of the exercise, in which students are instructed how to enter notes into the patient record. English translations by authors.

3.2 Initial User Experiences Based on the Feedback Survey

Of the course-enrolled students, 11 students had interacted with the Moodle activity of the exercise. Two first-year medical students completed at least one part of the exercise and took the feedback survey. Neither had previous experience in relevant working field nor previous experience with EMR systems.

The students' self-estimated competence in the respective course subject themes ("Electronic Health Records", "Components to EPR/EHR", and "Health Information Exchange and Kanta") varied from 4 and 8 before the exercise. After the exercise, the estimated confidence ranged from 6 to 7, meaning one of the students estimated their confidence lower by at least 1 point. The usefulness of Training Esko was evaluated

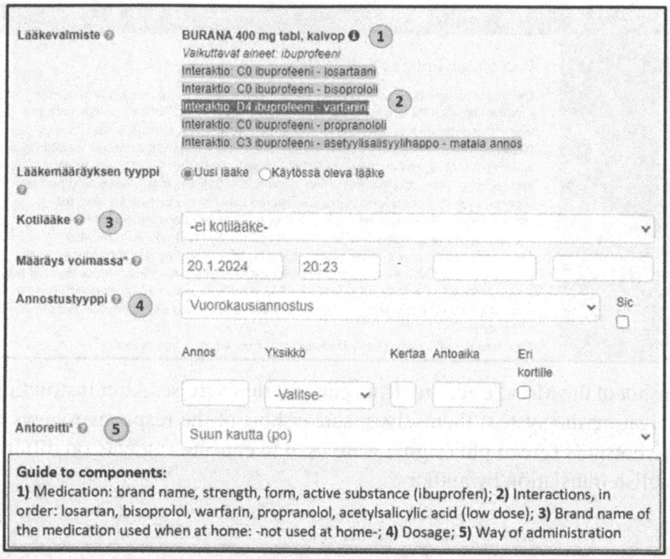

Guide to components:
1) Medication: brand name, strength, form, active substance (ibuprofen); 2) Interactions, in order: losartan, bisoprolol, warfarin, propranolol, acetylsalicylic acid (low dose); 3) Brand name of the medication used when at home: -not used at home-; 4) Dosage; 5) Way of administration

Fig. 5. Screenshot of the student's view in TrainingEsko as they practice entering medication orders in part 3 of the exercise. Following the instructions will result in a demonstration of several medical interaction warnings due to the patient's existing medication. System language Finnish, English translations provided by authors.

ranging from 5 to 9, and the students' readiness and eagerness to use the system in other courses varied from 5 to 8.

Part 1 of the exercise was assessed by one student, who assessed the Moodle-activity as moderately challenging (4) and the exercise-demanded use of TrainingEsko as suitably challenging (3). Likewise, part 2 of the exercise was assessed by one student, who found both the Moodle activity and the exercise-demanded use of the simulation environment as suitably challenging (3). Unfortunately, neither student filled the survey regarding exercise part 3.

4 Discussion

To our knowledge, this was the first EMR simulation environment piloted for medical education purposes in Finland. Globally, there have been a few initiatives to implement similar solutions in basic medical education, and the response to these initiatives has been mainly positive [12, 16, 17]. Recognized potential challenges include the availability of suitable systems meeting the technical requirements for educational use, the financial and human resources needed for the implementation and maintenance of these systems, resistance from faculty, educators, or students, and the already loaded curriculum of medical studies [12, 18, 19].

We report our experiences of successfully implementing an EMR simulation environment into a Finnish cross-institutional medical online course, and the collected preliminary experiences from students about the system and its use. Though our simulation environment focuses on only one Finnish EMR system, the connected exercise targets to teach about EMR systems, their functions and anatomy, at a universal level. The students who participated in the pilot exercise and the feedback survey expressed satisfaction with the performance of the simulation environment and the associated exercise. Students felt that the tasks supported their learning and perceived the EMR simulation environment as at least moderately useful for independent learning. They indicated readiness and eagerness to implement it in other courses, aligning with results found in literature [20, 21].

An interesting finding was that for at least one student, the self-assessed confidence level in using the EMR system decreased after completing the exercise. This might be attributed to increased awareness of the complexities and demands of recording patient data in EMR systems [22]. The sophistication of current systems may have been unexpected for participants with no prior EMR experience. However, due to the small number of participants, further conclusions on this topic are limited.

Another observation during the project was related to the published literature on EMR training and EMR simulation environments. More studies seemed to involve health care professionals or nursing students with relatively few focusing on undergraduate medical students [13]. This is noteworthy considering that medical students are a significant future user group of EMR systems. While the basic education in digital tools and eHealth was considered insufficient by doctors who graduated before 2016 [9], recent findings suggest that the self-reported competence level of fifth year medical students in Finland is at a good level, though there is room for improvement [23]. Globally, the situation may differ, as indicated by a study from Saudi-Arabia [24]. There is evidence that EMR teaching interventions can enhance students' competence levels and confidence in their skills [25].

Simulation-based teaching is at its core student-centered in nature, and directs the student to an active role [11]. Students' motivation can be increased by their learning having a direct transfer effect to the context of working life. More research is needed on the ways in which EMR teaching should be integrated into basic medical education. Developed frameworks, such as the one described by Borycki et al., are helpful for discussing ways and levels of EMR simulation integration [26]. The role of piloting is significant, as the models created with them can help to develop and promote teaching practices. We hope that our model of using a non-production copy of an EMR, combined with the flexibility of established educational environments like Moodle, will provide inspiration to others. However, the variety of technical solutions behind different EMRs may hinder or prevent their use in this manner.

Though the system and the associated exercise we have described demonstrates stand-alone learning, the system could potentially be used to supplement traditional medical education in the future, for example as a platform for clinical course material. Such integration would come with its own benefits, such as natural exposure to EMRs during basic studies while avoiding adding new course content to the curriculum. However, such use of the system could also introduce new requirements insure a smooth and seamless integration with other course education.

Based on the positive results we decided to make part 1 of the EMR simulation environment a compulsory exercise for all students in the "Basics in eHealth for Medical

Students" course, with minor modifications, while parts 2 and 3 remained optional. The EMR simulation system was also piloted on a clinical neurology course, receiving generally positive feedback from students. Many noted that the optimal timing for such a system would at the beginning of the clinical phase of their studies. As the "Basics in eHealth for Medical Students" is scheduled for the last year of pre-clinical studies, these comments reinforce our decision to continue implementing EMR simulation in this course.

4.1 Conclusions

According to the feedback, the students found the EMR simulation environment effective and the exercises beneficial for learning about EMR systems. Our experiences provide a solid foundation for the further use of the EMR simulation environment in future course implementations.

Acknowledgments. We would like to thank the students participating in the pilot exercise, Esko Systems Ltd and Oulu University Hospital (OYS) for providing the software environment, and the ICT specialists at Esko Systems Ltd, OYS, Istekki Ltd, and ICT Services of University of Oulu for their contribution and support in implementation of the system in medical education.

Disclosure of Interests. Authors PK, PV, TT and JR have been partly employed by MEDigi project financed by the Finnish Ministry of Education and Culture [Grant No. OKM/270/523/2017]. Authors TS ja PK have nothing to disclose.

References

1. Bichel-Findlay, J., et al.: Recommendations of the International Medical Informatics Association (IMIA) on education in biomedical and health informatics: second revision. Int. J. Med. Informatics **170**, 104908 (2023). https://doi.org/10.1016/j.ijmedinf.2022.104908
2. Levy, A., Reponen, J. (eds.) Digital transformation of medical education: MEDigi project report. University of Oulu (2021). https://urn.fi/URN:ISBN:9789526232454
3. Tuovinen, T., et al.: Sähköisten terveyspalveluiden opetus lääketieteessä. Duodecim **137**(17), 1807–1813 (2021)
4. Basics in eHealth for Medical Students (044113S) | Study Guide 2023–2024. https://opas.peppi.oulu.fi/en/course/044113S/7489?period=2023-2024. Accessed 12 Jan 2024
5. The National Alliance for Health Information Technology Report to the Office of the National Coordinator for Health Information Technology on Defining Key Health Information Technology Terms. US Department of Health and Human Services (2008)
6. Reponen, J., Kangas, M., Hämäläinen, P., Keränen, N.: Tieto- ja viestintäteknologian käyttö terveydenhuollossa vuonna 2014 - Tilanne ja kehityksen suunta [Use of information and communications technology in Finnish health care in 2014. Current situation and trends. In Finnish with an English abstract.] National Institute for Health and Welfare (THL) Report 12/2015. (2015). http://urn.fi/URN:ISBN:978-952-302-486-1
7. Jormanainen, V.: Kanta-palvelujen käyttöönotto vuosina 2010–2014. Duodecim **131**, 1309–1316 (2015)

8. What are the Kanta Services? https://www.kanta.fi/en/what-are-kanta-services. Accessed 04 Jan 2024
9. Mattila, P., et al.: Lääkäri 2018: kyselytutkimus vuosina 2007–2016 valmistuneille lääkäreille - Sosiaali- ja terveysministeriön raportteja ja muistioita 2019:69. Sosiaali- ja terveysministeriö (2019)
10. Lander, L., et al.: Self-perceptions of readiness to use electronic health records among medical students: survey study. JMIR Med Educ. **6**, e17585 (2020). https://doi.org/10.2196/17585
11. Nabovati, E., Jeddi, F.R., Ghaffari, F., Mirhoseini, F.: The effects of simulation training on learning of health information systems: a scoping review. J. Educ. Health Promot. **11**, 4 (2022). https://doi.org/10.4103/jehp.jehp_17_21
12. Herrmann-Werner, A., Holderried, M., Loda, T., Malek, N., Zipfel, S., Holderried, F.: Navigating through electronic health records: survey study on medical students' perspectives in general and with regard to a specific training. JMIR Med. Inform. **7**, e12648 (2019). https://doi.org/10.2196/12648
13. Samadbeik, M., et al.: Education and training on Electronic Medical Records (EMRs) for health care professionals and students: a scoping review. Int. J. Med. Informatics **142**, 104238 (2020). https://doi.org/10.1016/j.ijmedinf.2020.104238
14. Nurses' views on digitalisation - National Institute for Health and Welfare (THL). https://thl.fi/en/topics/information-management-in-social-welfare-and-health-care/what-is-inform ation-management-/follow-up-of-the-information-system-services-in-social-welfare-and-health-care/indicators-of-digitalisation/nurses-views-on-digitalisation. Accessed 19 Jan 2024
15. Physicians' views on digitalisation - National Institute for Health and Welfare (THL). https://thl.fi/en/topics/information-management-in-social-welfare-and-health-care/what-is-inform ation-management-/follow-up-of-the-information-system-services-in-social-welfare-and-health-care/indicators-of-digitalisation/physicians-views-on-digitalisation. Accessed 19 Jan 2024
16. Joe, R.S., Otto, A., Borycki, E.: Designing an electronic medical case simulator for health professional education. Knowl. Manage. E-Learning Int. J. **3**, 63–71 (2011). https://doi.org/10.34105/j.kmel.2011.03.007
17. Milano, C.E., Hardman, J.A., Plesiu, A., Rdesinski, R.E., Biagioli, F.E.: Simulated Electronic Health Record (Sim-EHR) curriculum: teaching EHR skills and use of the EHR for disease management and prevention. Acad. Med. **89**, 399–403 (2014). https://doi.org/10.1097/ACM.0000000000000149
18. Borycki, E.M., Kushniruk, A.W.: Educational electronic health records at the University of Victoria: challenges, recommendations and lessons learned. Stud Health Technol Inform. **265**, 74–79 (2019). https://doi.org/10.3233/SHTI190141
19. Hersh, W., et al.: From Competencies to Competence. In: Health Professionals' Education in the Age of Clinical Information Systems, Mobile Computing and Social Networks, pp. 269–287. Elsevier (2017). https://doi.org/10.1016/B978-0-12-805362-1.00013-9
20. Biagioli, F.E., et al.: The electronic health record objective structured clinical examination: assessing student competency in patient interactions while using the electronic health record. Acad. Med. **92**, 87–91 (2017). https://doi.org/10.1097/ACM.0000000000001276
21. Elliott, K., Judd, T., McColl, G.: A student-centred electronic health record system for clinical education. Stud Health Technol Inform. **168**, 57–64 (2011)
22. Haverinen, J., Kcränen, N., Tuovinen, T., Ruotanen, R., Reponen, J.: National development and regional differences in eHealth maturity in finnish public health care: survey study. JMIR Med. Inform. **10**, e35612 (2022). https://doi.org/10.2196/35612
23. Veikkolainen, P., et al.: eHealth competence building for future doctors and nurses - Attitudes and capabilities. Int. J. Med. Inform. **169**, 104912 (2023). https://doi.org/10.1016/j.ijmedinf.2022.104912

24. Jabour, A.: Knowledge of E-health concepts among students in health-related specialties in Saudi Arabia. Inform. Med. Unlocked. **25**, 100654 (2021). https://doi.org/10.1016/j.imu.2021.100654

25. Zavodnick, J., Kouvatsos, T.: Electronic health record skills workshop for medical students. MedEdPORTAL. **15**, 10849 (2019). https://doi.org/10.15766/mep_2374-8265.10849

26. Borycki, E., Kushniruk, A., Armstrong, B., Joe, R., Otto, T.: Integrating electronic health records into health professional and health informatics education: a continuum of approaches. Acta Inform. Med. **18**(1), 20–24 (2010)

How Does Human-Centred Extended Reality Support Healthcare Students' Learning in Clinical Conditions?

Kristina Mikkonen[1]([⊠]), Hany Ferdinando[1], Marta Sobocinski[2], Heli Kuivila[1], Sari Pramila-Savukoski[1], Tugba Vhitehead[2], Paula Ropponen[1], Teemu Myllylä[1,3], Jari Paunonen[1], Erson Halili[4], Joel Koutonen[4], Juha-Matti Taikina-Aho[4], Antti Siipo[2], and Sanna Järvelä[2]

[1] Research Unit of Health Sciences and Technology (HST), University of Oulu; Medical Research Center Oulu, Oulu University Hospital, Oulu, Finland
kristina.mikkonen@oulu.fi
[2] Learning and Educational Technology Research Unit (LET), University of Oulu, Oulu, Finland
[3] Optoelectronics and Measurement Techniques Unit (OPEM), University of Oulu, Oulu, Finland
[4] FrostBit Software Lab, Lapland University of Applied Sciences, Rovaniemi, Finland

Abstract. Healthcare education needs to be reformed to sustain quality, faster response to crises and ensure a rapid and efficient graduation path for future healthcare professionals. In this study, our multidisciplinary team has developed and tested a Human-centred extended reality (XR) to solve challenges in healthcare by connecting humans to technology in a human-centred, ethical way and by empowering end users through social innovation. In our study, we aimed to develop an intuitive XR virtual simulation environment with realistic scenarios and metahuman avatars, enabling team interaction to test and analyse participants' real-time adaptation through a combination of neurophysiological and behavioural data collected by wearable sensors. This novel research offers a solution to complement clinical placements of nursing and medical students and ensure that students achieve the required competencies even if unexpected situations or crises threaten to interrupt the practice of competencies in real-life environments. Furthermore, by utilising the neurophysiological data, we can assess the learning event based on analysis of the recorded signals. The XR solutions can reduce nursing and medical students' stress levels and enhance their resilience to work effectively in collaborative interprofessional teams.

Keywords: extended reality · XR · cultural and linguistic diversity · healthcare

1 Introduction

It is critical to promptly address issues contributing to the attrition of healthcare students and staff members, as we cannot afford to lose additional health professionals. WHO [1] and UN [2] predict international shortages will increase to 9.9 million healthcare workers

© The Author(s) 2024
M. Särestöniemi et al. (Eds.): NCDHWS 2024, CCIS 2083, pp. 181–188, 2024.
https://doi.org/10.1007/978-3-031-59080-1_13

by 2030. Higher education in healthcare enhances professionals' competence, which can positively impact staff retention and the overall quality of healthcare services [3]. For example, according to Directive 2013/55/EU [4], total nurses' education includes up to 50% of clinical practice, which is dysfunctional and ineffective because of the lack of healthcare staff to supervise students [5, 6]. As students cannot access necessary training because of a lack of healthcare supervisors at clinical placements, the pipeline of qualified healthcare professionals is compromised, exacerbating the broader healthcare workforce shortage. Addressing these challenges requires a comprehensive approach that involves increasing the healthcare workforce, enhancing support for educators and mentors, and finding innovative solutions to provide students with the necessary clinical experiences.

Healthcare education needs to be reformed to sustain quality, faster response to crises and ensure a rapid and efficient graduation path for future healthcare professionals. According to previous evidence, simulation-based extended reality (XR) education can partly replace healthcare clinical practice by supporting students' learning experiences in safe learning environments [7, 8]. Hybrid intelligence (including extended reality (XR) and artificial intelligence (AI)) is seen to be 'an effective way to augment traditional forms of pedagogy' [9] and offer new pedagogical methods for training opportunities.

2 Aim of the Study

Human-centred XR will empower end users and continuously involve healthcare students and educators in co-design and decision-making by aiming to respond to the objectives. This will be achieved by developing a) an intuitive extended reality (XR) virtual simulation environment with realistic scenarios, b) user experience analysis and real-time adaptation through a combination of neurophysiological and behavioural data collected by wearable sensors, and c) the creation of convincing digital humans (patients and mentors).

RQ1.: Does a human-centred XR support healthcare students' learning in clinical conditions?

RQ2.: How do students' cognitive and neural responses, as measured by fNIRS and EEG, differ during learning tasks in XR simulations compared to traditional learning?

H1: Human-centred XR will support students' learning in clinical conditions statistically significantly ($p \leq 0.05$).

3 Methodology

Two human-centred XR cases have been developed by integrating self-regulated learning [10], immersive technology principles [11] and interprofessional mentor competence framework [12]. The cases contained scenarios with an XR environment: a) discharging a patient by providing instructions and a home care plan, b) assessing a patient in anaphylactic reaction after administering intervenors antibiotics. In the XR technology, we have used game engine integration, e.g., rendering the full-body avatar of patients and nurses, implementing the single-user interaction design, integrating physical props, and the graphical content and scenario-specific sequences to comprise the whole simulation. The cases contained natural communication between real humans and avatar meta-human patients, making interaction seamless (see Picture 1). The development of XR technologies involved user-centred design and co-design by involving students, educators, and health professionals from the beginning until the testing phase. Expert panels have been used to assess the feasibility of the intervention, using design-thinking workshops to understand human needs, re-frame problems, and create ideas through brainstorming sessions and iterative low-cost rapid prototyping (Fig. 1).

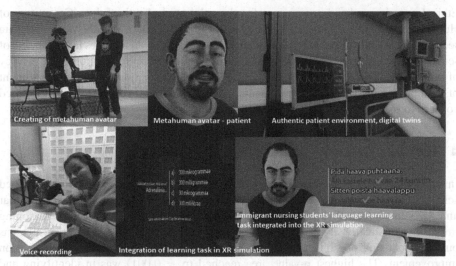

Fig. 1. Human-centred XR development

3.1 Data Collection and Analysis

The inclusion criteria for the pilot study were i) nursing students participating in English language degree programs at universities of applied sciences, ii) first-year students for cases of discharging a patient, and second/third-year students for cases of assessing patients in anaphylactic reactions. The effect of the human-centred XR environment was assessed using complex multimodal observational, behavioural, and neurophysiological outcome measures. The observational data included questions from validated scales of Nurse Clinical Reasoning (15 items,1–5 Likert scale) [13], Student Satisfaction and Self-Confidence in Learning Scale (13 items, 1–5 Likert scale) [14], and Simulation Design Scale (20 items, 1–5 Likert scale) [15]. Questionnaires were used before the XR and straight after and were analysed using the $\chi 2$ test and t-test.

Wearable sensors (functional near-infrared spectroscopy (fNIRS) brain monitoring device and Shimmer's wristband) were used to collect three types of neurophysiological signals: brain activity (fNIRS), heart activity (ECG), and electrodermal response from the skin (EDA) [16, 17]. A paired t-test examined any significant changes between the baseline and post-test scores.

Initially, students were introduced to the study and asked to respond to the first questionnaire at T0 measurement. After the questionnaire, wearable sensors were attached, and students had to sit calmly without any action for 5 min to take baseline measurements. After the baseline measurements, students were asked to read the Finnish terms included in the XR case for 10 min after completing the XR case, which lasted between 20 and 30 min. After the XR case, students complete a second questionnaire.

3.2 Ethical Issues

Ethical permission has been granted for the pilot study by the Ethics Committee of Human Sciences at the University of Oulu on 25.09.2023. In the study, we ensure data security, accessibility, and validation of results. Data generated includes large datasets of sensitive personal data (biometric data) and user-environment interactions. The privacy of individuals is protected according to GDPR [18] through monitoring and assessment of data processing activities. Participants received clear and comprehensive informed consent forms and could withdraw their consent at any point.

4   Results

In total, 30 subjects participated in the pilot study representing two universities of applied sciences in the Nordic part of Finland. 61% were first-year students, 36%- second year and 3% - third year. Preliminary results have shown that students' clinical reasoning improved statistically significantly (varying between $p = 0.028$ to $p < 0.001$) in all areas but two, focusing on collecting patient information and evaluating patient condition improvement. The highest p-value area reached ($p < 0.001$) was in identifying and communicating vital information clearly to the doctors based on the patient's current situation. Students evaluated that XR learning has increased their confidence in learning in all areas, mostly reporting enjoying how the instructor taught the simulation (mean 4.5, SD 0.73) and teaching methods used in the simulation were helpful and effective (mean 4.4., SD 0.62). Students evaluated simulation pedagogical design as having the highest instructor's support in their learning (mean 4.83, SD 0.46) and a clear understanding of the purpose and objectives of their learning (mean 4.50, SD 0.68). Students evaluated the lowest in the simulation, allowing them to analyse their behaviour and actions (mean 3.87, SD 0.86) and the opportunity to reflect with teachers to build their knowledge to another level (mean 3.93, SD 0.69).

Spectral entropy measures the complexity of the signal in the frequency domain; the higher the value, the more complex the signal. Figures 2, 3, and 4 show the response of oxy-, deoxy-, and total haemoglobin also with cerebrospinal fluid (CSF) in three different bands, very low frequency (0.008–0.1 Hz), respiratory (0.1–0.6 Hz), and cardiac (0.6–5 Hz) bands. P1 represents phase 1 and acts as a baseline for the measurement. P2 and P3 indicate reading and XR tasks. As the subjects only had a little knowledge of Finnish, they looked like they were struggling, and the spectral entropy scores during P2 were relatively high. Although the XR task seemed quite demanding in specific scenarios, the overall experience did not induce complexity in the signal.

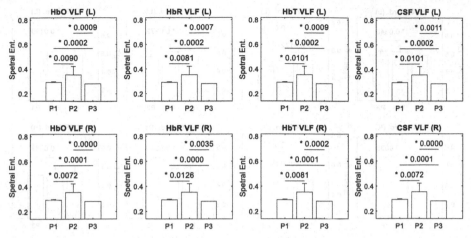

Fig. 2. Hemodynamic response in the very low-frequency band (0.008–0.1 Hz)

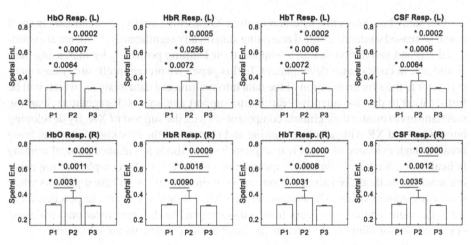

Fig. 3. Hemodynamic response in the very respiratory band (0.1–0.6 Hz)

5 Discussion and Conclusions

In our study, we aimed to develop an intuitive XR virtual simulation environment with realistic scenarios and metahuman avatars, enabling team interaction to test and analyse participants' real-time adaptation through a combination of neuro-physiological and behavioural data collected by wearable sensors. Until nowadays, formal healthcare training has focused predominantly on developing discipline-based knowledge, clinical expertise, and technical skills in non-adaptive designs [19]. Contemporary healthcare education needs to develop further solutions to enhance students' and future professionals' team-oriented competencies, such as non-technical skills, defined as situation awareness, decision-making, communication and teamwork.

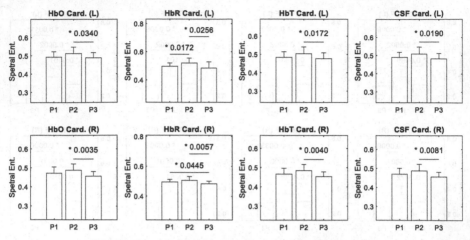

Fig. 4. Hemodynamic response in cardiac band (0.6–5 Hz)

Our study has shown that a human-centred XR learning environment already in short usage increased students' clinical reasoning statistically significantly. Students also evaluated XR and simulation design to support their learning positively by increasing their confidence in competence development. In this paper, we present preliminary data analysis prior to the synchronisation of the data into multimodal data analysis, which will be further used to develop adaptive learning to support students' self-regulatory learning mechanisms to master their clinical competencies with the support of XR. By developing human-centred XR with adaptive learning and mentoring, the new knowledge can bring breakthrough evidence of novel learning/teaching methods to enhance clinical training in healthcare. Students' clinical competence can be developed by complementing existing teaching methods, reducing the number of training hours with actual patients while increasing patient safety. The human-centred XR will allow students to practice clinical skills alone and/or with peers from a distance and in different locations, widening opportunities for clinical and interprofessional training in healthcare education.

5.1 Limitations

The study faced several challenges. Firstly, the XR learning environment caused motion sickness for few participants. It has been observed to happen to participants who participated in the study while hungry. Researchers were trained to react sensitively to the physical discomfort of the participants by providing drinks and snacks to the participants in that case and allowing to discontinue the testing if symptoms did not get better. Secondly, XR technology sometimes failed due to a slow internet connection, which disrupted participants' learning experience. Researchers assisted participants in that case by manually speeding up avatars' communication. Thirdly, the fNIRS sensors caused some participants discomfort, slightly pressing their forehead due to the XR headsets, which may affect the analysis results.

Acknowledgements. This study has been funded by 6GESS Profile 6 and Medical Research Center and supported by Hybrid Intelligence Profile 7, funded by the Research Council of Finland and the University of Oulu.

Disclosure of Interests. The authors have no competing interests to declare relevant to this article's content.

References

1. World Health Organization. Data and statistics [Internet] (2023). https://www.euro.who.int/en/health-topics/Health-systems/health-workforce/data-and-statistics
2. United Nations. Good health and well-being. the sustainable development goals report 2023: Special Edition (2023). https://unstats.un.org/sdgs/report/2023/Goal-03/
3. Niskala, J., et al.: Interventions to improve nurses' job satisfaction: a systematic review and meta-analysis. J. Adv. Nurs. **76**(7), 1498–1508 (2020). https://doi.org/10.1111/jan.1434
4. EUR-Lex. Directive 2013/55 (2014). https://eur-lex.europa.eu/legal-content/EN/TXT/?uri=CELEX%3A32013L0055&qid=1697718620788
5. Lau, S.T., Ang, E., Samarasekera, D.D., Shorey, S.: Development of undergraduate nursing entrustable professional activities to enhance clinical care and practice. Nurse Educ. Today **87**, 104347 (2020). https://doi.org/10.1016/j.nedt.2020.104347
6. Ulenaers, D.: Clinical placement experience of nursing students during the COVID-19 pandemic: a cross-sectional study. Nurse Education Today, 1 (2021)
7. Jimenez, Y.A., Gray, F., Di Michele, L., Said, S., Reed, W., Kench, P.: Can simulation-based education or other education interventions replace clinical placement in medical radiation sciences? A narrative review. radiography (London, England: 1995) **29**(2), 421–427 (2023). https://doi.org/10.1016/j.radi.2023.02.003
8. Quqandi, E., Joy, M., Drumm, I., Rushton, M.: Augmented reality in supporting healthcare and nursing independent learning: narrative review. Comput. Inform. Nursing: CIN **41**(5), 281–291 (2023). https://doi.org/10.1097/CIN.0000000000000910
9. Brown, M.: Educause Horizon Report Teaching and Learning. Educause, Louisville, CO (2020)
10. Järvelä, S., Hadwin, A., Malmberg, J., Miller, M.: Contemporary perspectives of regulated learning in collaboration. In: Fischer, F., Hmelo-Silver, C.E., Goldman, S.R., Reimann, P. (eds.) International Handbook of the Learning Sciences, pp. 127–136. Routledge, New York, NY: Routledge, 2018. (2018). https://doi.org/10.4324/9781315617572-13
11. Suh, A., Prophet, J.: The state of immersive technology research: a literature analysis. Comput. Hum. Behav. **9**, 77–90 (2018)
12. Ropponen, P., Tomietto, M., Kuivila, H., Koskenranta, M., Halili, E., Mikkonen, K.: The effects of educational interventions using VR simulations to develop nursing students' competence. PROSPERO 2023 CRD42023395095 (2023). https://www.crd.york.ac.uk/prospero/display_record.php?ID=CRD42023395095
13. Liou, S.-R., et al.: The development and psychometric testing of a theory-based instrument to evaluate nurses' perception of clinical reasoning competence. J. Adv. Nurs. **72**(3), 707–717 (2016). https://doi.org/10.1111/jan.12831
14. Unver, V.: The reliability and validity of three questionnaires: the student satisfaction and self-confidence in learning scale, simulation design scale, and educational practices questionnaire. Contemp. Nurse **1**, 60–74 (2017)

15. Franklin, A.E., Burns, P., Lee, C.S.: Psychometric testing on the NLN student satisfaction and self-confidence in learning, simulation design scale, and educational practices questionnaire using a sample of pre-licensure novice nurses. Nurse Educ. Today **34**(10), 1298–1304 (2014)
16. Chiossi, F., Welsch, R., Villa, S., Chuang, L., Mayer, S.: Virtual reality adaptation using electrodermal activity to support the user experience. BDCC **6**(2), 55 (2022)
17. Shukla, S.N., Marlin, B.M.: Integrating physiological time series and clinical notes with deep learning for improved ICU mortality prediction. Computer Science (2021)
18. EUR-Lex. General Data Protection Regulation (2016). https://eur-lex.europa.eu/search.html?scope=EURLEX&text=GDPR&lang=en&type=quick&qid=1697719513028
19. Jallad, S.T., Işık, B.: The effectiveness of virtual reality simulation as a learning strategy in the acquisition of medical skills in nursing education: a systematic review. Irish J. Med. Sci., 1–20 (2021). https://doi.org/10.1007/s11845-021-02695-z

Digital Health Innovations

Digital Empathic Healthcare: Designing Virtual Interactions for Human-Centered Experiences

Amy Grech(✉) ⓘ, Andrew Wodehouse ⓘ, and Ross Brisco ⓘ

University of Strathclyde, Glasgow G1 1XJ, UK
amy.grech.2020@uni.strath.ac.uk

Abstract. The evolution of the relationship between healthcare professionals and patients towards patient-centered care has emphasized the importance of understanding patients' perspectives, values, and needs. This shift has transformed decision-making from a technical standpoint to a more holistic approach integrating moral influences, driven by empathy. This research explores the transformative role of empathy, facilitated by Virtual Reality (VR) technology, in healthcare practitioners' interactions with patients. Inspired by VR's immersive capabilities, the novel specification entitled the Digital Empathic Design Voyage is presented as a foundation for operational virtual environments that empower humans to experience empathy. Through outcomes from literature and a qualitative study, this paper determines appropriate digital environment interactions relevant to a healthcare scenario. The research envisions a deeper understanding of patients, fostering human-oriented healthcare practices and solutions.

Keywords: Empathy · Virtual Reality · Digital Healthcare

1 Introduction

The relationship between the healthcare professional and the patient has been evolutionary. Patient-centered healthcare has led to increased empowerment of patients in decisions related to their medical care [1]. This entails healthcare professionals to fully understand the patients' perspectives, values, and needs [2] that have shifted the decision-making process from being merely based on technical expertise to a more holistic approach that integrates moral influences [3]. In fact, empathy is indicative to play a transformative role within the field of healthcare [4] which has led to increased patient satisfaction and treatment adherence [5, 6]. This could be attributed to the reduction in pain and anxiety associated with enhanced healthcare practitioner empathy [5, 7]. This not only improves the quality of the patient experience [8] but consequently enhances the well-being of professionals [9], which is also fundamental for empathy care to thrive in the first place [10]. Ostensibly, empathy in healthcare is therefore cost-effective [8]; for instance, in reducing medico-legal related risks [11].

Technology has often posed limitations to the development of empathic interactions [12]. In the past decades, psychology has highlighted simulation as a crucial process for comprehending the beliefs and perspectives of others [13, 14]. It has also been implied

M. Särestöniemi et al. (Eds.): NCDHWS 2024, CCIS 2083, pp. 191–206, 2024.
https://doi.org/10.1007/978-3-031-59080-1_14

that empathizing and 'mirroring' people's behaviors and feelings was a critical mechanism for understanding others [15]. Virtual Reality (VR) technology has the potential to emotionally engage users and foster empathy, leveraging the technology's interactive and visual elements that enable complete immersion in a virtual space and the embodiment of a digital self [16]. Particularly within the medical field, VR has proven effective in empathy training, utilizing simulation to provide a secure environment for trainees to reproduce clinical scenarios. This approach not only elicits empathic responses but also enhances behavioral skills through practical experiences [17]. Using multi-disciplinary approaches stemming from psychology and empathic design, this paper is an initial exploration of how the empathy experienced by healthcare practitioners towards patients can be augmented via a virtual environment simulation. This is achieved by determining the appropriate design requirements for an empathy-based virtual environment applicable to a healthcare setting, which is the aim of this paper. The foundation for designing the virtual experience follows the specification entitled the Digital Empathic Design Voyage [18], targeted to elicit empathic responses. The research outcome involves a novel design guideline developed as an extension of the Digital Empathic Design Voyage [18] placing focus on healthcare practitioner empathy towards patients in healthcare facilities. The goal is to reach a step further in patient-oriented healthcare practices and solutions.

1.1 Empathy in Design

For healthcare professionals to be exposed to a virtual environment simulation designed to allow them to experience the optimal level of empathy towards their patients, designers constructing that same virtual environment would also need to empathize with the users who would use the virtual environment, hence the healthcare practitioners, and the patients themselves. Duan and Hill [19] categorize empathy into two key dimensions. Cognitive empathy concerns understanding another human's situation, whilst affective empathy refers to the emotional reaction. Research suggests that designer empathy can be optimally experienced when a balance is generated between cognitive and affective empathy responses [20, 21]. Numerous methods and techniques are employed to support designer empathy in existing design processes. One approach involves observing end-users in their environments [22], while personas and journey mapping contribute to focusing on the users' standpoint [23]. Designers have also employed empathic modeling to simulate user experiences, particularly when seeking to comprehend unfamiliar situations influenced by users having diverse physical or cognitive abilities [23]. This modeling aligns with principles from psychology, where simulation is a crucial process in grasping other people's beliefs and perspectives [13, 14]. Strickfaden and Devlieger [24] underscore the importance of practical experiences that involve both the physical and emotional aspects of designers, leading to successful design solutions. This suggests that simulation allows designers to grasp users' thoughts and feelings from a first-person perspective, facilitating empathy.

Role-play serves as a simulation technique that deepens sensory engagement [25] and, consequently, positively influences empathic connections [26]. What sets role-play apart from other simulation methods is its incorporation of the narrative. Narratives, serving as a means of representation and reasoning [27], can be deemed plausible even in less immersive scenarios, such as when watching a video [28], indicating their ability to captivate viewers. Additionally, narratives contribute to the learning process, attributed to the active involvement of designers in constructing knowledge and decision-making processes as they progress toward their predefined objective [29]. The Digital Empathic Design Voyage [18] explores the power of the narrative to elicit empathy. This paper aims to apply the above methods to develop the requirements of a virtual environment that are targeted to augment healthcare practitioner empathy toward patients by eliciting a combination of cognitive and affective empathy responses.

1.2 Empathy in Virtual Spaces

Virtual Reality (VR) denotes the digital recreation of an environment [30]. In addition to the increased accessibility resulting from the decreased costs of Head-Mounted Displays (HMD) [31], VR offers various advantages applicable to empathic virtual environments. VR allows access to situations that are hazardous, expensive, and time-consuming [32]. Research indicates a positive correlation between elevated levels of graphical and audio quality and the subjective feeling of environmental presence [33, 34]. For instance, Kisker, Gruber, and Schöne [35] demonstrated that the incorporation of environmental and haptic cues could induce physiological responses akin to those in real-life interactions. Moreover, Gromer *et al.* [36] discovered that a participant's subjective sense of presence in a VR experience could predict their emotional response to it. Immersion and presence, fundamental to the effectiveness of mediated virtual environments across various applications [37], extend beyond empathic experiences to include learning and education [38]. Table 2 outlines Slater and Wilbur's [39] definitions of immersion and presence (Table 1).

Table 1. Definitions of Immersion and Presence [39]

Phenomena	Description
Immersion	The degree to which VR stimulates the sensory receptors of users
Presence	The psychological extent to which the human denotes the virtual environment as real

By embodying the viewer, virtual reality (VR) has been shown to improve perspective-taking, particularly in situations involving empathic concern [40]. The term "embodiment" denotes the viewer's capacity to project their body onto that of the avatar within the virtual environment [41]. Schutte and Stilinović [42] claim that VR's ability to evoke empathy stems from the interactive and immersive experience attained when embodying the perspective of someone else.

Empirical case studies have explored what facilitates empathy in VR in healthcare-related applications. Zhang *et al.* [43] replicated the experience of individuals, both children and adults, including adults in wheelchairs by aligning the participants' viewpoints with the intended perspective of the user. This was achieved through the dynamic scaling of the user's virtual eye height (EH) and virtual interpupillary distance (IPD).

Therefore, the perspective of the user, through spatial scale manipulation of EH and IPD could be a critical tool to simulate the experiences of multiple user groups of different ages [43]. Li *et al.* [44] added narrative elements by developing a game prototype that helped patients suffering from depression and their caregivers obtain an understanding of each other's emotional states. Character archetypes were used for the participants to virtually interact with. Additionally, sound and music positively influenced immersion, whilst the stereo vision was crucial for emotional stimulation and embodiment effects. The effect of narrative elements was also analyzed in Hu *et al.*'s [45] study which developed two virtual environments with different levels of contextual detail that simulated scenes of people having red-green color vision deficiency (CVD). The aim was to explore the effect of contextual depth and to demonstrate whether viewers can develop empathy towards this target user group. The rich contextual elements that contribute to the narrative positively influenced the accuracy, and relevance and reduced the misconceptions of the perception of the difficulties of CVD which suggests positive influences on empathy. However, for empathy to be elicited, further explicit instructions for perspective-taking were required.

Therefore, the mechanisms applied in the above studies that fostered empathy which were related to the perspective taken combined with narrative elements including rich contextual detail are further developed in this research. Other future areas of investigation include how empathy can be experienced in VR, whether it is cognitive or affective, and how it can be evaluated. Gerry *et al.* [17] claim that current research on empathy in VR lacks extensive longitudinal analysis and recommends a mixed-method approach to evaluate changes in behavior between that observed in the virtual experience and actual circumstances. In the above studies [43–45] self-reporting was one effective approach to evaluate empathy, however further exploration and standardization of evaluation methods are required for enhanced reliability.

2 Methodology

The Digital Empathic Design Voyage [18] specification was created to empower designers to experience the optimal level of empathy towards their users in a virtual space through a combination of cognitive and affective responses. To determine the applicability of the Digital Empathic Design Voyage specification to healthcare, a guideline was developed as an extension of this specification to determine detailed environment interactions of the empathic virtual space for this context. The guideline was developed by combining knowledge from The Empathy Tool Design Strategies Framework developed by Pratte, Tang, and Oehlberg [46] that encompasses empathy tools for design, the taxonomy developed by Fisher [47] for empathy in VR scenarios, and a qualitative study conducted as part of this research to explore empathic interactions towards people living with visual impairment [48]. This paper aims to develop a novel guideline that is specific to designing mechanisms for empathy in virtual environments.

The Empathy tool design strategies framework developed by Pratte, Tang, and Oehlberg [46] is a descriptive framework developed for designers that depicts how empathy was achieved within the field of human-computer interactions and classifies them according to three dimensions: agency, perspective, and sensations. Whilst Pratte, Tang, and Oehlberg [46] explored empathic design in the field of human-computer interaction, Fisher [47] sought to understand a more generalized form of empathy, but specifically for Virtual Reality mirroring design strategies through case studies. The strategies revolved around the role taken by the viewer, ranging from the viewer being a bystander to what is happening in VR to the viewer having the autonomy to make choices and affect the outcome of the VR experience. The guideline takes inspiration from the agency classification proposed by Pratte, Tang, and Oehlberg [46] which depicts the level of interactive and narrative control of the designer over the experience.

The qualitative study [48] involved conducting workshops with 57 participants from the fields of engineering design and product design. A significant majority (74%) were male, 14% were female, and one participant identified as gender diverse. Half of the students were affiliated with the United Kingdom, while the remaining participants came from various countries in Europe, Asia, Africa, and North America. The students were in the senior stage of their studies, with 77% being familiar with empathic design. Although most students (76%) were not acquainted with the lived experiences of visually impaired users, 53% expressed a willingness to learn more. The remaining participants (24%) had a closer connection to visual impairment either through personal experience or through people they know.

The participants were invited to role-play a situated interaction in pairs for 5–10 min, involving a visually impaired client sitting in a restaurant and a participant with no visual impairment who represented the server. The goal of the role play was to take an order from a menu and analyze empathic responses. The visual impairment condition was simulated through empathic modeling using glasses that represented a severe blurred vision that presented a challenge for the participant to interact with the surroundings and read the menu. This approach of integrating empathic modeling and role-play is referred to as Empathic Empowerment [48]. After Empathic Empowerment, participants were invited to enter a multi-user virtual space that provided an initial exploration of how the restaurant scenario can be virtually transformed. The environment was accessed via Oculus Quest 2 headsets and was created using ShapesXR® which is a free-to-use 3D prototyping environment for VR. The students were instructed to explore the environment for approximately 5 min by observing, interacting with objects, and engaging with each other. The visual impairment condition was not simulated in the virtual environment as the purpose of this virtual exposure was to provide students a basis of how the interaction could be represented in VR and to expose them to technological capabilities.

Following exposure to a virtual experience, the students were then invited to visualize and reflect on the transformation of the scenario into a virtual setting. The responses were gathered through a worksheet, which contained questions related to how they would imagine themselves interacting with the space considering VR's technological feasibility. The questions were inspired by multi-disciplinary knowledge by Pratte, Tang, and Oehlberg [46], Fisher [47], and literature on empathy, empathic design, and empathy in VR. Participants were asked to reflect on multiple aspects including entering and leaving the virtual space, navigation, realism, embodiment, and social interactivity.

A mixed-method approach was applied to analyze the data obtained from the worksheets. Multiple-choice questions and those answered on a Likert scale were analyzed quantitatively, whilst open-ended questions, were analyzed qualitatively through coding.

2.1 Methodology Applied to Healthcare Scenario

The interaction involved in the qualitative study was mirrored from a restaurant environment to a healthcare facility to obtain a broader perspective of how The Digital Empathic Design Voyage [18] applies to healthcare. In this case, the scenario involved an interaction between a healthcare practitioner and a visually impaired patient in a hospital bed while having a meal. A 3D space using ShapesXR® was created for a healthcare setting that served as a basis for exploration of the interactions involved in a hospital room, as shown in Fig. 1. In the environment, the viewer takes the perspective of the patient in a healthcare facility.

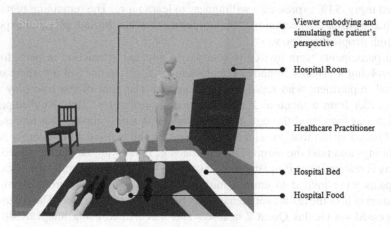

Fig. 1. First-person Perspective of Patient in Hospital accessed through ShapesXR®

The authors of this research explored the hospital room from the eyes of a patient sitting on a hospital bed by observing the surroundings and interacting with objects in front of them. The worksheet applied in the qualitative study for the restaurant scenario was adjusted for the healthcare setting. Following the exploration of the virtual environment, the worksheet was filled, to determine what would be the appropriate environment interactions for the virtual empathic environment that would facilitate healthcare practitioners to empathize with their patients.

3   Results

This section presents results obtained from the qualitative study for the restaurant scenario which were subsequently broadened to a healthcare scenario.

3.1 Restaurant Scenario Results

Table 2 presents the main results of the restaurant scenario obtained from the questionnaires submitted by the participants at the end of the study.

Table 2. Restaurant Scenario Results Obtained from the Qualitative Study

Requirements for Empathy in VR		Describing the Restaurant Scenario
▷	Gradual entering and leaving the space	"I want to visualize myself entering the restaurant from outside in VR"
🧭	Freedom of Navigation	"It depends on the person or scenario, a fixed position whilst sitting at the table would be useful." "Head movement is key for immersion because you tend to look around in a new space."
✋	Haptic Feedback	"I want realistic interactions whilst still being aware that I am in VR."
🌾	Vision and Sound Realism	"I want it to feel real and believable but not too realistic." "I want to hear other clients talking." "Lower realism may be helpful when the situation gets overwhelming."
👤	Embodiment Level	"It depends on the scenario. Embodiment of hands is sufficient when seated." "If a visually impaired person could make an outline of humans, full embodiment of the server is required."
🧍	Human Characteristics of Viewers in VR	"I am comfortable embodying someone of a similar age as me." "It is hard to embody someone with a higher mental ability."
⧂	Communication Level	"Dynamic communication is important but physical touch would be unprofessional between a client and a server

Participants generally preferred a gradual entry into the virtual space, either through a fading animation or an opening sequence with instructions. Head movement supported immersion, however, the level of navigation and embodiment is dependent on the context and perspective taken. Most participants desired the object interactions, visuals of the surrounding environment, and sound to be highly realistic for immersion purposes, however, certain participants noted that they wanted to feel aware they were in a virtual space. One participant noted that certain scenarios that may be difficult to engage with in real life, due to their emotional intensity, may benefit by having less realistic visuals. Background noise would ideally match the real environment, and many wanted to have the option to switch off the noise when needed in cases where a higher focus on the interaction is desired. Several participants could relate more with a client having similar characteristics as themselves, including age, gender, and physical and mental ability.

Future work requires further exploration of embodying others having different characteristics from the viewers in VR. Dynamic communication involving gestures, body language, facial and emotional recognition, and social openness were deemed highly beneficial, although these would be challenging for the visually impaired client. Physical touch, eye contact, and mimicry which involve the subconscious mirroring process of interaction leading to the imitation of speech patterns and body language [49] with a virtual agent were questionable amongst participants since this might lead to awkwardness, also because this depends on the type of contextual relationship. Physical touch between the server and client may be unprofessional. The results presented in Table 2 are therefore highly dependent on the contextual narrative and the perspective taken by the viewer.

Other requirements that the participants desired were a virtual companion to be with them in the virtual environment for operational instructions and a 2D user interface for various functionalities such as regaining access to the real world whenever necessary, troubleshooting, accessing VR environment settings, recording interactions through snapshots, videos, voice notes, text notes, and getting access to information sources. Participants also desire to replay or rewind the experience to pause and reflect, to observe themselves from a different perspective, and to improve their interactions and reactions and try alternative ones. Several participants desired feedback on the type and intensity of empathy experienced as a means of learning and improvement. However, others noted the subjectivity element of such a measure which might be detrimental to the empathy experienced since this would be viewed as a target and may be subject to creating false interactions to obtain more positive feedback and results.

3.2 Healthcare Scenario Results

Table 3 summarizes key results obtained from the worksheet for the healthcare application involving a patient with visual impairment in a hospital room which was presented in Sect. 2.1.

By mirroring results from Sect. 3.1, the appropriate environment interactions were determined for the healthcare scenario. A gradual entry into the virtual space, perhaps from outside the hospital room would be applicable as part of an opening sequence with background information. Freedom of head movement is required to mimic realistic scenarios. A highly realistic manipulation and control of objects is desirable, and a partial embodiment of hands would be sufficient due to the patient's fixed position. If the experience involves an interaction with a healthcare practitioner, full embodiment of the practitioner would be desirable. A semi-level of realism would be appropriate ensuring viewers are immersed in a 3D environment whilst still being aware that they are in a virtual space. Background noise would ideally match the real environment, with the option to switch off the noise when needed in cases where a higher focus on the interaction is desired. Dynamic communication is highly valuable, whilst also considering the professional relationship between the patient and caregiver. Other requirements including a virtual companion, a 2D user interface, the option to replay or rewind the experience, and taking the perspective of someone else such as the caregiver are all deemed to add value to the experience.

Table 3. Requirements for Empathy in VR Results Applied for Healthcare Scenario

Requirements for Empathy in VR		Describing the Healthcare Scenario
▷	Gradual entering and leaving the space	Visualizing the journey helps the viewer gradually immerse in the scene
🧭	Freedom of Navigation	Natural head movement is required; however, the patient in the hospital bed requires a fixed position
✋	Haptic Feedback	Realistic interactions are desirable whilst still being aware of the virtual space
🌾	Vision and Sound Realism	High visual realism but not to the extent of photorealism. Contextual background noise is required
👤	Embodiment level	Partial embodiment of hands is sufficient for the patient's perspective
🧍	Human Characteristics of Viewers in VR	Similar characteristics between viewer and patient apply, except vision
⸭	Communication level	Dynamic communication is critical in maintaining a professional relationship with the healthcare practitioner

4 Discussion

When comparing a visually impaired client in a restaurant and a visually impaired patient in a hospital, results demonstrate common elements in the environment interactions such as the level of navigation, embodiment, and object interactivity. However, the contextual narrative of both scenarios is very different. The hospital environment may subject the viewer to a more vulnerable state of mind. The narrative presented to the viewer as they gradually enter the hospital room may elicit stronger emotions. The communication in the interaction between a healthcare practitioner and a patient versus that of a restaurant server and a client would also differ significantly. This implies that a lower level of vision and sound realism may be required in the healthcare scenario to prevent the viewer from feeling overwhelmed. Therefore, the context plays a critical role the designing an empathic virtual space. Future work requires further development on how the narrative influences the resulting empathic responses. In this case, the narrative should be built around how healthcare professionals and servers are trained to communicate with people living with visual impairment to serve as learning experiences for practitioners needing to develop empathy towards visually impaired patients in a hospital setting.

Different scenarios and user conditions may present different design requirements in VR. The qualitative study performed in this research helped determine the requirements for a visually impaired client in a restaurant. However, performing studies in physical settings for other scenarios including other human conditions and environments might be time-consuming and costly. This paper broadened the knowledge obtained from the qualitative study to another scenario by transforming the restaurant environment into a hospital room. By combining knowledge developed by Pratte, Tang, and Oehlberg [46],

Fisher [47], and the outcomes of the qualitative study [48] conducted in this research which led to the results presented in this paper, a novel guideline was developed to support designers in determining the appropriate design requirements for any specific scenario targeting empathy in VR. The guideline, presented in Table 4, describes the specific environment mechanisms for empathy in VR and is presented as an extension to the Digital Empathic Design Voyage specification [18]. Such design requirements are listed in the 'Design Factors' column and are applied at a certain level of intensity. The intensity depends on the application itself, including the perspective taken by the viewer, the narrative role of the viewer, and the contextual narrative. The intensity of each factor is categorized according to three levels: High, Mid, and Low; however, these represent a spectrum of different levels of intensity that can be intermixed and combined as deemed most appropriate for the application. The intensities for each design factor determined for the healthcare scenario being considered in this paper are presented in Bold format below.

In this analysis, the environment interactions were determined for experiencing the perspective of visually impaired patients from a first-person perspective. The design guideline presented in Table 4 may differ depending on the perspective taken, therefore the design requirements would need to be determined for every role taken by the viewer in the same application. Relevant design requirements would also need to be established for any virtual agents that the viewer would be interacting with, such as their level of embodiment and realism. According to the Digital Empathic Design Voyage specification [18] the viewer is encouraged to embody multiple perspectives of the same scenario to holistically experience a combination of cognitive and affective responses. In this case, after the viewer takes the perspective of the patient, the same scenario is repeated by embodying the perspective of the healthcare caregiver.

Besides embodying multiple perspectives, this guideline strengthens further the balance between the prescribed narrative of the scenario and the viewer's level of agency and empowerment over the outcome of that scenario, which were key contributors to eliciting empathy in the qualitative study performed [48] and is relevant to healthcare scenarios as demonstrated in Sect. 3.2. The extent to which the viewer's agency determines the outcome of the scenario requires further empirical analysis, including in the field of healthcare, however, this guideline provides the required support for designers to achieve the right balance applicable to their scenario through enhanced structure and visualization, whilst also considering technological characteristics determined by VR. Pre-trials in VR are recommended to ensure the right balance is achieved between what the narrative communicates to the viewer and the viewer's level of autonomy whilst also determining the implications for healthcare practices. This guideline is subject to development following further research and technological advancements.

Limitations of this qualitative study are associated with potential biases from participants due to the relatively small sample size and cultural heterogeneity [50]. Future studies should be conducted to expand both the size and diversity of the sample. A challenge in designing the virtual environment is related to the acquisition of sufficient information from real patients and healthcare practitioners to construct the narrative. The Empathic Empowerment Scale [48] presents a novel evaluation system for analyzing empathic responses during the virtual experience. Future work of this research

Table 4. The Digital Empathic Design Voyage: Environment Interactions Guideline

Design Factors	High/ +	Mid	Low/−
Navigation Factors			
Navigational Agency	Full Freedom: Navigation of the virtual environment as in the real scenario. **Freedom of head motion**	Partial Freedom: Navigation of the space using controllers. **A virtual companion assists with navigation**	Fixed Position: **Navigation is fully guided by a virtual companion or by the narrative**
Narrative Factors			
Narrative Agency	Full Dramatic Agency: Choices have a consequence on the outcome. Full manipulation of the outcome	**Mixed Approach: The VR environment has partial control of the outcome**	Passive Witness: The VR environment has full control of the outcome. Highly structured narrative
Realism of Narrative	**High Contextual Depth: High level of contextual richness communicated by the environment**. Use of multi-sensory engagement such as aromas and spatial diegetic sound that matches the real scenario. High level of spatial depth through lighting and shadows. The narrative occurs in real-time. The narrative is related to real-life scenarios or based on facts. The narrative involves high emotional engagement	Mid Contextual Depth: Good level of contextual depth and multi-sensory engagement. Use of virtual and audio cues that support the narrative. The narrative may not happen constantly in real time. **Presence of virtual companion. Partial use of user interface during the experience**	Low Contextual Depth: Limited contextual depth and multi-sensory engagement. High use of virtual and audio cues to guide the viewer. High dependency on virtual companion and user interface. The narrative does not occur in real-time. The narrative involves low emotional engagement
Sensory Factors			
Visual Agency	**Full visual exploration: Limited by the size of the physical space**	Medium visual exploration: Limited by 1–2 obstacles in the real or virtual environment	Limited visual exploration: Obstacles in the real or virtual environment limit exploration
Object Agency	**Full manipulation and control: In the same manner as the user's reference population**	Medium manipulation and control: High level of realism achieved via controllers	Limited manipulation and control: Low level of realism with controllers

(*continued*)

Table 4. (*continued*)

Design Factors	High/ +	Mid	Low/−
Realism of Visuals	High Realism: The environment is photorealistic, denoted by high graphic resolution, realistic forms, materials, textures, and stereo vision. Avatars' appearance is highly realistic	**Semi-Realism: The environment and avatars' appearance are not realistic but have 3D form and some implementation of materials and textures**	Low Realism: The environment and avatars' appearance are not realistic and may be abstract or in 2D form. Limited use of materials and textures
Realism of Interactions	High Realism: Interactions are matched with real objects. **Multi-sensory interactions include tactile and haptic feedback,** ground vibrations, temperature, and humidity conditions. **Dynamic interactivity with other avatars**	**Mixed Realism: A combination of high and low realism of interactions is achieved**	Low Realism: Interactions are virtual. Limited multi-sensory and physiological interactions. Low interactivity with other avatars
Embodiment Factors			
Role Agency	Full Embodiment: Full body visualization and interaction. Possibility of appearance customization. Option to control the level of embodiment	**Partial Embodiment: Head, torso, and hands visualization and interaction. Possibility of appearance customization. Option to control the level of embodiment**	Limited embodiment: No visualization but may include interaction via controllers. No possibility of appearance customization
Role Characteristics	Fully Matched: Physical and cognitive characteristics between the viewer and the role taken are very similar	**Partially Matched: Few physical and cognitive characteristics between the viewer and the role taken differ**	Not Matched: Physical and cognitive characteristics between the viewer and the role taken are not similar

involves conducting an empirical analysis of The Digital Empathic Design Voyage with this evaluation system in VR.

5   Conclusions

This research explores The Digital Empathic Design Voyage specification [18] to support the development of a virtual environment to elicit empathy by healthcare practitioners toward their patients. By combining knowledge by Pratte, Tang, and Oehlberg [46], Fisher [47], and the outcomes of the qualitative study [48] conducted as part of this research to analyze empathy in VR, this paper presents a unique design guideline, presented as an extension of The Digital Empathic Design Voyage [18], to determine the most appropriate environment interactions for any application driven by empathy. The guideline was applied for one scenario involving a virtual environment that would empower healthcare practitioners and caregivers to obtain a deep understanding of visually impaired patients' experience in a healthcare facility. The outcome of this paper serves as a foundation for the exploration of other patients in different scenarios and of other applications requiring empathy. Other scenarios include having remote patient-physician consultations, telemedicine settings, physical outpatient clinic consultations, or procedure simulations. This research aims to take a significant stride toward developing the next generation of patient-centered healthcare practices intended to augment inclusivity and social value through practical and empowering experiences. Future work involves conducting empirical analysis in collaboration with healthcare professionals and visually impaired individuals to obtain a deeper understanding of healthcare scenarios. The resulting empathy will be also analyzed using the Empathic Empowerment Scale [48]. Therefore, the Digital Empathic Design Voyage [18] combined with the Empathic Empowerment Scale [48] provide the groundwork for designing and evaluating future virtual empathic experiences in industrial, research, and pedagogical settings across multiple disciplines including design, architecture, computer science, and any other field that requires a deep understanding of others, particularly those having different characteristics, such as age, physical and cognitive ability, and are therefore deemed highly valuable within the domain of digital healthcare.

Acknowledgments. The research is funded by the National Manufacturing Institute of Scotland (NMIS).

References

1. Kerasidou, A.: Artificial intelligence and the ongoing need for empathy, compassion and trust in healthcare. Bull. World Health Organ. **98**, 245–250 (2020). https://doi.org/10.2471/BLT. 19.237198
2. Emanuel, E.J., Emanuel, L.L.: Four models of the physician-patient relationship. JAMA **267**(16), 2221–2226 (1992). https://doi.org/10.1001/jama.1992.03480160079038
3. Bauchat, J.R., Seropian, M., Jeffries, P.R.: Communication and empathy in the patient-centered care model—why simulation-based training is not optional. Clin. Simul. Nurs. **12**(8), 356–359 (2016). https://doi.org/10.1016/j.ecns.2016.04.003
4. Howick, J., Rees, S.: Overthrowing barriers to empathy in healthcare: empathy in the age of the Internet. J. R. Soc. Med. **110**(9), 352–357 (2017). https://doi.org/10.1177/014107681771 4443
5. Kelley, J.M., Kraft-Todd, G., Schapira, L., Kossowsky, J., Riess, H.: The influence of the patient-clinician relationship on healthcare outcomes: a systematic review and meta-analysis of randomized controlled trials. PLoS ONE **9**(4), e94207 (2014). https://doi.org/10.1371/jou rnal.pone.0094207
6. Joffe, S., Manocchia, M., Weeks, J.C., Cleary, P.D.: What do patients value in their hospital care? An empirical perspective on autonomy centred bioethics. J. Med. Ethics **29**(2), 103–108 (2003). https://doi.org/10.1136/jme.29.2.103

7. Howick, J., et al.: Effects of changing practitioner empathy and patient expectations in healthcare consultations **11** (2015), https://doi.org/10.1002/14651858.CD011934

8. Mercer, S.W., et al.: The CARE Plus study–a whole-system intervention to improve quality of life of primary care patients with multimorbidity in areas of high socioeconomic deprivation: exploratory cluster randomised controlled trial and cost-utility analysis. BMC Med. **14**(88), 10 (2016). https://doi.org/10.1186/s12916-016-0634-2

9. Thomas, M.R., et al.: How do distress and well-being relate to medical student empathy? A multicenter study. J. Gen. Intern. Med. **22**(2), 177–183 (2007). https://doi.org/10.1007/s11 606-006-0039-6

10. Kang, E.S., Di Genova, T., Howick, J., Gottesman, R.: Adding a dose of empathy to healthcare: What can healthcare systems do? J. Eval. Clin. Pract. **28**(3), 475–482 (2022). https://doi.org/10.1111/jep.13664

11. Heydarian, A., Becerik-Gerber, B.: Use of immersive virtual environments for occupant behaviour monitoring and data collection. J. Build. Perform. Simul. **10**(5–6), 484–498 (2017). https://doi.org/10.1080/19401493.2016.1267801

12. Barbot, B., Kaufman, J.C.: What makes immersive virtual reality the ultimate empathy machine? Discerning the underlying mechanisms of change. Comput. Hum. Behav. **111**, 106431 (2020). https://doi.org/10.1016/j.chb.2020.106431

13. Keysers, C., Gazzola, V.: Integrating simulation and theory of mind: from self to social cognition. Trends Cogn. Sci. **11**(5), 194–196 (2007). https://doi.org/10.1016/j.tics.2007.02.002

14. Kampis, D., Southgate, V.: Altercentric cognition: how others influence our cognitive processing. Trends Cogn. Sci. **24**(11), 945–959 (2020). https://doi.org/10.1016/j.tics.2020.09.003

15. Iacoboni, M.: Mirroring People: The Science of Empathy and How We Connect with Others. Picador, New York (2009)

16. Markowitz, D., Bailenson, J.: Virtual reality and communication. Hum. Commun. Res. **34**, 287–318 (2019). https://doi.org/10.1093/obo/9780199756841-0222

17. Gerry, L.J., Billinghurst, M., Broadbent, E.: Empathic skills training in virtual reality: a scoping review. In: 2022 Conference on Virtual Reality and 3D User Interfaces Abstracts and Workshops (VRW). pp. 227–232. IEEE (2022)

18. Grech, A., Wodehouse, A., Brisco, R.: Designer empathy in virtual reality: transforming the designer experience closer to the user. In: IASDR 2023: Life-Changing Design. 119. IASDR (2023)

19. Duan, C., Hill, C.E.: The current state of empathy research. J. Couns. Psychol. **43**(3), 261–274 (1996). https://doi.org/10.1037/0022-0167.43.3.261

20. Battarbee, K., Suri, J.F., Howard, S.G.: Empathy on the edge: Scaling and sustaining a human-centered approach to innovation. Harvard Bus. Rev., 1–14 (2015)

21. Hess, J.L., Fila, N.D.: The development and growth of empathy among engineering students. In: 2016 ASEE Annual Conference and Exposition, pp. 26–29. ASEE (2016)

22. Patnaik, D.: Wired to Care: How Companies Prosper When They Create Widespread Empathy. FT Press, New Jersey (2009)

23. Raviselvam, S., Hwang, D., Camburn, B., Sng, K., Hölttä-Otto, K., Wood, K.L.: Extreme-user conditions to enhance design creativity and empathy-application using visual impairment. Int. J. Design Creat. Innov. **10**(2), 75–100 (2022). https://doi.org/10.1080/21650349.2021.2024093

24. Strickfaden, M., Devlieger, P.: Empathy through accumulating techné: designing an accessible metro. Des. J. **14**(2), 207–229 (2011). https://doi.org/10.2752/175630611X12984592780041

25. Altay, B., Demirkan, H.: Inclusive design: developing students' knowledge and attitude through empathic modelling. Int. J. Incl. Educ. **18**(2), 196–217 (2014). https://doi.org/10.1080/13603116.2013.764933

26. Moody, L., Mackie, E., Davies, S.: Building empathy with the User. In: Karwowski, Soares, Stanton (eds.) Human factors and ergonomics in consumer product design: Uses and applications, Boca Raton, pp. 177–198. CRC Press (2011)
27. Bruner, I.: Acts of meaning. Psychol. Med. **22**(2), 531–531 (1990). https://doi.org/10.1017/s0033291700030555
28. Cummings, J.J., Tsay-Vogel, M., Cahill, T.J., Zhang, L.: Effects of immersive storytelling on affective, cognitive, and associative empathy: the mediating role of presence. New Media Soc. **24**(9), 2003–2026 (2022). https://doi.org/10.1177/1461444820986816
29. Bell, P., Davis, E.A., Linn, M.C.: The knowledge integration environment: theory and design. In: International Conference on Computer Support for Collaborative Learning (CSCL), pp. 14–21 (1995)
30. Meyer, O.A., Omdahl, M.K., Makransky, G.: Investigating the effect of pre-training when learning through immersive virtual reality and video: a media and methods experiment. Comput. Educ. **140**, 103603 (2019). https://doi.org/10.1016/j.compedu.2019.103603
31. Neo, J.R.J., Won, A.S., Shepley, M.M.: Designing immersive virtual environments for human behavior research. Front. Virtual Real. **2** (2021). https://doi.org/10.3389/frvir.2021.603750
32. Bailenson, J.: Experience on Demand: What Virtual Reality is, How it Works, and What it Can Do. W.W. Norton & Company, New York (2018)
33. Makransky, G., Lilleholt, L., Aaby, A.: Development and validation of the multimodal presence scale for virtual reality environments: a confirmatory factor analysis and item response theory approach. Comput. Hum. Behav. **72**, 276–285 (2017). https://doi.org/10.1016/j.chb.2017.02.066
34. Shu, Y., Huang, Y.-Z., Chang, S.-H., Chen, M.-Y.: Do virtual reality head-mounted displays make a difference? A comparison of presence and self-efficacy between head-mounted displays and desktop computer-facilitated virtual environments. Virtual Reality **23**, 437–446 (2019). https://doi.org/10.1007/s10055-018-0376-x
35. Kisker, J., Gruber, T., Schöne, B.: Behavioral realism and lifelike psychophysiological responses in virtual reality by the example of a height exposure. Psychol. Res. **85**, 68–81 (2021). https://doi.org/10.1007/s00426-019-01244-9
36. Gromer, D., et al.: Height simulation in a virtual reality CAVE system: validity of fear responses and effects of an immersion manipulation. Front. Hum. Neurosci. **12**, 372 (2018). https://doi.org/10.3389/fnhum.2018.00372
37. Cummings, J.J., Bailenson, J.N.: How immersive is enough? A meta-analysis of the effect of immersive technology on user presence. Media Psychol. **19**(2), 272–309 (2016). https://doi.org/10.1080/15213269.2015.1015740
38. Monahan, T., McArdle, G., Bertolotto, M.: Virtual reality for collaborative e-learning. Comput. Educ. **50**(4), 1339–1353 (2008). https://doi.org/10.1016/j.compedu.2006.12.008
39. Slater, M., Wilbur, S.: A framework for immersive virtual environments (FIVE): speculations on the role of presence in virtual environments. Presence: Teleoperators Virtual Environ. **6**(6), 603–616 (1997). https://doi.org/10.1162/pres.1997.6.6.603
40. Hasler, B.S., Spanlang, B., Slater, M.: Virtual race transformation reverses racial in-group bias. PloS One **12** (2017). https://doi.org/10.1371/journal.pone.0174965
41. Villalba, É.E., Azócar, A.L.S.M., Jacques-García, F.A.: State of the art on immersive virtual reality and its use in developing meaningful empathy. Comput. Electrical Eng.**93** (2021). https://doi.org/10.1016/j.compeleceng.2021.107272
42. Schutte, N.S., Stilinović, E.J.: Facilitating empathy through virtual reality. Motiv. Emot. **41**, 708–712 (2017). https://doi.org/10.1007/s11031-017-9641-7
43. Zhang, J., Dong, Z., Bai, X., Lindeman, R.W., He, W., Piumsomboon, T.: Augmented perception through spatial scale manipulation in virtual reality for enhanced empathy in design-related tasks. Front. Virtual Reality **3** (2022). https://doi.org/10.3389/frvir.2022.672537

44. Li, Y.J., Huang, A., Sanku, B.S., He, J.S.: Designing an empathy training for depression prevention using virtual reality and a preliminary study. In: IEEE Conference on Virtual Reality and 3D User Interfaces Abstracts and Workshops (VRW), pp. 44–52. IEEE (2023)
45. Hu, X., Casakin, H., Georgiev, G.V.: Bridging designer-user gap with a virtual reality-based empathic design approach: contextual information details. Proc. Design Soc. **3**, 797–806 (2023). https://doi.org/10.1017/pds.2023.80
46. Pratte, S., Tang, A., Oehlberg, L.: Evoking empathy: a framework for describing empathy tools. In: International Conference on Tangible, Embedded, and Embodied Interaction (TEI), vol. 25, pp. 1–15 (2021)
47. Fisher, J.A.: Empathic actualities: toward a taxonomy of empathy in virtual reality. In: International Conference on Interactive Digital Storytelling (ICIDS). pp. 233–244 (2017)
48. Grech, A., Wodehouse, A., Brisco, R.: Empathic empowerment: an exploration and analysis of a situated interaction through empathic modelling and role-play. In: International DESIGN Conference (DESIGN) (2024)
49. Salmi, A., Li, J., Hölttä-Otto , K. Facial expression recognition as a measure of user-designer empathy. In: International Design Engineering Technical Conferences and Computers and Information in Engineering Conference (IDETC), 34th International Conference on Design Theory and Methodology (DTM), vol. 6, p. 10 (2022)
50. Li, J., Hölttä-Otto, K.: The influence of designers' cultural differences on the empathic accuracy of user understanding. Des. J. **23**(5), 779–796 (2020). https://doi.org/10.1080/14606925.2020.1810414

Developing a Digital Gaming Intervention with Yetitablet® to Improve Older People's Functioning and Activity in Long-Term-Care – a Feasibility Study

Saara Kukkohovi[1]([⊠]) [iD], Heidi Siira[1] [iD], and Satu Elo[2] [iD]

[1] University of Oulu, Aapistie 5 A, 90220 Oulu, Finland
`saara.kukkohovi@oulu.fi`
[2] Oulu University of Applied Sciences, Kiviharjuntie 4, 90220 Oulu, Finland

Abstract. Long-term care (LTC) residents often have many health problems and functional limitations, and their sedentary behavior is common. Playing digital games is one way to improve the well-being, functioning, and activity of older people. The purpose of this study was to test a digital gaming intervention with a new device in an LTC environment before the larger effectiveness study. The aim was to produce information on the benefits of the digital gaming intervention for residents, the success of the implementation of the intervention and the factors affecting it. One LTC facility for older people participated in the study. The data was collected with a semi-structured thematic interview after an eight-week intervention. The interview data was analyzed using inductive content analysis. Staff experiences of the benefits of the intervention were classified into three main categories: The intervention enabled a new kind of physical activity, the intervention increased the social activity and brought residents together and the intervention brought joy and variety to the residents. Success of the intervention implementation was classified into three main categories: active participation of the residents in the gaming sessions, low involvement of staff in the implementation of the intervention and variable success of implementing the intervention protocol in the everyday life of LTC facility. Factors affecting the implementation formed nine main categories. This feasibility study highlighted important factors related to the implementation of the intervention, which must be considered in the future for the success of the effectiveness study.

Keywords: Digital games · functioning · activity · long-term care · older people

1 Introduction

1.1 Background

Long-term care (LTC) residents often have many health problems and functional impairments. It has been noticed that physical activity of care dwelling older people is significantly lower than community dwelling older people [1] and older women living in LTC

© The Author(s) 2024
M. Särestöniemi et al. (Eds.): NCDHWS 2024, CCIS 2083, pp. 207–222, 2024.
https://doi.org/10.1007/978-3-031-59080-1_15

have been observed to spend over 70% of their time sitting or lying during daytime [2]. Lower level of physical activity is associated with more symptoms of anxiety and depression and lower physical performance [3, 4]. Time spent in weight bearing positions and activities is associated with better balance and physical performance while sedentary time is associated with reduced muscle strength, balance, and physical performance [2]. Sedentary time and functional impairments weaken ability to cope with daily activities and the quality of life, and thus cause an increased need for care and caring resources.

One of the promising ways to improve the well-being, functioning and activity of older people is digital gaming which is traditionally used as a leisure activity for younger people. Digital games are played on a digital device such as a tablet computer or a video game console. Nowadays the term serious games is also used, which means that playing has a serious purpose such as exercise, health, or rehabilitation [5]. The effectiveness of digital gaming on the functioning and activity of older people has been studied over the past ten years, and the results have been promising. Digital gaming has been found to improve balance, mobility, and gate [6, 7], promote social interaction [8], and reduce loneliness [9] and depression also on older people with memory disorder [10].

Despite the benefits of digital gaming, the implementation of it in LTC's everyday life can be challenging. The cost of these games is usually not very high [6] but there might be other barriers for implementation of digital games in LTC. These are for example lack of space, lack of the time required for staff to introduce games to residents and older people's lack of competence in using technology [6, 8]. Healthcare professionals may feel insecure about their own digital skills [11] and attitudes towards new technologies may be rejective, which reduces motivation to adopt new technologies [12]. Also, all the games and devices are not designed for the use of older people [8] and may therefore require quick response, hand-eye coordination, jumping, reaching, or other activities that can be challenging for the older people and require repetition and practice to successfully complete the game.

Mostly used and studied gaming device in LTC environment is Nintendo Wii [13] but in addition, new games and devices are designed and developed for the older people to meet their special needs [14–16]. There is not much scientific research evidence yet available on the effectiveness of these new technologies on the functioning and activity of older people. Also, the focus of digital game research has been on independently living and healthy older people, so there is a need for game research conducted in the context of long-term care and with population who already has functional decline in many areas. In many previous interventions games have been guided for LTC residents mainly by research staff but this study is carried out in the everyday life of a LTC facility, and the staff implements the digital gaming intervention. Previous digital gaming research has also focused on physical performance, and there is still only little research that considers the social and psychological aspects of gaming [13, 17].

1.2 Objectives

The aim of this study was to test the implementation of digital gaming intervention on a small scale before the full-scale effectiveness study to detect its possible problems. The objective was to obtain information on the feasibility of the intervention and the factors influencing the successful implementation of it, obtain preliminary information on the benefits of the intervention on long-term care residents' functioning and activity, and test the performance of functional capacity measurements for LTC-residents. We also wanted to test the use of activity monitors with this population which will be used in the future effectiveness study to gain information about changes in physical activity. Research questions were:

1. What benefits does the digital gaming intervention have on the functioning and activity of the residents?
2. How does the implementation of the intervention succeed?
3. What factors influence the implementation of the intervention?

2 Methods

2.1 Study Design, Setting and Participants

This was a qualitative feasibility study. One long-term care facility located in Northern Finland participated in this study. The LTC facility and participants were selected by purposeful sampling. Both residents of the facility and the staff were invited to participate in the study. Facility residents were invited to participate in the intervention and staff were invited to participate in the post-intervention interview. Participants of the intervention were selected between February and March 2023 according to the inclusion and exclusion criteria by the personnel of the facility who knew the residents well. Inclusion criteria to participate in this study were: 1) able to walk (independently) at least 10 m with or without walking aid 2) sufficient cognitive ability to understand the purpose of the study and instructions for the gaming 3) does not have any disease that would prevent light exercise 4) does not have any acute severe disease 5) living permanently in the facility. Exclusion criteria were: 1) not able to walk independently or with walking aid 2) severe memory disorder or other severe or acute illness 3) too poor vision to play games 4) is receiving some other treatment which may affect the change in functioning or activity. The researcher introduced the study to suitable residents, distributed the research information forms and inquired about their interest in participating in the study. The intern working in the facility contacted the relatives of the residents and delivered the consent forms to sign. Facility staff and interns who participated in the intervention's implementation were invited to participate in the post-intervention interviews.

2.2 Intervention

Eligible residents participated in an eight-week digital gaming intervention with a Finnish innovation, a Yetitablet (picture 1). Yetitablet is a large tablet computer with 55–65″ screen utilizing Android operating system. Yetitablet has a touch screen and a mobile stand on wheels, which allows the screen to be raised and lowered, as well as tilted as needed, all the way to a desk position. Large screen size enables group activities and social interaction. Yetitablet includes YetiCare software which gives Yetitablet an accessible user interface and has many stimulating applications for entertainment, rehabilitation, and physical exercise [18] (Fig. 1).

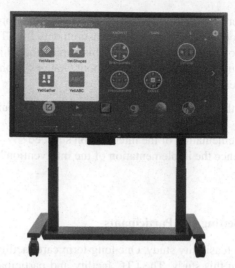

Fig. 1. Yetitablet and YetiCare applications

The development of the intervention started by conducting a systematic literature review on the previously implemented digital game interventions and their effectiveness on the functioning and activity of older people in a long-term care setting [13]. The dosage and duration of the intervention were determined based on this review.First, a one-hour training session was held for the facility staff. A member of the YetiCare company introduced the Yetitablet and advised how to use it remotely via Teams. After the introduction the principal investigator presented the intervention and guided staff in testing the Yetitablet and its games. During the intervention, study participants could choose the games and the amount of gaming because it better reflects the real-life situation and gives a true picture of the effects in a long-term care environment on this population. However, facility personnel were instructed to organize three gaming sessions per week, lasting for about half an hour to one hour. The personnel were instructed to consider the players' physical and cognitive functioning and coping when directing the games and to adjust the game session according to the participants' resources. Games were encouraged to be played with about four participants or more. As the intervention progressed, instructions were given to consider the progression of participants so that a more challenging level was selected for the games, and playing would take place as much as possible in a standing position. All persons working in the unit could carry out the intervention. A logbook was given for the facility and gaming session instructors were asked to mark down every playing sessions' date, duration, participants, and games played during the session. The logbook also contained instructions for the intervention, for example what games could be played, how to make progress to the program, playing in a standing position and in groups. The Yetitablet and logbook were placed in a large multiuse room next to the dayroom.

YetiCare applications (later: games) were classified into the following categories in the Yetitablet: coordination, motor skills, smart games, and entertainment. YetiCoordination included games like darts, bowling and YetiCups (picture 2). These games are played by throwing soft balls at the screen. Also, YetiReaction, YetiCups and YetiBubbles were included in the coordination category, but those games are played by touching the screen. These games require reaction ability, body and movement control and balance if games are played in a standing position. Motor skills category included games like YetiForms, YetiGather and YetiMaze. In these games a player must use fine motors skills in the upper limbs to reach the goal of the game such as moving an object from the starting point to the finish line through a labyrinth. YetiBrain Games included games like a memory game, guess the word –game and a word grid. These games require short term memory, attention, and perceptiveness. Entertainment category included games like table hockey or football, tic-tac-toe, and trivia. Although these games are classified as entertainment, playing them requires for example concentration, quick reactions, body control and weight shifting if played standing up. The staff were instructed to use the YetiCare gamified applications, but they were also allowed to use other content downloaded to the tablet such as Google Maps, newspapers, card games, sudoku and sensory applications. The staff and/or residents could choose the games played during the gaming sessions (Fig. 2).

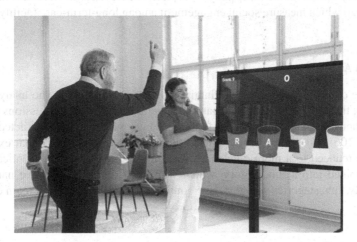

Fig. 2. Example of YetiCare coordination game, YetiCups

2.3 Data Collection

Qualitative data was collected during this study to obtain information on the intervention's benefits to the residents and its feasibility. Data was collected from the facility staff through a semi-structured thematic interview [19]. Two interns working at the facility at the time of the intervention and one permanent facility staff member participated. The interviewees were a nurse, an occupational therapist student and a geronomy student. Interviews were carried out after an eight-week intervention period in June 2023 via Teams and recorded with the permission of the participants. Two participants were interviewed together and one alone for scheduling reasons. The group interview lasted

59 min and the interview with one participant lasted 28 min. The interviews proceeded according to pre-planned themes which were attitudes towards the intervention and new technology, benefits of intervention for residents, the strain caused by the intervention on staff and residents, implementation of the intervention and usability of the Yetitablet. In addition, the personnel were asked for their thoughts and suggestions for changes related to the intervention protocol. The interview questions were based on earlier research about technology acceptance [20] and ICF framework [21]. The material was transcribed and the total number of transcribed material was 16 pages with the text type Times New Roman, with font 12 with a line spacing of 1.5.

Functioning measurements were done to the residents participating in the intervention before and after the eight-week intervention to test the suitability of the measurements for the target group. Testing data was not analyzed in this study due to the small sample size. Measures done were Short Physical Performance Battery (SPPB) which measures the mobility of older people, and it combines the results of balance tests, gait speed and chair stand [22], Timed Up and Go test (TUG) which measures mobility and balance [23], Geriatric depression scale (GDS-15) which is developed for identifying depressive symptoms in the older people [24] and The Revised Index for Social Engagement (RISE) which measure social engagement among long-term-care facility residents [25].

2.4 Data Analysis

Qualitative data was analyzed by inductive content analysis [26]. The analysis began by reading through the transcribed material several times. Next, expressions (sentence or set of thoughts) that corresponded to the research questions were extracted from the data (n = 106) and grouped according to the research question. Original expressions were then reduced to a more condensed form and expressions with identical content were combined into a subcategory, which were named with descriptive names (n = 36). Finally, subcategories with the same content were grouped to form main categories (n = 15).

3 Ethical Considerations

The study was approved by the regional medical research ethics committee of the Wellbeing services county of North Ostrobothnia (reference number: 49/2021) and research permission was requested from the facility. The aim, objective and procedure of the study were presented to the eligible subjects and their relatives/close ones. After informing eligible subjects and their close ones, written informed consent was obtained from participants or their trustee. Participants had the right to withdraw from the study at any time.

4 Results

4.1 Characteristics of the Residents Participating in the Intervention

Out of 18 residents in the facility eight were eligible to participate in the study based on the inclusion criteria and one refused to participate due to old age. Four residents who participated in the intervention were men and three were women. The mean age of participants was 86 years (range 8198 years). Participants had multiple physical, sensory, and cognitive impairments. All participants had a diagnosed memory disorder, one had poor vision and two had osteoarthritis. Male participants did not have walking aids, but all participating women used a walker. A summary of baseline characteristics of the residents participating in the intervention is presented in Table 1.

Table 1. Baseline characteristics of the residents participating in the intervention

Variable	Sub-category	
Age in years, mean (SD)		86.1 (6.4)
Gender, n (%)	Male	4 (57.1)
	Female	3 (42.9)
Walking aid, n (%)	No	4 (57.1)
	Yes	3 (42.9)
Memory disorder	No	0 (0.0)
	Yes	7 (100.0)

4.2 Implementation of Functioning Measurements and Intervention

Functioning measures could have been performed on the research participants. One participant refused to do the Timed Up and Go (TUG) and Short Physical Performance Battery (SPPB) measures in pretest and posttest and one refused to do Geriatric depression Scale (GDS-15) in the posttest. All seven participants finished the eight-week intervention program without any injuries. Gaming sessions lasted from five (5) minutes to two hours with an average of 30 min and participants played games from zero to four times per week based on the logbook.

4.3 Benefits of the Intervention for the Residents

Staff experiences of benefits of the digital gaming intervention were classified into three main categories: The intervention enabled a new kind of physical activity, the intervention increased the social a0ctivity and brought residents together and the intervention brought joy and variety to the residents. The intervention was described as enabling residents to engage in new kinds of physical activities by increasing residents' physical activity and requiring different body movement from the player for example compared to walking exercise. One resident who rarely left his room became more active and he started moving in the common areas of the LCT facility. Some of the residents liked playing games like bowling while standing, and that required weight shifting, reaching out in different directions, and picking balls from the floor. *"He surprised me by throwing balls and picking them up from the floor by himself."* Interviewee 2.

The intervention increased the social activity of the residents and brought them together, as the intervention increased the social interaction of the residents, created a connection between them, and acted as a joint activity and increased interaction. Part of the gaming sessions were held in pairs or in small groups and residents who usually do not interact with each other's played together and had a conversation. *"They started playing together and talked to each other on the side, in a way the ones that don't usually get closer to each other."* Interviewee 3. One resident often encouraged other players and became friends with others. Gaming was said to bring the residents together, which created a sense of community.

The intervention brought joy and variety to the residents, as the games delighted and increased residents' alertness and it was seen as a meaningful and varied activity. Residents had fun while playing games and one resident laughed and giggled while playing. *"...this is funny, she giggled, and she had so much fun."* Interviewee 1. One resident who never participated in activities found himself meaningful activity through gaming (Table 2).

Table 2. Qualitative analysis

Subcategory	Main category
Benefits of the intervention	
Playing increased residents' physical activity	The intervention enabled a new kind of physical activity
Playing required different body movement	
Intervention increased social interaction among residents	The intervention increased the social activity and brought residents together
Intervention created a connection between residents	
Gaming worked as a joint activity and increased interaction	
The intervention delighted and increased residents' alertness	The intervention brought joy and variety to the residents
Gaming as a meaningful and varied activity	
Success of implementing the intervention	
The staff showed little interest in the Yetitablet	Low involvement of staff in the implementation of the intervention
Few of the staff used the Yetitablet	
Residents participated in the game when requested	Active participation of the residents in the gaming sessions

(continued)

Table 2. (*continued*)

Subcategory	Main category
Gaming physical and mental load suitable for residents	
Residents were able to concentrate on playing well	
Game sessions can be arranged regularly	Variable success of implementing the intervention protocol in the everyday life of LTC facility
Varying success of playing while standing up	
The challenges of playing together	
Group play implementation challenging	
Filling out the game log challenging	
Factors affecting the implementation	
Staff motivation to do new things affects implementation	Positive attitude and motivation of staff important in implementation
Staff enthusiasm to try new things	
Staff struggling to adopt new technology	Staff attitude towards technology can challenge implementation
Negative attitude of staff towards learning to use new technology	
Yetitablet's easy use supported its use	Staff competence in using Yetitablet
The challenges of using Yetitablet	
Practical orientation and user support help the implementation	Practical training, clear instructions and an example of use support the implementation
Example of using a new device for staff	
The need for the clearer user instructions	
Insufficient guidance on suitable games	
Placing the Yetitablet in a separate space reduced its use	Proper placement of the device is essential to use
Choosing the type of device and placing the device in common areas would have increased use and enabled communal social events	
Residents' enthusiasm for intervention	Residents' attitude towards participating in activities
A challenge of involving some residents in activities general	
Poor memory challenged the adoption of new technology	Poor cognition as a challenge
Poor cognition challenged gaming	
Yetitablet games liked by residents	Identifying individually suitable games for residents
Lack of suitable games	
Problems with using the touch screen	Success of using the touchscreen
Residents were able to use the touchscreen successfully	

4.4 Implementation of the Intervention

Success of intervention implementation was classified into three main categories: active participation of the residents in the gaming sessions, low involvement of staff in the implementation of the intervention and variable success of implementing the intervention protocol in the everyday life of LTC facility. The interviewees felt that the staff showed little interest in Yetitablet and few of them used Yetitablet. Instructing residents how to play the games was mainly the responsibility of interns, and therefore few of the permanent staff used the Yetitablet.

The residents participated actively in the gaming sessions. They participated in the game when requested, gaming physical and mental load was suitable for residents, and they were able to concentrate on playing well. Some of the residents were always happy to play, but some had to be motivated sometimes. Watching others play encouraged participation, and some found it difficult to stop playing once they started playing.

The implementation of the intervention protocol in the everyday life of the LTC varied. Regular gaming sessions were organized but playing while standing up varied. To gain changes in physical functioning like balance and physical activity, games were supposed to be played standing up as much as possible. However, it was challenging to motivate some residents to play in a standing position and some of them usually wanted to sit down while playing. There were also challenges associated with playing together and playing as a group. To gain social and psychological changes, games were encouraged to be played together with other residents in small groups. However, some residents wanted to play alone or only with the staff member, not with another resident. Sometimes residents were insecure about their own skills while playing with another resident and they had to be encouraged to play together. Forming a group was sometimes challenging. *"It is one challenge to get them to play at the same time. One refuses, one goes to bed, one is sick. That group is sometimes hard to form."* Interviewee 1. Filling out a game log was challenging, and not all the gaming sessions were marked down.

4.5 Factors Influencing the Implementation

Factors affecting the implementation formed nine main categories: positive attitude and motivation of staff important in implementation, staff attitude towards technology can challenge implementation, staff competence in using Yetitablet, practical training, clear instructions and an example of use support the implementation, proper placement of the device is essential to use, residents' attitude towards participating in activities, poor cognition as a challenge, identifying individually suitable games for residents and successful use of the touchscreen.

In implementing the intervention, the staff must have a positive attitude and be motivated. The staff's motivation to do new things and the staff's enthusiasm to try new things affected the implementation. The staff's attitude towards technology can challenge its implementation, and the staff struggled to adopt new technology. Using the new device requires effort in the beginning, and the staff did not remember to use or put effort into using the Yetitablet. During the intervention, it was observed that the staff did not incorporate the Yetitablet into the daily activities, such as instructing stimuli activities, but instead acted as they were used to. *"Especially all such technological devices. Those are often more difficult to implement."* Interviewee 3. Staff may have a negative attitude towards learning to use new technology. The interview revealed that staff may find learning to use technical equipment annoying and that they think they will not learn how to use it. These beliefs can prevent usage.

The staff's competence in using Yetitablet influenced its use. Easy use of Yetitablet supported its use and staff members who did not participate in the Yetitablet training were able to use it. The device was also handy to use so using it was not time consuming. On the other hand, there were some challenges in using Yetitablet. Sometimes the power button was hard to find and navigating the tablet, for example, from the game back to the home screen was challenging for some of the staff.

Practical training, clear instructions, and an example of using Yetitablet supports the implementation of the intervention. The interviewees hoped for practical orientation and user support. Training of the staff should not be too theoretical, instead, it should encourage staff to try different games themselves to lower the threshold for using Yetitablet. *"It would need a really good hands-on orientation so that people could see what they could do with it, so maybe it would be easier to approach."* Interviewee 2. The interviewees also suggested holding Teams meetings to support the use of Yetitablet during the intervention. Interviewees also needed an example of using the new device as it would have a positive impact on the attitude of the rest of the staff, as they would see an example of using the new device and its benefits for residents. There was a need for clearer instructions for using the Yetitablet, and the guidance of suitable games was insufficient. The placement of the Yetitablet in the LTC premises is essential for its use. Placing the Yetitablet in a separate space reduced its use, and the interviewees felt that choosing the type of device and placing the device in common areas would have increased use and enabled communal social events.

The residents' attitude towards participating in activities affected participation in the intervention. The residents were enthusiastic about this intervention, but it was challenging to involve some residents in activities in general. One nurse said the residents participated surprisingly well and they really liked the intervention and Yetitablet. Some residents always participated in the activities of LTC, and they also participated in this intervention happily. Some of the residents did not normally participate in the LTC activities, but they too got excited about playing on the Yeti tablet. *"Many residents who don't usually participate in anything liked it. They liked to play with it a lot. So, I think it's nice that we got something to do with them."* Interviewee 3.

The poor cognition of the residents was a challenge. Poor memory challenged the adoption of new technology and for many residents, the purpose of the Yetitablet and the instructions for the games always had to be repeated, and they could not remember what the Yetitablet was, even though they had used it before. This challenged the learning of how to use it. In addition, poor memory affected the use of the activity monitor. Many residents took it off because they couldn't remember its purpose. *"Then that monitor was taken off the wrist pretty quickly. I guess it just felt weird and they wondered what it is, and then just took it off."* Interviewee 2. A poor cognition also challenged gaming. Two residents had problems concentrating on gaming and could leave in the middle of the session. Also changes in medication, for example, caused confusion in a resident, which prevented participation in the intervention.

Identifying individually suitable games for residents affects the use of Yetitablet. The games were mostly liked by the residents and Yetitablet had interesting games for most of the residents. *"All those word games were his favorites, but he also played all the other games, even though he thought they were too easy, he still got excited about them. He wouldn't quit playing those games on his own."* Interviewee 2. For some of the residents, there was a lack of suitable games. Some residents thought the games were childish and pointless.

The success of using the touchscreen contributed to the success of the residents' gaming. There were some problems with using the touch screen, but mainly the residents were able to use the touchscreen successfully. First the use of the touch screen was new for the residents but once they learned to use it was easy. Residents learned the use individually and for some it was easy and for some learning took more time. *"In my opinion, it depended on the person (success of using the touch screen). Others were just doing really well."* Interviewee 2.

5 Discussion

This study gave information about the feasibility of the intervention and Yetitablet and preliminary information about its benefits which helps the implementation of this intervention in the future. Based on this study, it seems that intervention can have benefits especially on social functioning and social activity. A previous study of older people living independently also found that playing a digital bowling game in a group reduces loneliness and increases social connection between players [27]. Again, this study found social interaction between players during gaming and improved social relationships between players. Benefits on mood were observed in this study, and these are in line with previous research findings [28, 29]. As in this study, also in the Keogh et al. [28] study it was found that older gamers have fun playing digital games. Jahouh et al. [29] found out digital exergames generate higher positive emotions in institutionalized older players than traditional exercise what helps reduce symptoms of depression.

In an earlier digital gaming usability study, it was noticed that facilitators of new technology adoption in LTC facilities were ease of use of the technology and versatility of the technology [30]. These same factors also helped in the implementation of the Yetitablet, as the Yetitablet was considered easy to use and its content was diverse, which made it possible to find suitable games for each player. It was also possible to modify the Yetitablet for both the purpose of individual rehabilitation and group activities. However, despite the ease, the staff had a high threshold to start using the Yetitablet. This has been noticed also in previous studies implementing new gaming technology to LTC facilities. In Jbilou et al. [31] pilot study strike, staffing shortage and competing research projects limited staff engagement in using new technology. At the beginning of this intervention, the LTC facility had an intern whose training tasks included guiding game sessions on a Yetitablet. Permanent staff probably felt that implementing the intervention was not their task because of the intern, so they did not use the Yetitablet much. Staffing shortage probably did not affect this study, but it will be great risk for recruiting facilities for future effectiveness study and for implementing the intervention.

User training of Yetitablet should be more hands on in the future. Based on this experience it is important that the staff get used to using Yetitablet, they know what can be done with it and what games work well with their residents. Jbilou et al. [31] suggested providing recurring training and information sessions for the staff and this same thing came up in this study as well. It was also challenging for the staff to find or choose suitable games for residents individually. In the future, the arrangement of applications and games on Yetitablet's home screen should be considered so that it would be easy for staff to choose suitable games for residents. Also, managers' support for the staff to implement the intervention should be better considered. It has been noticed that if health care leaders do not support implementation of new technology, it struggles to succeed [32]. It is also important to identify those staff members who have a strong interest in using the Yetitablet and implementing the intervention and who also have the ability to use new technology. Those people could support and train other staff members in the use of Yetitablet [31, 33].

During the study we noticed the Geriatric Depression Scale 15 was not suitable for this population because all the participants had severe memory disorder. Participants were unable to respond to all items consistently. Furthermore, it would be better to measure the effects of gaming on the mood before and after the game session, not before and after the intervention. The Short Physical Performance Battery was very difficult for those participants who used walking aid. Older people who already need the walker to support their movement already have balance issues and weakness in the muscles of the lower limbs so performing the balance test and chair raise test were impossible. The use of that measurement should be carefully considered in the future trial.

Although we received information about the feasibility of the intervention and the Yetitablet, some uncertainty remains. First, due to timetable issues, we were not able to test the activity monitors properly. The participants had activity monitors during the last two weeks of the intervention so we got some information about the usability of the monitors, but we could not test the data collection and reliability of the data. Commercial wearable monitors are often designed for healthy adults, and there is uncertainty about reliable measurement of activity data in older people with mobility problems [34]. Based on this trial there are challenges in the use of activity monitors if participant has a severe memory disorder, but activity data could be collected from participants with better cognitive capacity. However, the success of collecting activity data using activity monitors is uncertain.

This study has some limitations and sources of bias. First, this study was carried out only in one small long-term care facility which may limit generalizability of the intervention protocol to other facilities. The small number of participants is clearly a limitation since the literacy states that pilot trials should include about 30 participants [35]. For this reason, we did not analyze the results of the functioning measurements and thus did not obtain information on the intervention's effectiveness on functioning. Also, the number of people who used the Yetitablet and implemented the intervention in the facility was small and therefore the interview data remained limited.

6 Conclusions

Based on this feasibility study, the intervention was well received by the residents, and the staff responded positively to it. The intervention was beneficial for the residents as gaming had a positive impact on their mood, sociability, and physical activity assessed by the staff. Yetitablet and its games were also well suited for the residents. Based on this experience, intervention is therefore feasible for LTC residents. Yetitablet was suitable for the environment, but the challenge in implementing the intervention was the success of standing play, which would specifically promote the development of physical functioning, such as balance. In the future, attention must be paid to the commitment of staff to the implementation of the intervention and to the instructions for the use of the device and games, so that the use of Yetitablet becomes a part of everyday life at LTC facilities. This study highlighted important factors related to the implementation of the intervention, which will help the successful implementation of the intervention in future effectiveness study.

Disclosure of Interests.   The authors have no competing interests to declare that are relevant to the content of this article.

References

1. Sudhir, K., Sudheera, K., Demonge, K.A.: Physical activity levels among community dwelling and care home dwelling elderly population. Indian J. Physiotherapy Occupational Therapy **16**(1), 143–149 (2021). https://doi.org/10.37506/ijpot.v16i1.17787
2. Ikezoe, T., Asakawa, Y., Shima, H., Kishibuchi, K., Ichihashi, N.: Daytime physical activity patterns and physical fitness in institutionalized elderly women: An exploratory study. Arch. Gerontol. Geriatr. **57**(2), 221–225 (2013). https://doi.org/10.1016/j.archger.2013.04.004
3. Jantunen, H., Wasenius, N., Salonen, M.K., Perälä, M., Osmond, C., Kautiainen, H., et al.: Objectively measured physical activity and physical performance in old age. Age Ageing **46**(2), 232–237 (2017). https://doi.org/10.1093/ageing/afw194
4. de Oliveira, L., Souza, E.C., Rodrigues, R., Fett, C.A., Piva, A.B.: The effects of physical activity on anxiety, depression, and quality of life in elderly people living in the community. Trends Psychiatry Psychother **41**(1), 36–42 (2019). https://doi.org/10.1590/2237-6089-2017-0129
5. Wiemeyer, J., Kliem, A.: Serious games in prevention and rehabilitation—a new panacea for elderly people? Eur. Rev. Aging Phys. Act. **9**(1), 41–50 (2012). https://doi.org/10.1007/s11556-011-0093-x
6. Chu, C., Quan, A., Souter, A., Krisnagopal, A., Biss, R.: Effects of exergaming on physical and cognitive outcomes of older adults living in long-term care homes: a systematic review. Gerontology (Basel) **68**(9), 1044–1060 (2022). https://doi.org/10.1159/000521832
7. Taylor, L.M., Kerse, N., Frakking, T., Maddison, R.: Active video games for improving physical performance measures in older people: a meta-analysis. J. Geriatric Phys. Therapy **41**(2), 108–123 (2018). https://doi.org/10.1519/JPT.0000000000000078
8. Martinho, D., Carneiro, J., Corchado, J.M., Marreiros, G.: A systematic review of gamification techniques applied to elderly care. Artif. Intell. Rev. **53**(7), 4863–4901 (2020). https://doi.org/10.1007/s10462-020-09809-6
9. Li, J., Erdt, M., Chen, L., Cao, Y., Lee, S., Theng, Y.: The social effects of exergames on older adults: systematic review and metric analysis. J. Med. Internet Res. **20**(6), e10486 (2018). https://doi.org/10.2196/10486
10. Saragih, I.D., Everard, G., Lee, B.: A systematic review and meta-analysis of randomized controlled trials on the effect of serious games on people with dementia. Ageing Res. Rev. **82**, 101740 (2022). https://doi.org/10.1016/j.arr.2022.101740

11. Jarva, E., et al.: Healthcare professionals' perceptions of digital health competence: a qualitative descriptive study. Nurs. Open **9**(2), 1379–1393 (2022). https://doi.org/10.1002/nop2.1184

12. Nilsen, E.R., Dugstad, J., Eide, H., Gullslett, M.K., Eide, T.: Exploring resistance to implementation of welfare technology in municipal healthcare services – a longitudinal case study. BMC Health Serv. Res. **16**, 657 (2016). https://doi.org/10.1186/s12913-016-1913-5

13. Kukkohovi, S., Siira, H., Arolaakso, S., Miettunen, J., Elo, S.: The effectiveness of digital gaming on the functioning and activity of older people living in long-term care facilities: a systematic review and meta-analysis. Aging Clin. Exp. Res. **35**(8), 1595–1608 (2023). https://doi.org/10.1007/s40520-023-02459-y

14. Swinnen, N., et al.: The efficacy of exergaming in people with major neurocognitive disorder residing in long-term care facilities: a pilot randomized controlled trial. Alzheimer's Res. Therapy **13**(1), 70 (2021). https://doi.org/10.1186/s13195-021-00806-7

15. Delbroek, T., Vermeylen, W., Spildooren, J.: The effect of cognitive-motor dual task training with the biorescue force platform on cognition, balance and dual task performance in institutionalized older adults: a randomized controlled trial. J. Phys. Ther. Sci. **29**(7), 1137–1143 (2017). https://doi.org/10.1589/jpts.29.1137

16. Soares, A.V., Borges, N.G., Hounsell, M., Marcelino, E., Rossito, G.M., Sagawa, Y.: A serious game developed for physical rehabilitation of frail elderly. Neurophysiol. Clin. **46**(4), 281 (2016). https://doi.org/10.1016/j.neucli.2016.09.109

17. Va´zquez, F.L., Otero, P., Garcı´a-Casal, J.A., Blanco, V., Torres, A.J., Arrojo, M.: Efficacy of video game-based interventions for active aging. A systematic literature review and meta-analysis. PLoS ONE **13**(12), e0208192 (2018). https://doi.org/10.1371/journal.pone.0208192

18. Yeticare homepage. https://yeticare.fi/fi/. Accessed 05 Jun 2023

19. Kallio, H., Pietilä, A., Johnson, M., Kangasniemi, M.: Systematic methodological review: developing a framework for a qualitative semi-structured interview guide. J. Adv. Nurs. **72**(12), 2954–2965 (2016). https://doi.org/10.1111/jan.13031

20. Yang, H., Yoo, Y.: It's all about attitude: revisiting the technology acceptance model. Decis. Support. Syst. **38**, 19–31 (2004). https://doi.org/10.1016/S0167-9236(03)00062-9

21. World Health Organization (WHO). International Classification of Functioning, Disability and Health: ICF. https://iris.who.int/bitstream/handle/10665/42407/9241545429.pdf?sequence=1 (2001)

22. Guralnik, J.M., Simonsick, E.M., Ferrucci, L., Glynn, R.J., Berkman, L.F., Blazer, D.G., et al.: A short physical performance battery assessing lower extremity function: association with self-reported disability and prediction of mortality and nursing home admission. J. Gerontol. **49**(2), 85–94 (1994). https://doi.org/10.1093/geronj/49.2.m85

23. Podsiadlo, D., Richardson, S.: The Timed "Up & Go": a test of basic functional mobility for frail elderly persons. J. Am. Geriatr. Soc. **39**(2), 142–148 (1991). https://doi.org/10.1111/j.1532-5415.1991.tb01616.x

24. Kurlowicz, L., Greenberg, S.A.: The geriatric depression scale (GDS). Am. J. Nurs. **107**(10), 67–68 (2007). https://doi.org/10.1097/01.NAJ.0000292207.37066.2f

25. Gerritsen, D.L., Steverink, N., Frijters, D.H.M., Hirdes, J.P., Ooms, M.E., Ribbe, M.W.: A revised index for social engagement for long-term care. J. Gerontol. Nurs. **34**(4), 40–48 (2008). https://doi.org/10.3928/00989134-20080401-04

26. Elo, S., Kyngäs, H.: The qualitative content analysis process. J. Adv. Nurs. **62**(1), 107–115 (2008). https://doi.org/10.1111/j.1365-2648.2007.04569.x

27. Schell, R., Hausknecht, S., Zhang, F., Kaufman, D.: Social benefits of playing Wii bowling for older adults. Games Culture **11**(1–2), 81–103 (2016). https://doi.org/10.1177/1555412015607313

28. Keogh, J.W.L., Power, N., Wooller, L., Lucas, P., Whatman, C.: Physical and psychosocial function in residential aged-care elders: effect of Nintendo Wii sports games. J. Aging Phys. Act. **22**(2), 235–244 (2014). https://doi.org/10.1123/japa.2012-0272
29. Jahouh, M., González-Bernal, J., González-Santos, J., Fernández-Lázaro, D., Soto-Cámara, R., Mielgo-Ayuso, J.: Impact of an intervention with wii video games on the autonomy of activities of daily living and psychological-cognitive components in the institutionalized elderly. Int. J. Environ. Res. Public Health **18**(4), 1570 (2021). https://doi.org/10.3390/ijerph 18041570
30. Chu, C., Biss, R., Cooper, L., Quan, A., Mantulis., H.: Exergaming platform for older adults residing in long-term care homes: user-centered design, development, and usability study. JMIR Serious Games **9**(1), e22370 (2021) https://doi.org/10.2196/22370
31. Jbilou, J., El Bouazaoui, A., Zhang, B., Henry, J., McDonald, L., Hall, T. et al.: Evaluating and motivating activation in long term care: lessons from a pilot study. In: International Symposium of Human Factors and Ergonomics in Healthcare 2021, vol. **10**(1), pp. 42–46. Sage (2021). https://doi.org/10.1177/2327857921101016
32. Laukka, E., Huhtakangas, M., Heponiemi, T., Kanste, O.: Identifying the roles of health-care leaders in hit implementation: a scoping review of the quantitative and qualitative evidence. Int. J. Environ. Res. Public Health **17**(8), 2865 (2020). https://doi.org/10.3390/ijerph 17082865
33. Dugstad, J., Eide, T., Nilsen, E.R., Eide, H.: Towards successful digital transformation through co-creation: a longitudinal study of a four-year implementation of digital monitoring technology in residential care for persons with dementia. BMC Health Serv. Res. **19**(1), 366 (2019). https://doi.org/10.1186/s12913-019-4191-1
34. Teixeira, E., Fonseca, H., Diniz-Sousa, F., Veras, L., Boppre, G., Oliveira, J., et al.: Wearable devices for physical activity and healthcare monitoring in elderly people: a critical review. Geriatrics (Basel) **6**(2), 38 (2021). https://doi.org/10.3390/geriatrics6020038
35. Lewis, M., Bromley, K., Sutton, C.J., McCray, G., Myers, H.L., Lancaster, G.A.: Determining sample size for progression criteria for pragmatic pilot RCTs: the hypothesis test strikes back. Pilot Feasibility Stud. **7**(1), 40 (2021). https://doi.org/10.1186/s40814-021-00770-x

Orchestrating Customer-Oriented Public-Private Ecosystem

Satu Nätti, Hanna Komulainen, Saila Saraniemi[✉], and Pauliina Ulkuniemi

Oulu Business School, University of Oulu, P.O. Box 4600, 90014 Oulun Yliopisto, Finland
saila.saraniemi@oulu.fi

Abstract. The way public procurers interact with the supply market is developing from purely transactional towards more resource focused and collaborative exchanges. Still, what seems to be missing in the public procurement culture is knowledge of how to connect to a wider network of resource providers. We do not have adequate understanding about customer orientation in public sector, nor about customer-centric ecosystem. This is especially true in public health services; systems that are under huge transformation. In this paper, we have followed that development to understand: *How can public health care transformation towards customer-oriented ecosystems be orchestrated?* We had a unique opportunity to follow the renewal of the healthcare system in Finland, having access to interview those involved in planning the system. In total 17 in-depth interviews enabled us to create understanding of this challenge.

Keywords: Customer Orientation · Digital Transformation · Ecosystem · Orchestration · Health Care · Marketing

1 Introduction

Increasing number of Western countries are riding the wave of public sector modernization and approaches are ranging from cost-cutting, productivity and privatization strategies to quality assurance, personnel development and devolving central state responsibilities to civil society [1]. This is particularly relevant in the context of healthcare services, which are continuously facing a demand to improve access to primary care, to tackle ever-growing costs, and to change the focus from curing disease to preventing illness [2, 3]. Moreover, healthcare services are constantly being developed by the new solutions and opportunities offered by digitalization with the aim of creating a more efficient, patient-centric, and sustainable healthcare system. Systemic changes needed in the future for public health and social service provision are so remarkable, that the process can also be seen as a real possibility to renew customer-orientation in public health care. Likewise, the change will hopefully boost development of more customer-centric ecosystems. Our aim in this article is to create an in-depth understanding of how transformation of a public health care system towards customer-oriented ecosystem could be orchestrated.

M. Särestöniemi et al. (Eds.): NCDHWS 2024, CCIS 2083, pp. 223–230, 2024.
https://doi.org/10.1007/978-3-031-59080-1_16

Presumably, these initiatives may face many challenges. Customer-centric i.e. customer-oriented ecosystem formation is to some extent against traditional outsourcing culture characteristic to the public sector, where focus has been on dyadic relationships and contracts with single actors, administered by public sector representatives. Likewise, constructing interfaces between public and private actors needed to act in the ecosystem can also be challenging in the competitive setting. Thus do the changes of culture and perspective from an individual service provision to a service ecosystem, that enable also for a customer more empowered role.

In addition, public actors responsible for organizing health care services follow the regulative framework of public procurement deriving from the EU and national legislation. Accordingly, transparency, fair treatment and competition are nurtured in the decisions resulting typically in transactional exchange and arm's length relationships between public and private organizations [4]. The role of contracts and formal exchange in public procurement relationships has been emphasized although lately also the need for more collaborative engagements between public actors and supplier companies have been put forward [5]. This has especially been connected to the development of new public procurement procedures, focusing on innovative public procurement and seeing the role of public procurement as generating innovations [6]. Pre-commercial public procurement, for example, refers to procurement that is connected to a R&D phase of the actual object of exchange [e.g. 7], and life-cycle procurement in which long-term partnerships around service business model is created between the public procurer and supplier, instead of large infrastructure procurements. The way public procurers are interacting with the supply market is thus developing from purely transactional towards more resource focused and collaborative exchanges, but the outsourcing remains still highly dyadic and the focus for interaction with the surrounding market resources is highly concentrated on managing single relationships between the public buyer and specific suppliers. Thus, what seems to be missing in the public procurement culture is the way public procurement connects to a wider network of resources providers. Likewise, although research on this matter is emerging, current literature still does not provide adequate understanding about customer orientation in public sector, nor about customer-oriented ecosystem view or its applicability to the new, reorganized public-private collaboration. This is especially true in our empirical context, public health services. These systems are under transformation, and we have followed that development to understand: *How can public health care transformation towards customer-oriented ecosystems be orchestrated?* First, we need to understand the starting point of developments, and core actors in the system. Thus, we need to answer: *Who are nodal actors influencing ecosystem development?* Second, many aspects of prevailing culture and structures in public health care need to be transformed to change the system. Thus, we need to answer the question: *How can variety of orchestration activities be implemented to influence and transform existing system (towards customer-oriented ecosystem)?* Finally, because the core aim is to create a customer-centric ecosystem, we must create an understanding of the inner meaning of this concept in this specific context: *How customer-orientation could be realized in the ecosystem?*

We had a unique opportunity to follow the renewal of the healthcare system in Finland, having access to interview those involved in planning the system. This reform as our case, we conducted in total 17 in-depth interviews that enabled us to create understanding of this challenge.

2 Theoretical Background

2.1 Customer-Oriented Ecosystem

The idea of customer dominant logic emphasizes that customer's process should be a starting point of any service development: Service providers' role is to identify ways to connect to customer's real life challenges, and offer resources needed for customer value creation [see 8]. One service provider can seldom meet all these needs in the long run, but a variety of actors are needed to combine their resources in order to support customer health and wellbeing. We need customer-oriented ecosystems. Therefore, instead of the focus being on how service systems are arranged and organized from the service providers' point of view, the interest should be also in what constitutes the customer's ecosystem providing resources for customer value creation process [e.g., 9]. In this kind of ecosystem, customers may also take a more active role, in some cases even orchestrating the ecosystem for his or her own value creation.

To meet this challenge of customer-orientation, ecosystem dynamics in this new situation and setting should be understood, and we should be able to form customer-oriented ecosystems where private and public actors act as seamlessly as possible to link their resources for customer purposes. This happens by taking different positions and roles in the network, by influencing other actors. In other words, network orchestration is conducted.

2.2 Ecosystem Orchestration

According to Dhanaraj and Parkhe [10], network orchestration refers to taking deliberate, purposeful actions for initiating and managing collaboration processes. Network orchestration is a dynamic, emergent process, where actor roles and orchestration activities can change in time [11].

Examining these dynamics is critical in understanding service ecosystem and related value creation potential, or inhibitors for it. When formation, or transformation of ecosystem takes place, mobilization of variety of actors needed is not without challenges. Network mobilization presumes some actors taking initiative. As our first sub research question presumes, first we need to understand who are those nodal actors that can act as net weavers when promoting ecosystem formation in health care sector. We assume that in the present situation those actors are often public organizations that hold sufficient legitimacy and regional power/influence to take the orchestration initiative [12, 13]. After defining nodal actors, the basis to form the ecosystem should be understood. Actors needed for integrated service paths should be attracted and mobilized for these networks to form value-creating ecosystem. For example, nodal actors should be able to create an attractive agenda for collaboration and communicate that agenda for potential service providers to mobilize them for the collaboration [14]. Network orchestration mechanisms when forming the ecosystem, also in existing service ecosystem, can relate to many practicalities, like how nodal actors can influence knowledge transfer between organizations in the ecosystem, between customers and service providers, for example. Or how to influence identity of the network in question, so there would be a strong basis for keeping up the long-term motivation to collaborate? Network orchestration can also relate to appropriability issues, especially when collaboration contributes new innovations; Influencing appropriability means defining common norms and principles to share benefits gained are needed on the collaboration. Network orchestration is also about plain coordination and organization. Someone must take care of practicalities and organize platforms of interaction for customers and service providers maintaining the collaboration. Defining roles and responsibilities for different actors is important [10, 15].

Building customer-centric ecosystem may presume customer participation in the ecosystem already in the transformation phase, thus, customers as participatory actors in the ecosystem should be recognized. Indeed, it is crucial to understand how ecosystem structure and resources it can offer meets customer value creation, seeing customer as an active member of the ecosystem, contributing to its resource constellation. Thus, in addition to understand nodal actors and orchestration mechanisms implemented to form and transform the system, we want to create understanding of the inner meaning of customer-centricity of an ecosystem in this specific context [e.g., 16].

2.3 Levels of Change

What is characteristic to public context are many friction forces there can be on a way when forming the ecosystem and transforming the existing dyadic approach to ecosystems. Indeed, transforming the health care system towards a new approach can include many challenges due to specific characteristics of public procurement and culture in public organizations, for example. Thus, in addition to understanding orchestration activities we can use, and the path of customer centricity we want to follow, there are many "levels of change" we must consider when trying to understand how and what we should transform in existing system.

Remarkable transformation always presumes organizations and systems to develop new, actionable mental models. In the public sector creating flexibility needed in new approach can be challenging because of strong traditions, history, certain stagnation of the strategic environment, and earlier mentioned procurement conventions and legislation, to mention few. Under influence of these "friction forces", these organizations have developed strong dominant logic which is a challenging starting point for disruptive change and ecosystem formation. Furthermore, the difficulty of the dominant logic is that these mindsets are usually tacit, even subconscious, and although they become dysfunctional, organization is not able to question or renew these assumptions [e.g., 17]. Even though changes may make good sense, existing emotional attachments and even fear may stimulate considerable resistance towards development initiatives. When the aim is to form customer-oriented ecosystem, how to tackle this challenge by means of orchestration? The same question relates to renewing organizational culture(s), which refers to the shared values and beliefs that are held by actors [e.g., 18]. How orchestration can facilitate cultural change needed to form ecosystems or later, how common identity for ecosystems can be strengthened to facilitate customer-oriented activities? If culture is coherent, customer-oriented values are commonly understood and they can form a basis for everyday work and choices in the service ecosystem, contributing to higher service quality and customer satisfaction.

Radical change is also needed in organizational design and incentives [19]. By creating a suitable organizational design, and further ecosystem design, organizations can provide forums for knowledge sharing and discussion. By facilitating organizational dialogue and questioning, also change in above mentioned deeper structures of culture and dominant logic is enabled. Related to structural issues, developed incentives can profoundly influence activities in the ecosystem. For example, the presence of structural barriers and competitive attitudes between different activities in the ecosystem (forced by incentives) can raise problems from the transformation standpoint, hampering integration efforts. Our aim is to understand how these factors can be influenced by means of orchestration.

Digital transformation is relevant in almost any environment nowadays, and that is also the case in public health care. However, it is critical to understand that functioning digital system is only the tip of the iceberg. All the above presented influence how we can alter our attitudes and work processes to the new mode needed also in digital transformation. Naturally, development of digital systems is needed. However, developing systems only is not enough to create facilitative conditions for health care transformation and related change needed. In the following tentative framework (Fig. 1), key concepts of our research are combined.

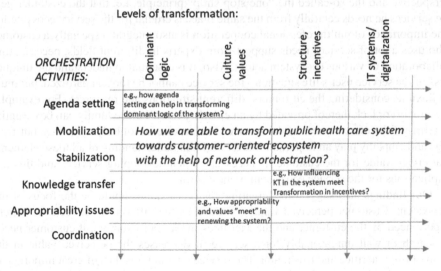

Fig. 1. Tentative framework for the study (adapted from e.g., Hurmelinna-Laukkanen et al., 2011)

3 Methodology

We collected primary data through 17 interviews with regional health care service developers. Those informants were senior managers and experienced officers in regional health care authorities, hospitals, and health care centers. The informants were chosen based on them being part of the group responsible for developing a new regional, more centralized organization of health and social services at the time when new system was under construction in Finland. Interviews were conducted using an open-ended interviewing technique to allow informants to express their perceptions without restrictions. We discussed following themes in the interviews: concept of customer in social and health care, concept of customer-orientation, different interests and actors in health care system, challenges in service development, organizing of service development, collaboration and networks in health care system and service integration in the system. The interviews stayed at a general level, covering management perspective, and not going to anyone's specific health issues; thus, no ethical permission was needed. The interview data were transcribed and analyzed using the abductive approach, which enables a profound dialogue between the theoretical understanding and insights arising from the empirical data [20].

4 Findings and Conclusions

Our research emphasized the importance of managing the service system so that providing flexible and individually designed services is enabled. Also, taking a holistic perspective and the so-called the "one stop shop" principle, i.e. that the customer gets the services he needs centrally from the same place is crucial for the service ecosystems. The importance of multiprofessional cooperation is also integral; especially a customer who uses a lot of services needs support from experts in different fields, necessitating collaboration of various ecosystem actors. Also, it is essential to understand the uniqueness of the service user's life situation - the service cannot be too standardized, but must be flexible, considering the customers' different situations and resources. For example, the support or lack thereof provided by an elderly person's close family can be essential in terms of the effectiveness of the service. The service is not only measures, but feelings and empathy play an important role as well. An understanding of all these elements that create value for the customer is necessary when developing services and this has implications for the service ecosystem orchestration.

Our findings also suggest that creating customer value should be the focus of the ecosystem. Customer perceived value is formed as the difference between the benefit experienced by the customer and the sacrifices made. For example, if customer needs to search or wait unreasonably for a service, it decreases the perceived value in the form of time sacrifice and frustration. The service encounter is thus of great importance, but so is what happens after the actual service encounter, e.g. does the service really improve the customer's situation. The service ecosystem thus needs to be able to tackle the customer's value creation on a longitudinal basis.

The present study also brings forth the role of digitalization in the service ecosystem orchestration, from the customer's perspective. Digitalization has been offered as a solution for creating more efficient and tailored service solutions. However, it is crucial to examine and understand, what kind of opportunities, skills, know-how and resources a health care customer has for participating in such co-creation of value. Digitalization and online, remote services can serve some target groups well, but not all, thus suggesting need for relevant segmentation of customers, as well as integration of systems and services, including smooth knowledge transfer, for example [see 15, 21], also providing a lot of potential for development.

To conclude, in public health care systems, resources are scarce. However, the decision-making related to the organization of services should be possible under the conditions of long-term effectiveness. For organizing and orchestrating the service ecosystem to be more customer-oriented, a genuine customer perspective is central, emerging alongside resource thinking and financial optimization. By organizing according to customer needs, even scarce resources can be used wisely.

Disclosure of Interests. The authors have no competing interests to declare that are relevant to the content of this article.

References

1. Naschhold, F.: New Frontiers in the Public Sector Management. Trends and Issues in State and Local Government in Europe. de Gruyter Studies in Organization, Reprint ed. (2017)
2. Komulainen, H., Nätti, S., Saraniemi, S., Ulkuniemi, P.: Towards a holistic customer value approach in managing public health care services: a developers' view. Int. J. Public Sect. Manag. **36**(1), 46–63 (2023)
3. Palumbo, R.: Contextualizing co-production of health care: a systematic literature review. Int. J. Public Sect. Manag. **29**(1), 72–90 (2016)
4. Lian, P.C.S., Laing, A.W.: Public sector purchasing of health services: a comparison with private sector purchasing. J. Purch. Supply Manag. **10**(6), 247–256 (2004)
5. Keränen, O.: Roles for developing public–private partnerships in centralized public procurement. Ind. Mark. Manage. **62**, 199–210 (2017)
6. Edquist, C., Zabala-Iturriagagoitia, J.M.: Public Procurement for Innovation as mission-oriented innovation policy. Res. Policy **41**, 1757–1769 (2012)
7. Edquist, C., Zabala-Iturriagagoitia, J.M.: Is PCP a demand- or a supply-side innovation policy instrument? R&D Manage **45**, 147–160 (2015)
8. Heinonen, K., Strandvik, T.: Reflections on customer's primary role in markets. Eur. Manag. J. **36**, 1–11 (2018)
9. Jacobides, M.G., Cennamo, C., Gawer, A.: Towards a theory of ecosystems. Strateg. Manag. J. **39**, 2255–2276 (2018)
10. Dhanaraj, C., Parkhe, A.: Orchestrating innovation networks. Acad. Manag. Rev. **31**(2), 659–669 (2006)
11. Davis, J.P., Eisenhardt, K.M.: Rotating leadership and collaborative innovation: recombination processes in symbiotic relationships. Adm. Sci. Q. **56**, 159–201 (2011)
12. Hurmelinna-Laukkanen, P., Nätti, S.: Orchestrator types, roles and capabilities – a framework for innovation networks. Ind. Mark. Manage. **74**, 65–78 (2018)
13. Pikkarainen, M., Ervasti, M., Hurmelinna-Laukkanen, P., Nätti, S.: Orchestration roles to facilitate networked innovation in healthcare ecosystem. Technol. Innov. Manag. Rev. **7**(9), 30–43 (2018)

14. Möller, K., Rajala, A.: Rise of strategic nets—new modes of value creation. Ind. Mark. Manage. **36**, 895–908 (2007)
15. Hurmelinna-Laukkanen, P., Möller, K., Nätti, S.: Innovation orchestration – matching network types and orchestration profiles. In: Proceedings of 27th IMP Conference, Glasgow, Scotland, 30 August–3 September 2011 (2011)
16. Aarikka-Stenroos, L., Ritala, P.: Network management in the era of ecosystems: systematic review and management framework. Ind. Mark. Manage. **67**, 23–36 (2017)
17. Bettis, R.A., Prahalad, C.K.: The dominant logic: retrospective and extension. Strateg. Manag. J. **16**, 5–14 (1995)
18. Barney, J.B.: Organisational culture: can it be source of sustained competitive advantage? Acad. Manag. Rev. **11**(3), 356–665 (1986)
19. Birkinshaw, J., Nobel, R., Ridderstråle, J.: Knowledge as a contingency variable: do the characteristics of knowledge predict organization structure. Organ. Sci. **13**(3), 274–289 (2002)
20. Dubois, A., Gadde. L.: Systematic combining: an abductive approach to case research. J. Bus. Res. **55**(7), 553–560 (2002)
21. Lähteenmäki, I., Nätti, S., Saraniemi, S.: Digitalization-enabled evolution of customer value creation: an executive view in financial services. J. Bus. Res. **146**, 504–517 (2022)

Near-Infrared Spectroscopic Study Towards Clinical Radiotherapy Treatment Monitoring

Priya Karthikeyan[1,3]([📧]), Hany Ferdinando[2,3], Vesa Korhonen[1,3,4,5], Ulriika Honka[1,3], Jesse Lohela[1,3,5], Kalle Inget[1,3,5], Sakari Karhula[1,3,4,5], Juha Nikkinen[1,3,4,5], and Teemu Myllylä[1,2,3,4]

[1] Research Unit of Health Science and Technology, University of Oulu, Oulu, Finland
priya.karthikeyan@oulu.fi
[2] Optoelectronics and Measurement Techniques Unit, University of Oulu, Oulu, Finland
[3] Department of Diagnostic Radiology, Oulu University Hospital, Oulu, Finland
[4] Medical Research Center (MRC), Oulu, Finland
[5] Department of Oncology and Radiotherapy, Oulu University Hospital, Oulu, Finland

Abstract. This study used near-infrared spectroscopy to monitor dynamic spectral effects to radiotherapy aiming to monitor spectral response for clinical radiotherapy. Twenty-four patients with total fractions of 96 measurements were measured to evaluate the dynamic spectral status of radiotherapy response. Dynamic responses from absorbance measurement were found to be associated with effects of induced radiation to skin and it linearly correlates to the dose given. Whereas significantly no response was found in ex vivo samples. A spectrometer was used in near infrared range between 650 nm and 1100 nm wavelength in absorbance mode. The absorbance spectral dynamics were measured using one light source-detector probe attached to the forehead in human patients and chicken samples to compare their responses to irradiation. The absorbance measurements of the forehead (skin) show absorbance increase throughout the spectra during irradiation in patients and confirmed with repeatability whereas in corresponding irradiation of ex vivo chicken samples, no absorbance changes were detected. Since spectral range of 650 nm–950 nm is dominantly affected by hemodynamical changes in tissue this indicates the oxygenation of blood in patients is strongly affected by irradiation. Furthermore, the irradiation caused absorbance changes also between 950 nm to 1100 nm range which is dominated by water in tissue, however in ex vivo chicken no visible effects of irradiation were detected in this range either.

Keywords: Radiotherapy · Near-infrared Spectroscopy · Skin · Haemodynamics · Lipid · Water

1 Introduction

Cancer is one of the leading causes of death in the world. The International Agency for Research on Cancer (IARC) reported in 2020 that 10.0 million deaths worldwide were due to cancer and 63% of cancer deaths are reported to be from developing countries [1]. Radiation therapy (RT) is one of the well-established and effective methods for many

© The Author(s) 2024
M. Särestöniemi et al. (Eds.): NCDHWS 2024, CCIS 2083, pp. 231–239, 2024.
https://doi.org/10.1007/978-3-031-59080-1_17

cancer treatments. In particular, for brain tumor RT is used to treat approximately 50% of all patients and for cure or palliation it has been shown to be cost effective. However, on the down side, RT can often affect patient's quality of life due to possible harmful late effects [2]. For instance, the radiation toxicity of normal tissue may lead to brain radiation necrosis (BRN) primarily includes inflammation and angiogenesis in which account for the breakdown of the blood–brain barrier (BBB), resulting in contrast-enhanced lesions and perilesional edema [2–6]. As severe toxicity in a some patients limits the doses that can be safely given to the majority, there is interest in developing a measurement method to assess individual's tissue response during the treatment [7].

At present, the development of advanced RT techniques aim to deliver radiation to cancerous areas, while avoiding healthy tissues. These techniques include image-guided RT, intensity-modulated RT, stereotactic body RT, and proton beam therapy. Magnetic resonance (MR) guided RT combines a magnetic resonance imaging (MRI) unit with a RT unit. This allows real-time analysis of target volumes before and during irradiation, providing an instant feedback for the treatment planning. Another method in clinical practice for treatment planning is conventional photon RT which involves utilizing a computed tomography (CT) scan of the treatment position, commonly known as CT-based treatment planning. However, none of these can provide instant radiation response from the tissue.

Ionizing radiation impacts the cells by direct and indirect effects. The indirect effects are more significant interaction in RT use, when 2/3 of the oxygen radicals rise from the radiolysis of water. Radiation ionizes water molecules which generates oxygen radicals. However, technology to detect the free oxygen radicals during RT is lacking. Such technology could improve the effectiveness of the RT when measuring the concentration of oxygen radicals that correlate with the dose of irradiation.

Recently, we demonstrated that cerebral hemodynamics can be measured by functional near-infrared spectroscopy (fNIRS) during RT [8]. Furthermore, we have verified that the technology based on fiber optics can be used also combined with MR guided RT. This study further investigates the spectroscopic response to radiation at range of 650 nm to 1100 nm. Within this NIR range, the primary light-absorbing molecules in tissue are metal complex chromophores: haemoglobin, cytochrome and water, where the absorption spectra of deoxyhaemoglobin (HbR) is dominated from 650 to ~810 nm, oxyhaemoglobin (HbO) from ~810 nm to 950, and water between 950 to 1100 nm. The isobestic point wavelength at which oxy- and deoxyhaemoglobin species have the same molar absorptivity for HbO and HbR is around 810 nm and this isosbestic absorption spectra reflects total haemoglobin (HbT). In addition, cytochrome oxidase (Caa3) has a broad peak at 820–840 nm [9].

1.1 Effects of Irradiation When Measured Using Optical Techniques

Previous optics based studies on chemoradiotherapy-effects in patients with head and neck tumors indicated increased blood flow and changes in tissue oxygenation [10–12]. Jakubowski et al. showed that the greatest changes in hemoglobin concentrations, water and lipid content in breast tumor occurred within the first week of neoadjuvant chemo RT [13]. It seems that tissue deoxygenates in few days after the first fraction of the RT [14]. A recent human RT study by Myllylä et al. showed that there is also immediate effect in cerebral hemodynamics, particularly tissue oxygenation index (TOI) drops as a direct effect of irradiation but starts to increase again immediately after the irradiation [15]. A study by Darren et al. showed using diffuse optical spectroscopy (DOS) a correlation between oxygen saturation and erythema of skin in mice [16]. Similarly, Lee et al. showed in a mice study increased hemoglobin after irradiation. Still, most of the studies on effects of irradiation are conducted using mice models [17, 18].

In this paper, we measured absorption effects of irradiation in human skin at near infrared (NIR) light range of 650 nm to 1100 nm (in vivo) and in chicken thigh skin (ex vivo) to compare in vivo vs. ex vivo tissue effects of irradiation. Based on light propagation studies in tissue, when using fiber source-detector distance of 10 mm placed on human forehead, the spectrometer measurement volume does not reach the brain cortex [19] however, it covers few millimeters depth in human skin, including stratum corneum (0.02 mm), epidermis (0.07 mm to 0.13 mm), dermis (1 mm) and subcutaneous fat (1.2 mm) [20, 21]. Within the NIR region, we can generally consider four substances to dominate the absorption of light in skin tissue at ~2 mm depth: hemoglobin (oxy and deoxy), and water (H_2O) and melanin in the range 620–720 nm [20] and their irradiation effects to NIR absorbance are discussed in this study.

2   Methodology

The spectroscopic measurements included patient (in vivo) measurements and store bought fresh chicken sample (ex vivo) measurements. All measurements were performed in Oulu University Hospital (Oulu, Finland) under the approval of the ethical committee of the North Ostrobothnia's Hospital district (Finland) (No. 237/2018). Irradiation was performed with the Oulu University Hospital's linear accelerators (Clinac iX and True beam, Varian medical systems). Figure 1 illustrates the measurement setup.

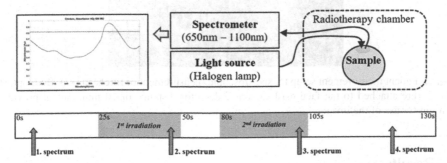

Fig. 1. Absorbance measurement setup used in the study. Optical fibres are guided to the RT chamber and attached at 1 cm source-detector distance to centre of the irradiated area (yellow) in the measured sample. (Color figure online)

For absorbance measurement, QE pro-ocean optics spectrometer system was used with a tungsten-halogen broadband light source (HL-2000-HP, Ocean Optics) having emission spectral range of 350 nm to 2400 nm. The optical fibers for both light source and spectrometer detector had a refractive index of approximately 1.58 and an internal transmittance of 0.999 in the range of 600 to 1100 nm, fabricated by Schott and then customized for RT environment usage. Fibre tip with a diameter of 2.5 mm and a length of 10 mm was attached perpendicular to the patient's skin and sample using 3D printed fibre probe holder. Both fibers had the same dimensions. Patients were measured in the treatment position under the medical linear accelerator and the fiber probes (tips touching skin) were attached to the face mask, which are typically used in RT (Fig. 2). Chicken leg sample was treated similarly. Prior to each data collection background and reference spectra measurements were performed using the standard procedures provided by the spectrometer manufacturer.

The study included 20 patients with total fractions of 80 measurements. Measured patients were undergoing whole brain RT (WBRT) for 20 Gy delivered in small doses called fractions in 4 Gy. Delivery of radiation dose implemented using forward-intensity modulated RT (FIMRT) and open field techniques. All the treatments were implemented with the dose rate of 600 monitor units (MU)/min. During the treatment session, the patient is in a supine position while two opposed radiation fields are targeted in the brain bilaterally, in 2 field setups of 1st irradiation of 25 s and 2nd irradiation of 24 s. For the tissue response comparison, chicken samples with skin were irradiated similarly, with same amount of treatment dose and setup as patient's measurement were implemented.

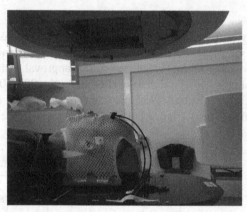

Fig. 2. Patient measurement setup for spectroscopic measurement of forehead skin. Both optical fibers were attached to the face mask at source-detector distance of 10 mm. Patient provided consent for use of the image.

3 Results

Figure 3 and 4 shows absorption effects of irradiation in the spectral range of 650 nm to 1100 nm when measured from patient's (on the left) and corresponding effects of irradiation measured from chicken sample (on the right). Both figures include four spectra responses representing average response before radiation, during irradiations, and after irradiation. In patient measurement, on the left, can be seen that absorbance increases as function of the irradiation. In chicken measurement there are no obvious changes in absorbance spectra caused by the irradiation.

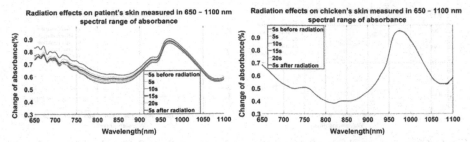

Fig. 3. Radiation effects on patient's skin (left) vs chicken skin (right) measured in 650–1100 nm spectral range of absorbance. Measurements were done during 1st irradiation continuously before, during and after irradiation. Spectra includes average of 5 s before radiation, average of 20 s of irradiation in 5 s period and average of 5 s after radiation.

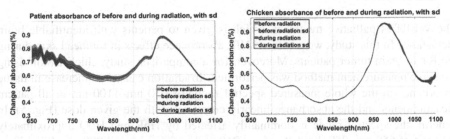

Fig. 4. Standard deviation of measured spectra from patient on the left and chicken sample on the right.

Figure 4 shows the change in absorbance due to irradiation. In the patient's measurement, as can be seen in the range 650 nm–800 nm absorbance starts to increase most strongly while between 800 nm–950 nm increase is slightly lower. In the range 950 nm–1100 nm where water is dominating the absorbance increase is lowest.

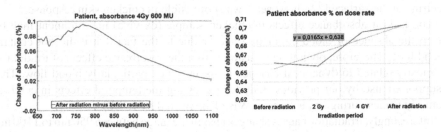

Fig. 5. Change of absorbance due to irradiation in patient RT. The absorbance increases due to irradiation, strongly from 700 nm to 800 nm and less in range of 800 nm to 1100 nm. On the right is shown dose dependent increase of absorbance at spectral range from 650 nm to 1100 nm.

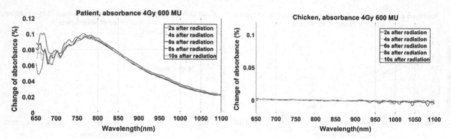

Fig. 6. Change of absorbance after irradiation in 2 s steps patients (left) and chicken (right). As can be seen after irradiation the absorbance starts to decrease back to its normal initial level, whereas no changes in absorbance can be seen in chicken sample.

4 Discussion

The WBRT is palliative treatment, which is given to patients with identifiable brain metastases. In this study, we measured NIR absorbance effects in forehead skin during the RT of brain tumor patients. Moreover, for a comparison study, chicken skin using the same measurement method was performed. Irradiation caused an increase in tissue absorbance in the whole measured spectral range of 650 nm–1100 nm in all patient measurements and the absorbance linearly correlates with the given dose (Fig. 5). In general, the spectral range is dominantly affected by HbR and HbO approximately at range of 650 nm–950, lipid at around 940 and water at around 980 nm. Significant changes from 650 nm to 800 nm indicate strong hemodynamic changes due to irradiation, which is interestingly visible only in patient's measurements (Fig. 5) and (Fig. 4). This indicates that oxygenation of blood in patients is strongly affected by irradiation. After irradiation the spectral response relaxes with time (Fig. 6).

Also, The LINACs used in radiation oncology that produce radiation in pulsed microseconds-long bursts, generated by the accelerator waveguide, and effects of Cherenkov radiation could be possible. Figure 5 (left) from patient's response shows similar to the radio dense tissue under 1 mm depth, effects of the Cherenkov emission spectrum at the surface [22], however it was not visible in chicken skin response.

The lack of absorbance effects in chicken sample (ex vivo) measurement may be due to the absence of blood circulation and/or due to the fact that it did not contain much blood. Therefore, obvious conclusion is that the absorbance effects of irradiation are mostly related to dynamical changes in tissue fluids particularly blood flow. This is supported also by our previous study [23] showing the temporal effects in cerebral haemodynamics during irradiations of WBRT measured by fNIRS.

Interestingly, irradiation causes changes also in the range between 950 nm to 1100 nm that is dominated by water absorbance, however, in chicken sample measurements there were in this spectral range neither visible effects of irradiation detected. The water absorbance effects in the patient measurements may be also related to blood circulation and particularly to the water bound with blood.

Prior research investigating tissue oxygenation and blood flow during RT indicates an association with increased blood flow and tissue oxygenation [10–12]. The efficacy of RT is known to be dependent on tumor oxygen status, as it enhances the free radicals which is responsible for DNA damage and cell death. Hence, the interaction of radiation in oxygenated tissue is more effective than the interaction in hypoxic cells. Usually tissue deoxygenates in few days after the first fraction of the radiation therapy [14]. However, there are studies reveal instances where some well-oxygenated tumors did not respond, while certain hypoxic tumors exhibited positive responses, possibly due to the dynamic changes during treatment in tumor oxygen status induced by radiation. Therefore, continuous monitoring of individual tumor hemodynamic status during therapy may provide valuable predictive information for treatment outcomes [11, 24]. In future, we aim to identify dose dependent absorbance response at selected NIR ranges during patient RT. The possibility to detect immediate tissue NIR absorbance changes during the RT can lead to different strategies in radiation dose planning and potentially improve the outcome of the RT when used in individual patient treatment planning.

Acknowledgments. This work was supported by Academy of Finland (grant 318347), EDUFI Fellowships and Finnish Cultural Foundation (Priya Karthikeyan).

References

1. LATEST GLOBAL CANCER DATA: CANCER BURDEN RISES TO 19.3 MILLION NEW CASES AND 10.0 MILLION CANCER DEATHS IN 2020 – IARC. https://www.iarc.who.int/featured-news/latest-global-cancer-data-cancer-burden-rises-to-19-3-million-new-cases-and-10-0-million-cancer-deaths-in-2020/. Accessed 23 May 2023
2. Furuse, M., et al.: Radiological diagnosis of brain radiation necrosis after cranial irradiation for brain tumor: a systematic review. Radiat. Oncol. **14**(1) (2019). https://doi.org/10.1186/S13014-019-1228-X
3. Li, Y.-Q., Ballinger, J.R., Nordal, R.A., Su, Z.-F., Wong, C.S.: Hypoxia in radiation-induced blood-spinal cord barrier breakdown 1. CANCER Res. **61**, 3348–3354 (2001)
4. Yoritsune, E., et al.: Inflammation as well as angiogenesis may participate in the pathophysiology of brain radiation necrosis. J. Radiat. Res. **55**(4), 803 (2014). https://doi.org/10.1093/JRR/RRU017
5. Nordal, R.A., Nagy, A., Pintilie, M., Wong, C.S.: Hypoxia and hypoxia-inducible factor-1 target genes in central nervous system radiation injury: a role for vascular endothelial growth factor. Clin. Cancer Res. **10**(10), 3342–3353 (2004). https://doi.org/10.1158/1078-0432.CCR-03-0426
6. Buboltz, J.B., Tadi, P.: Hyperbaric treatment of brain radiation necrosis. StatPearls, January 2023
7. Mehta, S.R., Suhag, V., Semwal, M., Sharma, N.: Radiotherapy: basic concepts and recent advances. Med. J. Armed Forces India **66**(2), 158–162 (2010). https://doi.org/10.1016/S0377-1237(10)80132-7
8. Karthikeyan, P., et al.: NIR spectroscopic immediate effects of irradiation on skin tissue: a comparison study of in vivo and ex vivo, vol. 12192, pp. 161–166, April 2022. https://doi.org/10.1117/12.2626362
9. Murkin, J.M., Arango, M.: Near-infrared spectroscopy as an index of brain and tissue oxygenation. Br. J. Anaesth. **103**(SUPPL.1), i3–i13 (2009). https://doi.org/10.1093/BJA/AEP299

10. Sunar, U., et al.: Noninvasive diffuse optical measurement of blood flow and blood oxygenation for monitoring radiation therapy in patients with head and neck tumors: a pilot study. J. Biomed. Opt. **11**(6), 064021 (2006). https://doi.org/10.1117/1.2397548

11. Dong, L., et al.: Diffuse optical measurements of head and neck tumor hemodynamics for early prediction of chemoradiation therapy outcomes. J. Biomed. Opt. **21**(8), 085004 (2016). https://doi.org/10.1117/1.jbo.21.8.085004

12. Oshtrakh, M.I.: Comparison of the oxyhemoglobin deoxygenation and radiolysis by γ-rays and electrons: study by Mössbauer spectroscopy. Nucl. Instruments Methods Phys. Res. Sect. B Beam Interact. with Mater. Atoms **185**(1–4), 129–135 (2001). https://doi.org/10.1016/S0168-583X(01)00815-1

13. Jakubowski, D.B., et al.: Monitoring neoadjuvant chemotherapy in breast cancer using quantitative diffuse optical spectroscopy: a case study. J. Biomed. Opt. **9**(1), 230 (2004). https://doi.org/10.1117/1.1629681

14. Rf, K.: The phenomenon of reoxygenation and its implications for fractionated radiotherapy. Radiology **105**(1), 135–142 (1972). https://doi.org/10.1148/105.1.135

15. Myllylä, T., Karthikeyan, P., Honka, U., Korhonen, V., Karhula, S.S., Nikkinen, J.: Cerebral haemodynamic effects in the human brain during radiation therapy for brain cancer, p. 76 (2020). https://doi.org/10.1117/12.2555892

16. Yohan, D., et al.: Quantitative monitoring of radiation induced skin toxicities in nude mice using optical biomarkers measured from diffuse optical reflectance spectroscopy. Biomed. Opt. Express **5**(5), 1309 (2014). https://doi.org/10.1364/BOE.5.001309

17. Chin, L.C.L., et al.: Early biomarker for radiation-induced wounds: day one post-irradiation assessment using hemoglobin concentration measured from diffuse optical reflectance spectroscopy. Biomed. Opt. Express **8**(3), 1682 (2017). https://doi.org/10.1364/BOE.8.001682

18. Chin, L., et al.: Diffuse optical spectroscopy for the quantitative assessment of acute ionizing radiation induced skin toxicity using a mouse model. J. Vis. Exp. **2016**(111), 53573 (2016). https://doi.org/10.3791/53573

19. Korhonen, V.O., et al.: Light propagation in NIR spectroscopy of the human brain. IEEE J. Sel. Top. Quantum Electron. **20**(2) (2014). https://doi.org/10.1109/JSTQE.2013.2279313

20. Finlayson, L., et al.: Depth penetration of light into skin as a function of wavelength from 200 to 1000 nm. Photochem. Photobiol. **98**(4), 974–981 (2022). https://doi.org/10.1111/PHP.13550

21. Bertout, J.A., Patel, S.A., Celeste Simon, M.: The impact of O2 availability on human cancer. Nat. Rev. Cancer **8**(12), 967–975 (2008). https://doi.org/10.1038/nrc2540

22. Alexander, D.A., Nomezine, A., Jarvis, L.A., Gladstone, D.J., Pogue, B.W., Bruza, P.: Color Cherenkov imaging of clinical radiation therapy. Light Sci. Appl. **10**(1), 1–7 (2021). https://doi.org/10.1038/s41377-021-00660-0

23. Myllylä, T., et al.: Cerebral tissue oxygenation response to brain irradiation measured during clinical radiotherapy. J. Biomed. Opt. **28**(1) (2023). https://doi.org/10.1117/1.JBO.28.1.015002

24. Brizel, D.M., Sibley, G.S., Prosnitz, L.R., Scher, R.L., Dewhirst, M.W.: Tumor hypoxia adversely affects the prognosis of carcinoma of the head and neck. Int. J. Radiat. Oncol. Biol. Phys. **38**(2), 285–289 (1997). https://doi.org/10.1016/S0360-3016(97)00101-6

Digital Twins for Development
of Microwave-Based Brain Tumor Detection

Mariella Särestöniemi[1,2]([✉]), Daljeet Singh[1], Charline Heredia[1], Juha Nikkinen[1,3,5], Mikael von und zu Fraunberg[5], and Teemu Myllylä[1,3,4]

[1] Health Science and Technology, Faculty of Medicine, University of Oulu, Oulu, Finland
mariella.sarestoniemi@oulu.fi
[2] Centre for Wireless Communications, Faculty of Information Technology and Electrical Engineering, University of Oulu, Oulu, Finland
[3] Medical Research Center, Oulu, Finland
[4] Optoelectronics and Measurements, Faculty of Information Technology and Electrical Engineering, University of Oulu, Oulu, Finland
[5] Oulu University Hospital, University of Oulu, Oulu, Finland

Abstract. Digital twins for different healthcare applications are currently being studied actively since they could revolutionize research on customized and personalized healthcare and enable realistic evaluations of new medical devices and applications in early phase. This paper presents a study on the development of digital twins aiming to be utilized for the development of microwave technique-based brain tumor detection. Realistic anatomical models of the digital twins were designed based on magnetic resonance images (MRI) scanned from the brain with brain tumor. These twins aim to correspond to the human brain and brain tumor in terms of size, shape, and tissue dielectric properties. Furthermore, developed digital twins include both phantom models for measurement emulation as well as corresponding simulation models designed using electromagnetic simulation software. By using the developed digital twins, our aim is to evaluate microwave-based sensing technique for brain tumor detection. Evaluations were carried out using flexible ultrawideband (UWB) antennas which would be beneficial for practical solutions. Our simulation and emulation results show that microwave technique with flexible antennas has high potential for brain tumor detection.

Keywords: Brain Tumor Detection · Digital Twins for Healthcare · Human Tissue Phantoms · Microwave Technique · Ultrawideband

1 Introduction

Digital twins in healthcare commonly refer to virtual representations or models of physical patients, organs, or processes. These virtual replicas can be created using data collected from various sources, including e.g. medical records and images or physiological measurements. Hence, digital twins aim to accurately mimic the behavior, characteristics, and responses of their real-world counterparts and they are considered to have

M. Särestöniemi et al. (Eds.): NCDHWS 2024, CCIS 2083, pp. 240–254, 2024.
https://doi.org/10.1007/978-3-031-59080-1_18

many potential and significant benefits in the research of medical diagnosis and therapies [1–5]. Digital twins serve for several different purposes: a) Simulation and predictive analysis, b) Personalized medicine, c) Medical training and education, d) Remote Monitoring and Telehealth, and e) Research and Development. For instance, digital twins have been proposed e.g., for research on drug delivery, arrythmia, detecting severity of carotid stenoses from head vibration [1, 5]. The proposed digital twins in the literature are mainly computer models without possibility to test diagnosis device or treatment in practice.

There exist few 3D phantom-based studies in the literature which aim at realistic appearance and tissue thickness [6, 7]. However, very limited number of studies have been presented how digital twins could be developed using magnetic resonance images (MRI) and how they could be used in realistic simulation and emulation platforms for assessments of new medical monitoring applications [8–10] Moreover, up to authors' knowledge, none of the previous studies have focused on brain tumor modelling.

1.1 Microwave-Based Brain Tumor Monitoring

Brain tumors are abnormal growth of cells in the brain which can be categorized to benign (noncancerous) or malignant (cancerous) [11]. Conventionally, brain tumors are detected by magnetic resonance imaging (MRI) scanning, computed tomography (CT) scans, and positron emission tomography (PET) [12, 13]. Recently, interest in using microwave sensing/imaging technology for brain cancer detection has increased since it enables a safe, rapid, low-cost, noninvasive solution which involves nonionizing radiation, and it can be realized with portable devices [14]. The microwave technique is based on detecting differences in radio channel responses caused by abnormalities having different dielectric properties than the surrounding tissues [14]. Microwave technique has been proposed for several different brain monitoring applications such as stroke detection [15, 16], brain temperature monitoring [17, 18], and cerebral circulation monitoring [19–21]. Additionally, its suitability for detection of brain tumors has been studied in [23–27].

1.2 Objectives and Contribution

The first aim is to show how realistic digital brain tumor twins are developed from gadolium enhanced T1 weighted MRI images. The second aim is to utilize digital twins to prepare a realistic emulation and simulation environments to evaluate microwave sensing based brain tumor detection technique. The emulation environment developed with the brain tumor digital twin and realistic human tissue mimicking phantoms, i.e. replicas of human tissues in terms of size, shape, and dielectric properties. The simulation environment is created in electromagnetic simulation software platform with the developed tumor simulation model embedded with anatomically realistic human head model. The third aim is to carry out evaluations with developed emulation and simulation platforms to investigate microwave sensing technique in brain tumor detection.

This paper is organized as follows: Sect. 2 describes in detail how the brain tumor digital twins can be prepared from MRI images. Section 3 describes the realistic simulation and emulation platforms. Section 4 presents results for measurements and simulations. Finally, Conclusions and future works in given in Sect. 5.

2   Preparation of Digital Twin of Brain Tumor from MRI

2.1   Tumor Mold Preparation

In this section, the procedure to prepare digital brain tumor twins is explained. It includes description how to develop brain tumor models from gadolium enhanced T1 weighted MRI images and how to prepare brain tumor phantoms as well as other relevant phantoms to be used in the realistic emulation platform. Additionally, use of brain twins in realistic simulation platforms is explained as well.

Realistic-shaped and -sized brain tumor digital twin is developed by using MRI images of real brain tumor (permission obtained from the patient), which is presented using *FSLeyes software* image in Fig. 1. The tumor is approximately 5 cm large and located on the left temporal lobe of the brain. The aim is to convert the MRI-image to a 3D model, which can be used directly in the simulation model and/or further convert a negation of the model to obtain a tumor mold which could be used for brain tumor phantom development.

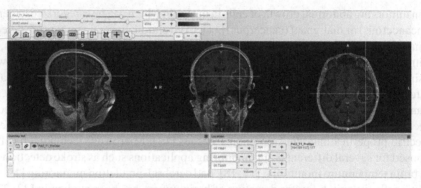

Fig. 1. Brain tumor image represented with the FSLeyes software.

Firstly, tumor's mask is created on each MRI slice image, as shown in Fig. 2a. Tumor is cropped from each MRI-image slice manually to isolate it from the rest of the image, as shown in Fig. 2b. As a result, the tumor model shown in Fig. 2c is obtained. The model is in.nii format, which is a raster format, with files generally containing at least 3-dimensional data: voxels, or pixels with a width, height, and depth. To convert this file to smoother format and suitable for 3D printing, the second software, *3DSlicer* is used.

With 3D slicer software, pixelization can be removed and unnecessary holes of the model can be filled. Figure 3 illustrates tumor model before and after smoothening with 3DSlicer. Additionally, the 3DSlicer converts the tumor model to.stl format which is suitable to be used for 3D printing or in simulation software.

Finally, *Fusion360* software is used to create a mold for phantom by performing the negation of the 3D model, as shown in Fig. 4. The mold is composed of two inter-locking parts including a hole which allows the insertion of the phantom mixture before solidification. Finally, the mold parts are printed with 3D printer. The mold halves are presented in Fig. 5.

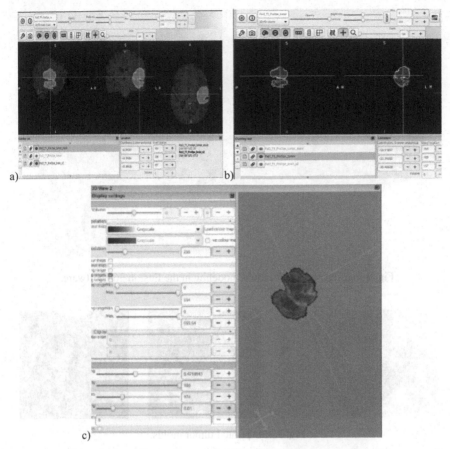

Fig. 2. a) Creation of a tumor's mask on each MRI slice image, b) isolation of the tumor from the rest of the MRI image, c) volume visualization of the tumor on the FSLeyes software.

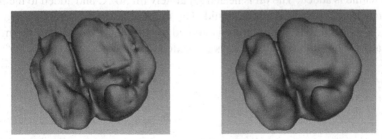

Fig. 3. Tumor model (on the left) before and (on the right) after the smoothening with 3DSlicer software.

2.2 Tumor Phantom Preparation

Tumor phantom mixture is prepared using the recipe presented in [7] and repeated in Table 1. The aim is to obtain the same dielectric properties as measured for brain tumor

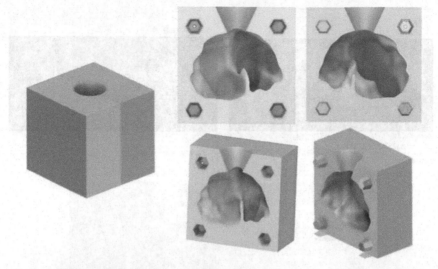

Fig. 4. Different views of mold modeling in the Fusion 360 software.

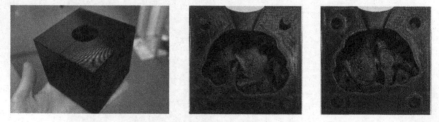

Fig. 5. 3D printed tumor molds.

in [29]. The cooking procedure is the following: First, the water is heated to 65 °C before gelatine is added. The oil is heated separately till 50 °C and added to the mixture at the same time with dishwashing liquid. The mixture is stirred smoothly and heated until 65 °C is achieved. The mixture is cooled slightly and poured into the mold for solidification. The solidified phantom is presented in Fig. 6.

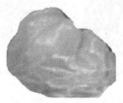

Fig. 6. Solidified brain tumor phantom with size of 5 cm.

3 Realistic Emulation and Simulation Platforms

3.1 Realistic Emulation Platform: Phantoms, Antennas, and Measurement Setups

3.1.1 Phantoms

The realistic emulation platforms include human tissue phantoms (skin and brain), tumor phantom, real human skull (borrowed from Pathology department), Vector Network Analyzer (VNA8720ES), and flexible ultrawideband (UWB) antennas.

Brain phantom is prepared using a realistic sized and shaped brain model retrieved from public 3D organ library The mold for brain phantom, illustrated in Fig. 7a, is prepared using Fusion360 software similarly to the brain tumor mold is prepared as explained in Sect. 2. The tumor and brain phantoms are prepared using the recipe depicted in Table 1 and which are originally presented in [7]. The solidified brain phantom is presented in Fig. 7b. Besides this average brain phantom, we also prepare a tumorous brain phantom in which the earlier developed tumor phantom is inserted inside the brain in the same location as depicted by MRI image. The skin phantom is also prepared based on the recipe given in [7] and summarized in Table 1. Solidified skin phantom is presented in Fig. 7c. The dielectric properties of the skin and brain phantoms are designed to closely match those of average human tissue at the selected frequencies, as outlined in ITIS foundation public datasheets [30].

Table 1. Recipes for skin, brain, and tumor phantoms [7].

Ingredients	Distilled water [ml]	Gelatine [g]	Oil [ml]	Distilled water [ml]
Skin	10	3.01	1.68	0.83
Brain	9	1.5	1.1	0.5
Tumor	20.3	1.63	1.1	0.9

3.1.2 Antennas

The antenna used in this study is a flexible monopole designed for in-body sensing for the frequency range 2–10 GHz covering both ISM band 2.5 GHz and UWB 3.1–10.6 GHz. The antenna is a slightly larger but improved version of the flexible antenna introduced in [31]. The size of the antenna is $x = 40$ mm, $y = 40$ mm, and $z = 0.125$ mm; it is fabricated on a thin flexible substrate Rogers5880 and is designed to be attached to the skin surface. Figure 8a–b presents the simulation model and the prototype of the antenna, respectively.

3.1.3 Measurement Setups

In this study, two measurements setups are required. The first one, consisting of Vector Network Analyzer (VNA) and SPEG's probe and depicted in Fig. 9a, is used to evaluate

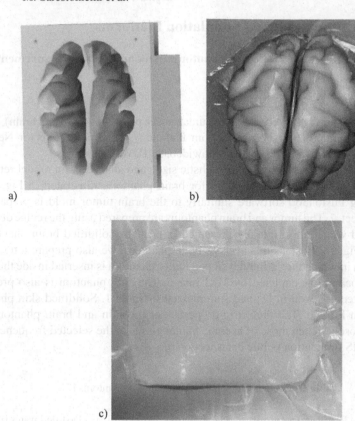

Fig. 7. a) Brain mold prepared with Fusion 360 software, b) solidified brain phantom, c) solidified skin phantom.

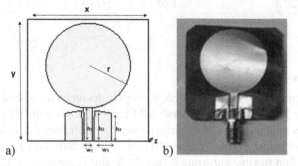

Fig. 8. The flexible UWB antenna used in the evaluations: a) simulation model, b) prototype.

dielectric properties of the phantoms before using them in the measurements. The second measurement setup consists of VNA, UWB antennas and absorber pieces which are built to avoid additional reflections to antennas from the surrounding items. The antennas are located around the voxel model's head similarly to a portable helmet or band type of scenario. Measurements with VNA are carried out for the frequency range 2–8 GHz to evaluate antenna reflection coefficients S11 and S22 as well as channel transfer function S21 and S12.

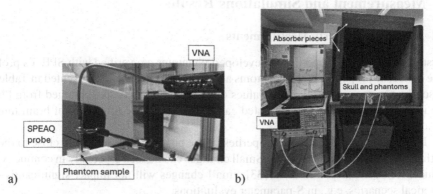

a)   b)

Fig. 9. a) measurements set up with VNA and SPEAG probe to evaluate dielectric properties of the developed phantoms, b) measurements set up with VNA, real human skull, phantoms, and antennas to evaluate microwave sensing technology in brain tumor detection.

3.2 Realistic Simulation Setup

The simulations are carried out using electromagnetic simulation software CST [32] which has several anatomically realistic human voxel models resembling humans having different sizes and body constitutions. For these evaluations, we chose the voxel model Hugo since it has the most realistic brain model. The antennas are located around the voxel model's head similarly to a portable helmet or band type of scenario. Firstly, the simulations are carried out in the reference case, i.e. without any abnormalities. Next, the realistic tumor model is inserted into the brain model in the same location as in MRI-image hence resembling fully realistic scenario. S-parameters simulations are conducted

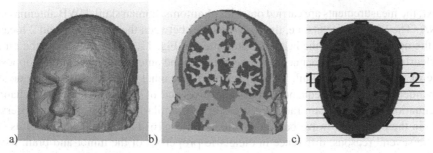

a)   b)   c)

Fig. 10. a) Realistic CST's Hugo-voxel model, b) vertical crosscut of the voxel's head, c) horizontal cross-section of the voxel's head illustrating the location of the realistic tumor model and antennas 1 and 2.

only up to 5.8GHz to save simulation time which usually increases remarkably with voxel models with higher frequencies.

4 Measurement and Simulations Results

4.1 Dielectric Property Measurements

Firstly, the dielectric properties of developed phantoms are verified with SPEG's probe. The dielectric properties of the phantoms at 2.5 GHz and 6 GHz are presented in Table 2. Also, the corresponding reference values of average human tissue, obtained from [30], are included for comparison. As stated earlier, the dielectric properties of brain tumor are obtained from [29].

It is found that the dielectric properties of the phantoms are relatively close to those of the average human tissue values. Small changes can be seen especially in conductivity values. However, as presented in [33], small changes will not impact significantly on practical scenarios, e.g., in S-parameter evaluations.

Table 2. Dielectric properties of the developed phantoms and average tissues [29, 30]

Frequency	2.5 GHz	6 GHz
Brain tumor phantom	59.1	56
Brain tumor	58.5/5.1	52.2/7.5
Brain phantom	42.8/2.1	39.5/4.8
Average brain	42.45/1.54	38.05/4.44
Skin phantom	38.2/1.96	34.1/3.76
Average skin	38.0/1.49	34.9/3.89

4.2 Measurement Results with Realistic Platform

Next, the measurements are carried out with phantoms, human skull, UWB antennas and VNA. The S21 parameters, i.e. the radio channel between the antennas 1 and 2 located on the opposite sides of the head, are presented in Fig. 11. As it can be seen the tumor is clearly visible in the channel response between the antennas located on the opposite side of the sides of the skull. The impact on the channel characteristics is frequency-dependent: at certain frequency ranges the presence of tumor increases the channel attenuation and the certain ranges decrease it. A similar tendency has been observed also in the other microwave-based detection studies [16, 17]. This phenomenon is due to the several reasons: difference in dielectric properties of the tumor and brain tissue vary with the frequency and thus the diffraction caused by tumor on the propagation signal may vary clearly. Additionally, antenna radiation characteristics may vary with frequency: at certain ranges there might be a radiation null towards the tumor and at certain ranges there could be a stronger lobe towards the tumor or on the sides of the tumor. All these aspects affect together on the propagation in vicinity of tumor and hence in general inside the tissue. Hence, careful study on optimal frequency range and optimal antenna locations with realistic models is essential for microwave-based detection applications.

When comparing the reference and tumorous results obtained from the measurements, there is always a small possibility of some uncertainties, e.g., due to unintentional movements of cables, or antennas. Thus, it is good to carry out comparative simulations in which these uncertainties are removed. The simulation results for a similar setup are presented in the next section.

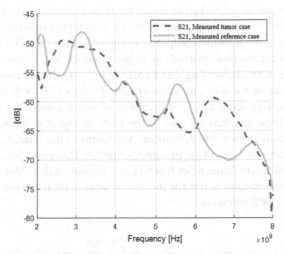

Fig. 11. Measured S21 results obtained with phantoms and real human skull.

4.3 Simulation Results

Finally, the simulations are carried out with CST and realistic brain tumor. The location of the tumor is set the same as with the measurement model and in MRI-images. In this case, the simulations are carried out only till 5.8 GHz to save simulation time which increases drastically as the frequency increases. Besides, at higher frequencies, the penetration of the radio signal through the whole head is not possible within due to higher propagation loss. The S-parameter results are presented in Fig. 12. It is found that also in this case, there is clear difference between the reference and tumorous cases: even up to 15 dB at 2.5 GHz. Channel attenuation decreases significantly after 3 GHz since the propagation loss in the tissue increases. Additionally. The flexible antennas are not directional and thus, less power can be directed towards the body than compared to the directive antennas. However, the advantage of the flexible antennas is excellent feasibility to the practical applications.

When comparing simulation and measurement results, it is noted that the channel attenuation is clearly stronger in the simulations than in the measurements. For instance, at 2.5 GHz, the level of S21 parameters is −60 dB in the simulations whereas only around −50 dB in the measurements. One reason for this is that the size of Hugo-voxel's head is larger than that of a real human skull. Additionally, as noted in Fig. 10b, Hugo -voxel clearly has thicker muscle and fat layers than average in that area of the head where antennas (and tumor) are located. Especially in muscle tissue, the propagation loss is high due to high relative permittivity [30] and thus excessively thick muscle layer effects on the results remarkably. However, the trend is similar in both results: tumor causes clear differences in the channel responses. At lower frequencies, 1–1.5 GHz, the channel attenuation is stronger in the presence of tumor, whereas between 2–4 GHz it is vice versa. In the measurement the trend was somewhat similar, but the S21 curves have more fluctuation and thus there are some exceptions in this trend.

The reason for this trend is that, at lower frequencies, where the microwave signal penetrates the whole head easily, the tumor tissue with higher relative permittivity than brain tissue impedes propagation compared to the reference case. This can be seen as increased channel attenuation. Instead, at higher frequencies, where the propagation inside the tissue is more challenging due to higher loss, significant amount of the radio signal propagates as on the skin surface as creeping waves [33] or though the fat layer. In this antenna location setup case, the presence of tumor causes stronger diffractions towards on-body area, and thus the part of the in-body signal is summed to the signal travelling on the skin surface which is more prominent in this case. Consequently, the channel appears to be stronger in the presence of tumor. However, the antenna radiation characteristics at different frequencies have a clear impact on this. More comprehensive analysis of this phenomenon is left for the future work with the evaluations of several different types of UWB antennas.

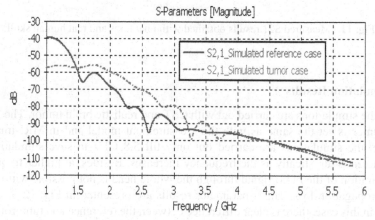

Fig. 12. S21 parameter results with Hugo-voxel model obtained with the simulation in the presence and absence of the realistic brain tumor model.

5 Summary and Conclusions

This paper presents a study on the development of digital twins for microwave sensing based brain tumor monitoring applications. The first aim was to show how realistic digital brain tumor twins can be developed from MRI and CT images. The second aim was to utilize digital twins to prepare a realistic emulation and simulation environment to evaluate microwave sensing based brain tumor detection technique. The emulation environment was developed with the brain tumor digital twin and realistic human tissue mimicking phantoms, the simulation environment was created in electromagnetic simulation software with the developed tumor simulation model embedded with anatomically realistic human head model.

This paper also presented realistic evaluations with the developed emulation and simulation platforms to investigate microwave sensing technique in brain tumor detection. Evaluations were carried out using flexible UWB antennas which are beneficial for practical solutions. The realistic simulation and emulation results show that microwave sensing is efficient in brain tumor detection also with flexible antennas. In order to have fully comparable simulation and measurement results, thicknesses of the tissues and also dimensions of the skull should be equal, otherwise there are clear differences in the S-parameter results especially if the antennas are located on the opposite sides of the head. Nevertheless, the trend was found to be similar in both cases: the presence of tumor clearly changes the radio signal propagation inside the brain which can be detected in S21 results. The changes are frequency dependent as is found also in previous studies [12].

The results presented in this paper are remarkable in several ways: the development of digital twins for healthcare is an important and timely topic since they could revolutionize research on medical/healthcare applications taking steps towards the future's customized and personalized health care. In addition, digital twins with authentic texture of target tissue could be used in the training of microsurgical skills to neurosurgery residents The results of this paper outline the importance of usability of adjustable digital twins in the evaluations: they help to understand how for instance frequency selection and antenna location has to planned carefully with realistic and adjustable models since the tissue thicknesses affect clearly on the results, especially if aiming to do whole head scanning using antennas located opposite sides of the head. Moreover, the detectability of brain tumor with flexible antennas is a promising result for the research on practical applications: flexible antennas are easily feasible even with a head band type of portable monitoring device.

In this paper, we presented only pure frequency domain S-parameter data. As our future work, we will analyze microwave sensing in different signal domains and study the efficiency of different imaging algorithms. Furthermore, we will start developing digital twins for multimodal monitoring applications which includes design and development of multimodal phantoms.

Acknowledgments. This research is funded by Academy of Finland Profi6 funding, 6G-Enabling Sustainable Society (University of Oulu, Finland) the Academy of Finland 6G Flagship, under Grant 318927, and by European Structural and Investment Funds - European Regional Development Fund (ERDF), EMUVALID, which are greatly acknowledged.

Disclosure of Interests. The authors have no competing interests to declare that are relevant to the content of this article.

References

1. Alazab, M., et al.: Digital twins for Healthcare 4.0—recent advances, architecture, and open challenges. IEEE Consum. Electron. Mag. **12**(6), 29–37 (2023). https://doi.org/10.1109/MCE. 2022.3208986
2. Angulo, C., Gonzalez-Abril, L., Raya, C., Ortega, J.A.: A proposal to evolving towards digital twins in healthcare. In: International Work-Conference on Bioinformatics and Biomedical Engineering, pp. 418–426 (2020)
3. Neghab, K.H., Jamshidi, M., Keshmiri Neghab, H.: Digital twin of a magnetic medical microrobot with stochastic model predictive controller boosted by machine learning in cyber-physical healthcare systems. Information **13**(7), 321 (2022)
4. Okegbile, S.D., Cai, J., Niyato, D., Yi, C.: Human digital twin for personalized healthcare: vision, architecture and future directions. IEEE Netw. **37**(2), 262–269 (2023). https://doi.org/10.1109/MNET.118.2200071
5. Shengli, W.: Is human digital twin possible? Comput. Methods Progr. Biomed. Update **1**, 100014 (2021). https://doi.org/10.1016/j.cmpbup.2021.100014
6. Särestöniemi, M., Dessai, R., Heredia, C., Hakala, J., Myllymäki, S., Myllylä, T.: Novel Realistic 3D phantom emulation platform for human torso and head at microwave range. MPDI Sens. (2024)
7. Pokorny, T., Vrba, D., Tesarik, T., Rodrigues, D.B., Vrba, J.: Anatomically and dielectrically realistic 2.5 D 5-layer reconfigurable head phantom for testing microwave stroke detection and classification. Int. J. Antenn. Propag. **2019**, 1–7 (2019)
8. Myllylä, T., et al.: Prototype of an opto-capacitive probe for non-invasive sensing cerebrospinal fluid circulation. In: Dynamics and Fluctuations in Biomedical Photonics XIV, vol. 10063, pp. 40–46. SPIE, March 2017
9. Korhonen, V.O., et al.: Light propagation in NIR spectroscopy of the human brain. IEEE J. Sel. Top. Quantum Electron. **20**(2), 289–298 (2013)
10. Myllylä, T., Popov, A., Korhonen, V., Bykov, A., Kinnunen, M.: Optical sensing of a pulsating liquid in a brain-mimicking phantom. In: European Conference on Biomedical Optics, p. 87990X. Optica Publishing Group, May 2013
11. RicardoMcFaline-Figueroa, J., Lee, E.Q.: Brain tumors. Am. J. Med. **131**(8), 874–882 (2018). https://doi.org/10.1016/j.amjmed.2017.12.039
12. Fink, J.R., Muzi, M., Peck, M., Krohn, K.A.: Multimodality brain tumor imaging: MR imaging, PET, and PET/MR imaging. J. Nucl. Med. **56**(10), 1554–1561 (2015). https://doi.org/10.2967/jnumed.113.131516
13. Mohammed, B.J., Abbosh, A.M., Mustafa, S., Ireland, D.: Microwave system for head imaging. IEEE Trans. Instrum. Meas. **63**(1), 117–123 (2014)
14. Ali, S., Li, J., Pci, Y., et al.: A comprehensive survey on brain tumor diagnosis using deep learning and emerging hybrid techniques with multi-modal MR image. Arch. Comput. Methods Eng. **29**, 4871–4896 (2022). https://doi.org/10.1007/s11831-022-09758-z
15. Särestöniemi, M., Myllymäki, S., Reponen, J., Myllylä, T.: Remote diagnostics and monitoring using microwave technique – improving healthcare in rural areas and in exceptional situations. Finnish J. eHealth eWelfare (FinJeHeW) **15** (2023)
16. Scapaticci, R., Di Donato, L., Catapano, I., Crocco, L.: A feasibility study on microwave imaging for brain stroke monitoring. Progr. Electromagnet. Res. B **40**, 305–324 (2012). https://doi.org/10.2528/PIERB12022006

17. Guo, L., Alqadami, A.S.M., Abbosh, A.: Stroke diagnosis using microwave techniques: review of systems and algorithms. IEEE J. Electromagnet. RF Microwaves Med. Biol. **7**(2), 122–135 (2023). https://doi.org/10.1109/JERM.2022.3227724

18. Särestöniemi, M., et al.: Detection of brain hemorrhage in white matter using analysis of radio channel characteristics. In: BodyNets2020, October 2020

19. Stauffer, P.R., et al.: Non-invasive measurement of brain temperature with microwave radiometry: demonstration in a head phantom and clinical case. Neuroradiol. J. **27**(1), 3–12 (2014). https://doi.org/10.15274/NRJ-2014-10001. Epub 2014

20. Shevelev, O., et al.: Using medical microwave radiometry for brain temperature measurements. Drug Discov. Today **27**(3), 881–889 (2022)

21. Moradi, S., Ferdinando, H., Zienkiewicz, A., Särestöniemi, M., Myllylä, T.: Book chapter "Current and emerging methods for monitoring cerebral circulation in human,". In: IntechOpen Book, titled Cerebral Circulation - Updates on Models, Diagnostics and Treatments of Related Diseases, January 2022

22. Ojaroudi, M., Bila, S.: Dynamic short-range sensing approach using MIMO radar for brain activities monitoring. In: 2020 14th European Conference on Antennas and Propagation (EuCAP), 15–20 March 2020, pp. 1–5. IEEE, Copenhagen (2020)

23. Ojaroudi, M., Bila, S.: Multiple time-variant targets detection using MIMO radar framework for cerebrovascular monitoring. In: 2021 15th European Conference on Antennas and Propagation (EuCAP), Dusseldorf, Germany, 22–26 March 2021, pp. 1–5. IEEE (2021)

24. Stancombe, A., Bialkowski, E., Abbosh, A.M.: Portable microwave head imaging system using software-defined radio and switching network. IEEE J. Electromagnet. RF Microwaves Med. Biol. **3**(4), 284–291 (2019)

25. Inum, R., Rana, Md.M., Shushama, K.N., Quader, Md.A.: EBG based microstrip patch antenna for brain tumor detection via scattering parameters in microwave imaging system. Int. J. Biomed. Imaging **2018**, 12 pages (2018). https://doi.org/10.1155/2018/8241438. Article ID 8241438

26. Velan, B., Marcilin, L.J.A., Sheeba, I.R., Mani, S., Sanju, M.S.: Design of microwave wideband antenna for brain tumor imaging applications. In: 2021 International Conference on Artificial Intelligence and Smart Systems (ICAIS), Coimbatore, India, pp. 906–910 (2021). https://doi.org/10.1109/ICAIS50930.2021.9396000

27. Sholeh, H.R., Rizkinia, M., Basari, B.: Design of microwave-based brain tumor detection framework with the development of sparse and low-rank compressive sensing image reconstruction. Int. J. Technol. **11**(5), 984–994 (2020)

28. Gao, Y.J., Liu, J.X., Ye, Q.Y.: Research on the detection of the brain tumor with the ultrawideband microwave signal based on the high-precision symplectic finite-difference time-domain electromagnetic algorithm and beam forming imaging algorithm. Int. J. RF Microwave Comput. Aided Eng. **30**, e22463 (2020)

29. Yoo, D.S.: The dielectric properties of cancerous tissues in a nude mouse xenograft model. Bioelectromagnetics **25**(7), 492–497 (2004). https://doi.org/10.1002/bem.20021. PMID: 15376246

30. https://www.itis.ethz.ch/virtual-population/tissue-properties/databaseM. Accessed 1 Oct 2023

31. Särestöniemi, M., Sonkki, M., Myllymäki, S., Pomalaza-Raez, C.: Wearable flexible antenna for UWB on-body and implant communications. Telecom. **2**(3), 285–301 (2021)

32. Dassault Simulia CST Suite. https://www.3ds.com/. Accessed 1 Nov 2022

33. Särestöniemi, M., Dessai, R., Myllymäki, S., Myllylä, T.: A novel durable fat tissue phantom for microwave based medical monitoring applications. In: Chen, Y., Yao, D., Nakano, T. (eds.) BICT 2023, pp. 166–177. Springer, Cham (2023). https://doi.org/10.1007/978-3-031-43135-7_16

34. Orfanidis, S.: Electromagnetic Waves and Antennas. http://www.ece.rutgers.edu/~orfanidi/ewa/

Digital Care Pathways 1

The Role of Digital Care Pathway for Epilepsy on Patients' Treatment Burden: Clinicians' Perspective

Manria Polus[1,2]([✉]) [iD], Pantea Keikhosrokiani[1,2] [iD], Johanna Uusimaa[3,4] [iD],
Jonna Komulainen-Ebrahim[3,4] [iD], Johanna Annunen[4,5,6] [iD], Sehrish Khan[1] [iD],
Woubshet Behutiye[1] [iD], Päivi Vieira[3,4,5] [iD], and Minna Isomursu[1,2] [iD]

[1] Faculty of Information Technology and Electrical Engineering, University of Oulu,
90570 Oulu, Finland
manria.polus@oulu.fi

[2] Faculty of Medicine, University of Oulu, 90014 Oulu, Finland

[3] Department of Children and Adolescents, Division of Pediatric Neurology,
Oulu University Hospital, 90029 Oulu, Finland

[4] Research Unit of Clinical Medicine and Medical Research Center, Oulu University Hospital
and University of Oulu, 90014 Oulu, Finland

[5] Member of ERN-Epicare, Oulu University Hospital, 90029 Oulu, Finland

[6] Neurocenter, Neurology, Oulu University Hospital, 90029 Oulu, Finland

Abstract. Epilepsy is a chronic neurological disorder, requiring long-term treatment. The workload and impact of treatment causes a significant burden to patients. Digital care pathways may have potential for reducing treatment burden, but there also may be concerns of additional burden caused by digital healthcare. The aim of this study is to investigate the role of digital care pathway on treatment burden for patients with epilepsy. This was a single case study with the digital care pathway for epilepsy in the Wellbeing Services County of North Ostrobothnia (Pohde), in Finland, as a unit of analysis. The data was collected by observing an expert meeting of three clinicians. The meeting focused on five pre-defined domains of treatment burden: Medication burden, Time and travel burden, Financial burden, Social and emotional burden, and Healthcare access burden. The data was analyzed qualitatively and organized based on the pre-defined categories. The results suggest that the digital care pathway supports patients with treatment burden for all the pre-defined domains. Reported benefits include reduced travel, options for remote appointments, providing informational support and easier ways to contact healthcare professionals (HCPs). The main concerns clinicians had was could the use of digital care pathway cause rushed treatment decisions, difficulties of building trust and seeking support from HCPs, and difficulties of using the digital systems. A new theme emerged from the data, Diverse burdens, highlighting the variety of patients with epilepsy with differing needs for treatment.

Keywords: Chronic Illness · Treatment Burden · eHealth · Digital health

© The Author(s) 2024
M. Särestöniemi et al. (Eds.): NCDHWS 2024, CCIS 2083, pp. 257–268, 2024.
https://doi.org/10.1007/978-3-031-59080-1_19

1 Introduction

Digital healthcare has been found to be effective, accessible, and cost-effective for treating many conditions [1–3]. One way of complementing traditional health care with digital and remote treatment is through digital care pathways. Digital care pathways are web- or mobile-based healthcare interventions, where multidisciplinary teams works together to deliver care to patients, usually in a structured evidence-based way [4, 5]. Digital care pathways are used, for example, for filling in surveys, receiving feedback, reading patient instructions, and communicating with healthcare providers [6]. Oulu University Hospital has been using a web based digital care pathway for the treatment of epilepsy since 2020, and in December 2022 a mobile version was introduced to adults with epilepsy. Currently the users of the digital care pathway can keep a digital seizure diary, contact healthcare professionals, receive their replies, and record their healthcare data regarding treatments, other diagnosis, daily functional capacity, and possible depressive symptoms.

The current evidence shows that digital care pathways can improve patient outcomes, quality of care, and healthcare resource utilization [5]. People with epilepsy may specifically benefit from dynamic remote care, as it gives them easier ways to reach out when needed, and it has been suggested this could potentially reduce the number of seizures [7]. Digital care pathways can therefore offer new opportunities for improving outcomes beyond what current medication and healthcare delivery can achieve.

However, for developing digital healthcare, it is necessary to understand the unique circumstances for patients with different conditions. Epilepsy is a chronic neurological disorder characterized by recurrent seizures. The treatment of epilepsy may last through lifetime [8]. Even though the long-term prognosis for seizure cessation tends to be better in children than adults, 1/3 of children don´t achieve remission [9]. To manage their condition, people with epilepsy need to adhere to their treatment and learn various self-management skills, including identifying and managing seizure triggers, minimizing seizure-related risks, and educating others what to do during a seizure [10]. These demands are often referred to as treatment burden [11]. Treatment burden can be divided on several domains, including taking medications, travelling to appointments, cost of treatments, impact to social life, and difficulties accessing healthcare services [12, 13]. Digital healthcare may support patients with their treatment burden by, for example, reducing travel and making communication with healthcare professionals (HCPs) easier [14, 15]. It can also create additional challenges and barriers, for example by being inaccessible to some patients or shifting too much responsibility of care to the patients [16, 17].

Although the development of digital healthcare aims to consider patients' needs, the research for epilepsy has been mostly focusing on health outcomes, such as medication adherence, reducing seizures, and quality of life [18–21]. Since epilepsy is a life-long disease and often requires daily long-term treatment [8], it is important that the digital care pathways support patients managing their treatment burden and promoting long term use of the program. Therefore, there is a need to evaluate how digital care pathways affect the workload and demands of treatment for the patients using the care pathway.

The objective of this study is to investigate the role of digital care pathway on the treatment burden on patients with epilepsy, from the clinicians' point of view. The study design, procedures, and data analysis will be explained in Sect. 2, and the findings will be reported in Sect. 3. The paper is wrapped up with concluding remarks and future directions in Sect. 4 and 5.

2 Methods

2.1 Design

The study design is a single case study based on the definition by Robert Yin [22], with the digital care pathway for epilepsy (see Fig. 1) in the Wellbeing Services County of North Ostrobothnia (Pohde), in Finland, as a unit of analysis. Pohde is the wellbeing services county responsible for organizing public health, social and rescue services in North Ostrobothnia area [23]. The digital care pathway is one part of the public health services Pohde provides for patients with epilepsy in North Ostrobothnia.

Case study is a suitable method for the present study, as there is currently limited research about the impact of digital care pathways on treatment burden, and case study can be used as an exploratory phase of research to gather qualitative data [24]. We examine the role of digital care pathway on the treatment burden on patients with epilepsy and identify the potential challenges.

We followed the University of Oulu ethics process as defined in the guidelines from Ethics Committee of Human Sciences [25]. Even though the research topic is health related, the method does not involve medical research as defined in Ethics Committee of Medical Sciences [26]. Therefore, the guidelines for human sciences were more suitable.

The case study used systematic participant observation of an expert meeting for data collection. In participant observation, the researcher is a member of the group they are researching and so can better understand their situation [27]. The first author and the sixth author, who attended the meeting as participant observers, have been collaborating in the same research project as the clinicians and therefore were already familiar with them and the meeting topic. Using participant observation was selected for the present study, since it allowed the researchers to further gain familiarity with the digital care pathway development.

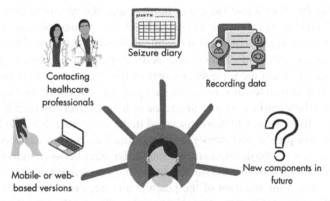

Fig. 1. Illustration of the components and functions of the digital care pathway for epilepsy in Pohde

2.2 Procedures

In December 2023, three experienced clinicians from Oulu University Hospital were invited to participate in an expert meeting. One clinician was working in the Neurocenter (Neurology) and two in the Pediatric neurology department. The purpose of the expert meeting was to discuss topics related to the treatment burden for patients and the sustainable design of the digital epilepsy care path. The invited clinicians treat patients with epilepsy in the Oulu University Hospital and have used the digital care pathway for epilepsy previously. For the purpose of this study, we have focused on the observed data relating to the treatment burden topic.

The meeting focused on five pre-defined domains of treatment burden: *Medication burden, Time and travel burden, Financial burden, Social and emotional burden*, and *Healthcare access burden*. These domains were identified based on two systematic reviews regarding treatment burden on people with chronic conditions [12, 13]. Prior to the meeting, the first author prepared a checklist to list and keep track of the relevant concepts discussed during the meeting. The checklist was reviewed and approved by three other authors from the research team. Clinicians were invited to discuss how the digital care pathway for epilepsy can impact these domains, considering both positive and negative impact.

2.3 Data Analysis

The online meeting was organized on Microsoft Teams. The meeting was recorded and automatically transcribed. The transcripts were analyzed with NVivo [28]. The transcripts were coded by the first author using deductive analysis approach [29] and organized according to the pre-defined categories. Inductive analysis approach [30] was used for adjusting existing categories and creating a new category from codes that did not fall under the pre-defined categories.

3 Results

Three clinicians attended the meeting on 8th December 2023. The collected data provided substantial content under five out of six pre-defined themes *Time and travel burden, Medication burden, Social and emotional burden*, and *Healthcare access burden*. The pre-defined theme *Financial burden* was moved under the theme *Time and travel burden*. The theme *Financial burden* consisted of treatment costs related to travel to appointments and other expenses, such as medications and medical operations. Even though non-travel related costs of treatment are a significant part of the overall treatment burden for the patients, the clinicians stated that the digital care pathway does not have direct impact on them. However, there can be a positive impact on reducing travel costs and loss of income due to absences from work, which are discussed in the *Time and travel burden* theme. In addition to the five pre-defined themes, a sixth theme *Diverse burdens* was discovered. *Diverse burdens* covers the discussion regarding differences between individual patients and special patient groups, that did not fall under the pre-defined themes. The findings are illustrated in a Venn diagram of the positive and negative impacts of digital care pathway on the treatment burden categories (see Fig. 2), and the identified impacts are listed in more detail in Table 1.

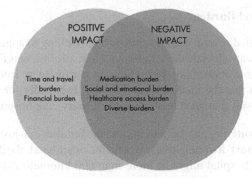

Fig. 2. A Venn diagram presenting the positive and negative impact of the digital care pathway regarding each category of treatment burden

Table 1. A list of the identified positive and negative impacts of digital care pathway on treatment burden

Treatment burden category	Positive impact	Negative impact
Time and travel burden	Less time spent on travelling to appointments Less absences from work or school	
Financial burden	Reduced cost of travel	
Medication burden	Informational support Increased effectiveness of care Faster resolving of problems	Potentially too fast decisions regarding medication
Social and emotional burden	Reduced negative emotions from hospital environment Reduced stigma and illness identity Remote appointments help to spend more time with family	Difficulties seeking support without face-to-face meetings Difficulties building trust and relationships with HCPs
Healthcare access burden	Contacting HCPs is easier Access to informational support	Inaccessibility of digital interventions to some patients Difficulties starting to use the digital care pathway
Diverse burdens	Suits some patients better than traditional care	Not suitable or accessible for all patients Life circumstances prevent the use of digital care pathway to some patients

3.1 Time and Travel Burden

The clinicians identified several burdens caused by travelling to appointments, and ways digital care pathway can alleviate those burdens. First, all clinicians discussed how travel to appointments is time consuming for patients living far away from the hospital. One clinician emphasizes that the distances can be long, especially for some patients with drug-resistant epilepsies that need treatment in a tertiary care hospital.

> "[Travel] can be quite easy, so the patients and the families can just live very near to our hospital, like next door neighbors. But on the other hand, the distance between the home and the hospital might be more than 600 kilometers if the patient lives up in the north."
>
> -Clinician 1.

The clinician 1 continued the discussion with how travelling impacts families: more time for travelling means children and adolescents will miss school, and people with jobs need to be absent from work, leading to loss of income. Travel can be especially challenging for parents of small children who must manage childcare during hospital visits, and for parents who must accompany their children to their appointments. Another clinician complemented this with the perspective of adult patients. For adults with epilepsy, travelling can also be difficult to organize, since at least for one year from diagnosis people with epilepsy are not allowed to drive. Additional risks from traveling were mentioned. Driving to appointments increases the risk of road accidents, especially in winter. Once in the hospital, there is a risk of viral infections spreading to patients and their families, causing additional burden by the possibility to increase the risk for seizures, and absences from work.

The clinicians agreed that the digital care pathway has addressed these burdens by reducing the need for travelling. Traditional appointments can be replaced by remote online appointments, and in some cases the issues can be solved through the digital care pathway with no need for physical checkups. For example, some medication changes can be feasible organized remotely, as described in the following quote:

> "Sometimes, maybe it would be easier if you can bring the situation to notice from the digital care path, and if there is no need for changing care, if it is quite stable situation, maybe it is unnecessary to come for a checkup. It is quite a big effort, and then it is easier maybe to say, just tell that yeah, it is fine. We can postpone it."
>
> -Clinician 3.

3.2 Medication Burden

Two clinicians suspected that the digital care pathway does not have a direct impact on the time and inconvenience of taking medication. However, they identified three ways the digital care pathway can support people with epilepsy with self-management and issues related to medication. First, the digital care pathway provides informational support. Better instructions can increase medication adherence and help people with epilepsy with self-management, dealing with medication side-effects, and a healthy lifestyle. The following quote illustrates the clinician's experience of improvement of patients' adherence:

"The adherence to the treatment has gone way up due to the digital eHealth path. The patients used to say to me that 'my treatment plan was, there was no plan', or 'my future is a black hole'. Nowadays they do have some kind of better treatment plan and they have a method to contact us. And they know that the changes are done, and they are going to be heard, if they only contact us … And I think that this is the like the best thing ever."

-Clinician 2.

Second, the digital care pathway may increase the effectiveness of care, which will consequently reduce the burden of self-management. Also, getting seizures during travel could be more dangerous than at home, and seizures may sometimes be triggered by mood changes, for example anxiety of going to hospital. Therefore, the option of remote appointments from home can make the management of seizures easier.

Third, two clinicians discussed that when a patient has a problem with medication, digital care pathway can help to resolve it faster. Patients can easily contact through the messaging systems and referrals and adjustments to medication can be done from there. On the other hand, reacting quickly to patients' concerns through the digital care pathway creates a risk of acting too fast. Medications can take a long time to start working, and initial side-effects can go away with time, so reactions too fast may lead to making changes to treatment when it is not necessary.

3.3 Social and Emotional Burden

Two clinicians discussed ways the digital care pathway might both increase and decrease the burden related to stigma, identity, and negative emotions. Going to hospital might cause negative feelings, such as anxiety, fear, and frustration. The digital care pathway can help by treating patients in their home, where they can feel safe and comfortable. The hospital environment might also enforce patients' identity as a sick person. When the treatment happens in a familiar environment, and it takes less time, they may feel that having epilepsy is less consuming part of their lives and therefore has less impact on their identity.

However, the clinicians also acknowledge that face-to-face meetings can be beneficial for building trust and good relationships between patients and HCPs. Having only remote appointments may make it more difficult for patients to seek and receive support from professionals, increasing their treatment burden. It can be beneficial to have some face-to-face appointments initially, for patients to build trust on HCPs and feel confident that they will take as good care of them online as face-to-face. The following quote discusses the complex impact of face-to face care on emotions:

"These negative emotions might be towards us as medical, healthcare and hospital, depending on what has happened with the person. I think all these emotional things are difficult when you're not face-to-face, but maybe it's important to see them and to be able to show them. And if you are not face-to-face, maybe it's not good. But if you think in that way that hospital brings negative emotions, and you're happy in your home surroundings, and then that's good. There is so many ways to think about this."

-Clinician 3.

Two clinicians discussed how epilepsy treatment can be a strain for family relationships, and the digital care pathway has potential of reducing that impact. When one or multiple family members must spend considerable time away from home travelling to appointments, it can burden the whole family. Online meetings can be a great option, as they save time and can be attended from home. However, the digital care pathway can also be an additional burden for parents whose lives are already full of responsibilities. One clinician mentioned a parent, who reported being so exhausted with their everyday life, that they felt unable to start using the digital care pathway. As children with epilepsy do not use the care pathway themselves, parents must take responsibility of learning and using the system, which will add to their workload.

3.4 Healthcare Access Burden

All clinicians estimated that the digital care pathway is easy to use, and it makes contacting HCPs easier for patients. There were some concerns of patients having difficulties starting to use the care path, especially for those who recently had their diagnosis and are not yet experienced with epilepsy self-management. When an individual gets familiar with the system, organizing appointments and messaging HCPs is easy and convenient for patients. However, to allow fast contact with HCPs, the professionals need sufficient working time allocated to answering messages through the digital care path. Currently the time schedule for HCPs working with the digital care pathway is quite tight, and there are concerns of how the work time arrangements will develop if the number of users of the digital care pathway increases.

"When there are more and more users of these digital care pathways, of course [lack of time] has to be taken into account in our time scheduling. Also, it helps us to focus on those patients where there is really a need for a face-to-face meeting."

-Clinician 1.

All clinicians discussed the informational support digital care pathway can provide to patients in addition to contacting HCPs. Currently the Finnish patients can access informational resources in public online services called Health Village [31], which already covers all general epilepsy related information patients need and is regularly updated by the health care professionals from the Finnish university hospitals. The clinicians suggest that the Health Village resources are sufficient for general information, but perhaps the digital care pathway could include individual instructions, for example, for treatment of prolonged seizures.

3.5 Diverse Burdens

All clinicians agreed that the digital care pathway is not suitable for all patient groups. There are patients with cognitive challenges and epilepsies related to progressive neurological diseases, which will require clinical examinations during appointments. There are also patients going through a changing period in their epilepsy care, such as the time of getting diagnosed, or when adolescents make a transition to adult care. In these cases, face-to-face meetings are usually more suitable. The patients may also have non-epilepsy related challenges and life-circumstances that prevent them from using the digital care path. However, one clinician reminded that there is also a group of patients that can be treated exclusively through the digital care pathway and remote appointments, with no need for face-to face meetings:

> "There are a group of patients that do not have needs for face-to-face meetings. So, all the things can be managed through the digital care pathway and remote visits. We have to just identify and optimize our services for different groups of patients."
> -Clinician 1.

One clinician suggested that the patient population should be seen as two groups, those that use the digital care pathway and those that do not use it. When the digital care pathway is developed, it should be done considering the needs of both groups, with understanding that not everyone can use the digital care path.

4 Discussion

The results show that the digital care pathway supports patients with treatment burden for all the pre-defined domains. Domain *Financial burden* was only relevant for travel-related costs of treatments; therefore, it was moved under *the Time and travel burden*. The clinicians had concerns for digital care pathway potentially causing additional treatment burden for the domains of *Medication burden, Social and emotional burden*, and *Healthcare access burden*. A new theme emerged from the data, *Diverse burdens*, highlighting the variety of people with epilepsy with differing needs for treatment. There is a considerable number of people with epilepsy to whom digital care pathway is not suitable.

Our results support the suggestions of previous research on virtual appointments [14, 15] emphasizing the advantages in alleviating patient burden by reduction of travel and easier contacting of HCPs. Additionally, we found that digital care pathway also supports patients with providing informational support, quick adjustments of medication, better treatment plan, reducing negative emotions and illness identity, and making accessing services and arranging appointments easier.

For the negative impact of digital care path, the clinicians shared the same concerns brought up in previous research [16, 17] about the digital care pathway being inaccessible to some groups of patients, and some patients having difficulties of using the care path. Clinicians strongly agreed that digital care pathways are not suitable for everyone and there should be an alternative to the traditional care path. There is a need for structured system, where sufficient time is allocated and divided between the digital care pathway users and patients who will not use it.

If the schedule is managed responsibly considering the increasing numbers of patients using the digital care path, there is a potential of not only supporting the digital care pathway users with their treatment burden, but also increasing resources to focus more on patients who need face-to-face care. Additionally, the clinicians raised concerns of making too quick changes to treatment, and difficulties with building trust and seeking support from HCPs. These are important factors that need to be evaluated when considering the need for face-to-face appointments.

There are some limitations in the current study. First, the number of experts attending the meeting was small. More extensive qualitative research with larger sample size would be needed to support the findings of this study. Second, due to the case study design, the scope of this study was limited to the clinicians' perspective in the unit of analysis, digital epilepsy care path in Pohde. For complement the findings from the current study, it would be particularly relevant to study the patient's perspective. Therefore, further research would be needed for extending findings to broader population.

This study is part of an EpiDigi-project, which is aiming to evaluate and further develop the digital care pathway for epilepsy in Pohde. Following the exploratory qualitative findings from the current study, we are planning to conduct more extensive qualitative study, including larger number of HCPs, patients who have personal experience of using the digital care path, and their caregivers. In addition to qualitative evaluation, EpiDigi will include quantitative survey study for the patients, and developing improvements to the digital care pathway for epilepsy based on the findings of the experience of patients, caregivers, and HCPs.

5 Conclusions

The results of this study indicate that digital care pathway can support patients with epilepsy with their treatment burden. The digital care pathway for epilepsy can reduce travel, provide options for remote appointments, informational support, and easier ways to contact HCPs. The main concerns clinicians had was how the use of digital care pathway may cause rushed treatment decisions, difficulties of building trust and seeking support from HCPs, and difficulties using the digital systems. Future research from patients' perspective would be needed to better understand the impact of digital care pathways on patients' treatment burden.

Acknowledgements. PK developed the initial research plan, and MP and MI organized the meeting. MP and SK prepared the materials for the meeting and attended as participant observers. JU, JKE, and JA attended the meeting and provided their expert knowledge. MP analyzed the data and wrote and edited the manuscript. JU, JKE, JA, PV, WB, and MI contributed to the editing and approved the final manuscript.

Disclosure of Interests. The authors have no competing interests to declare that are relevant to the content of this article.

References

1. Blandford, A., Wesson, J., Amalberti, R., AlHazme, R., Allwihan, R.: Opportunities and challenges for telehealth within, and beyond, a pandemic. Lancet Glob. Health **8**, e1364–e1365 (2020). https://doi.org/10.1016/S2214-109X(20)30362-4
2. Portnoy, J., Waller, M., Elliott, T.: Telemedicine in the era of COVID-19. J. Allergy Clin. Immunol. Pract. **8**, 1489–1491 (2020). https://doi.org/10.1016/j.jaip.2020.03.008
3. Sim, I.: Mobile devices and health. N. Engl. J. Med. **381**, 956–968 (2019). https://doi.org/10.1056/NEJMra1806949
4. Rotter, T., et al.: Clinical pathways: effects on professional practice, patient outcomes, length of stay and hospital costs. Cochrane Database Syst. Rev. (2010). https://doi.org/10.1002/14651858.CD006632.pub2
5. Neame, M.T., Chacko, J., Surace, A.E., Sinha, I.P., Hawcutt, D.B.: A systematic review of the effects of implementing clinical pathways supported by health information technologies. J. Am. Med. Inform. Assoc. **26**, 356–363 (2019). https://doi.org/10.1093/jamia/ocy176
6. Terveyskylä: digital care pathways. https://www.terveyskyla.fi/en/mypath/digital-care-pathways. Accessed 05 Jan 2024
7. Page, R., Shankar, R., McLean, B.N., Hanna, J., Newman, C.: Digital care in Epilepsy: a conceptual framework for technological therapies. Front Neurol. **9** (2018). https://doi.org/10.3389/fneur.2018.00099
8. World Health Organisation: Epilepsy. https://www.who.int/news-room/fact-sheets/detail/epilepsy. Accessed 08 Sep 2023
9. Wilfong, A.: Epilepsy in children: comorbidities, complications, and outcomes (2024). https://www.uptodate.com/contents/epilepsy-in-children-comorbidities-complications-and-outcomes?search=epilepsy%20prognosis&source=search_result&selectedTitle=2~150&usage_type=default&display_rank=2#H1084946935
10. Laybourne, A.H., Morgan, M., Watkins, S.H., Lawton, R., Ridsdale, L., Goldstein, L.H.: Self-management for people with poorly controlled epilepsy: participants' views of the UK Self-Management in epILEpsy (SMILE) program. Epilepsy Behav. **52**, 159–164 (2015). https://doi.org/10.1016/j.yebeh.2015.08.023
11. Eton, D., et al.: Building a measurement framework of burden of treatment in complex patients with chronic conditions: a qualitative study. Patient Relat. Outcome Meas. **39** (2012). https://doi.org/10.2147/PROM.S34681
12. Demain, S., et al.: Living with, managing and minimising treatment burden in long term conditions: a systematic review of qualitative research. PLoS ONE **10**, e0125457 (2015). https://doi.org/10.1371/journal.pone.0125457
13. Sav, A., et al.: Burden of treatment for chronic illness: a concept analysis and review of the literature. Health Expect. **18**, 312–324 (2015). https://doi.org/10.1111/hex.12046
14. Heckman, B.W., Mathew, A.R., Carpenter, M.J.: Treatment burden and treatment fatigue as barriers to health. Curr. Opin. Psychol. **5**, 31–36 (2015). https://doi.org/10.1016/j.copsyc.2015.03.004
15. Kelley, L.T., et al.: Exploring how virtual primary care visits affect patient burden of treatment. Int. J. Med. Inf. **141** (2020). https://doi.org/10.1016/j.ijmedinf.2020.104228
16. Mair, F.S., Montori, V.M., May, C.R.: Digital transformation could increase the burden of treatment on patients. BMJ. n2909 (2021). https://doi.org/10.1136/bmj.n2909
17. Henni, S.H., Maurud, S., Fuglerud, K.S., Moen, A.: The experiences, needs and barriers of people with impairments related to usability and accessibility of digital health solutions, levels of involvement in the design process and strategies for participatory and universal design: a scoping review. BMC Public Health **22**, 35 (2022). https://doi.org/10.1186/s12889-021-12393-1

18. Mohammadzadeh, N., Khenarinezhad, S., Gha-Zanfarisavadkoohi, E., Safari, M.S., Pah-Levanynejad, S.: Evaluation of M-Health applications use in epilepsy: a systematic review (2021)

19. Escoffery, C., et al.: A review of mobile apps for epilepsy self-management (2018). https://doi.org/10.1016/j.yebeh.2017.12.010

20. Hubbard, I., Beniczky, S., Ryvlin, P.: The challenging path to developing a mobile health device for epilepsy: the current landscape and where we go from here (2021). https://doi.org/10.3389/fneur.2021.740743

21. Alzamanan, M.Z., Lim, K.-S., Akmar Ismail, M., Abdul Ghani, N.: Self-management apps for people with epilepsy: systematic analysis. JMIR Mhealth Uhealth **9**, e22489 (2021). https://doi.org/10.2196/22489

22. Yin, R.K.: Case Study Research: Design and Methods (Applied Social Research Methods). Sage Publications, Thousand Oaks (2014)

23. Pohde: Information about the wellbeing services county of North Ostrobothnia, https://pohde.fi/en/about-us/. Accessed 05 Jan 2024

24. Eisenhardt, K.M.: What is the eisenhardt method, really? Strateg. Organ. **19**, 147–160 (2021). https://doi.org/10.1177/1476127020982866

25. University of Oulu: Ethics committee of human sciences. https://www.oulu.fi/en/university/faculties-and-units/eudaimonia-institute/ethics-committee-human-sciences. Accessed 09 Jan 2024

26. University of Oulu: Lääketieteellinen tutkimuseettinen toimikunta. https://oys.fi/tutkimus-ja-opetus/tutkijan-ohjeet/laaketieteellinen-tutkimuseettinen-toimikunta/. Accessed 09 Jan 2024

27. Gray, D.E.: Doing Research in the Real World. SAGE Publications Ltd (2021)

28. QSR International Pty Ltd: NVivo (Version 14) (2023)

29. Elo, S., Kyngäs, H.: The qualitative content analysis process. J. Adv. Nurs. **62**, 107–115 (2008). https://doi.org/10.1111/j.1365-2648.2007.04569.x

30. Braun, V., Clarke, V.: Using thematic analysis in psychology. Qual. Res. Psychol. **3**, 77–101 (2006). https://doi.org/10.1191/1478088706qp063oa

31. Terveyskylä, https://www.terveyskyla.fi/. Accessed 19 Jan 2024

Design Sustainability Goals for Digital Care Pathway for Epilepsy: A Healthcare Professionals' Perspective

Sehrish Khan[1]([📧]) [iD], Pantea Keikhosrokiani[1] [iD], Johanna Uusimaa[2,3],
Johanna Annunen[2] [iD], Jonna Komulainen-Ebrahim[4,5] [iD], Manria Polus[1] [iD],
Paivi Vieria[2,3], and Minna Isomursu[1] [iD]

[1] M3S, University of Oulu, 90570 Oulu, Finland
sehrish.khan@oulu.fi
[2] Research Unit of Clinical Medicine, University of Oulu, Oulu, Finland
[3] Medical Research Center Oulu, Oulu University Hospital and University of Oulu, 90570 Oulu,
Finland
[4] Department of Children and Adolescents, Division of Pediatric Neurology, Oulu University
Hospital, Oulu, Finland
[5] Oulu University Hospital, Member of ERN EpiCARE (Helsinki-Oulu ERNEpi Consortium),
90029 Neurocenter, NeurologyOulu, Finland

Abstract. The healthcare systems across the world are transitioning towards sustainable development of digital health solutions such as digital care pathway (DCP) to meet the growing needs of healthcare services. DCP is a digital health solution to provide facilities like making online appointments, ease of access to connect with a healthcare professional (HCP), sharing symptoms and tracking progress of the disease. In this paper, a team of researchers and healthcare professionals (HCP) examine and propose the sustainability goals for Digital Care Pathway for Epilepsy (DCPE) project from the economic, social, and environmental perspectives. The project is a DCPE for children, adolescents, and adult patients with epilepsy. The research methodology is a single case study approach based on the DCPE in Northern Ostrobothnia Wellbeing County (Pohde), in Finland as a unit analysis. Furthermore, the data was collected using feedback from a co-design session with four HCPs all working as clinicians in epilepsy care at Oulu University Hospital. The analysis from the co-design session resulted in various factors to achieve sustainability goals like reduction in travel to hospital, cost efficient, time saving, ease of access to connect with HCPs, and lower CO_2 emission. However, there are several challenges such as adaptation to the online treatment options, proper management, and scheduling of online appointments, and building trust in epilepsy patients for remote treatment. Despite the challenges, HCPs confirm that the DCPE can be useful for treating patients with epilepsy through remote consultation along with the traditional ways.

Keywords: Sustainability · Digital health solution · patients with epilepsy ·
Digital healthcare pathway · Healthcare professionals

M. Särestöniemi et al. (Eds.): NCDHWS 2024, CCIS 2083, pp. 269–283, 2024.
https://doi.org/10.1007/978-3-031-59080-1_20

1 Introduction

Around 70 million people worldwide suffer from epilepsy which is a non-communicable neurological illness [1]. It affects nearly 60,000 Finns, out of which 5000 are children [2]. Since 2020, there is a web based digital tool of DCPE for all age groups of patients with epilepsy in the Wellbeing Services County of Northern Ostrobothnia (Pohde) at Oulu University Hospital (OUH). Furthermore, a similar mobile based service is developed for adult patients since December 2022. Furthermore, the mobile based version will be developed for children and adolescents patients with epilepsy in future [3]. Thus, a lot of research and study is required to improve the DCPE. The DCP is a digital health solution which enables a healthcare system to provide healthcare services to the patients from the comfort of their homes [4]. It allows the patients to communicate their concerns about their disease, receive care and treatment from clinicians in a streamlined, proactive, and patient-centric way [5].

The healthcare systems across the globe are overburdened to treat patients suffering from different diseases, especially chronic diseases which require long-term care [6]. The conventional patient-care model is getting overwhelmingly demanding, expensive and less sustainable in this era of booming digitization [7]. Moreover, with the effects left by pandemic of COVID-19, the outpatient care model or remote-treatment has begun to be seen as resource efficient in terms of cost and capacities of healthcare systems, and environment [8]. Thus, more and more healthcare systems are drawing attention towards this new mode of service delivery because of its promising features of sustainability [9]. It inspires and necessitates to innovate and deploy novel methods of delivering healthcare services. Furthermore, there is an ever-increasing drive to achieve sustainability goals for the healthcare system. To meet this challenge, advancements in Information Communication Technology ICT and digitalization of healthcare services offer promising solutions.

When we design digital care pathways, one of the most important design goals is to make them sustainable. We want to design and develop digital solutions which do not increase the burden for the healthcare system, humans involved or our environment. In the past, sustainability was more associated to mitigating environmental hazards and reduce CO_2 emissions [10]. The World Commission on Environment and Development [11] defines sustainability as "meeting the needs of the present without compromising the ability of future generation to meet their own needs" and "entails protection of the environment and natural resources as well as to provide social and economic welfare to the present and to subsequent generations" [12]. In healthcare sector, sustainability is further assessed through social, economic, and environmental dimensions [13, 14]. Therefore, digital healthcare services like digital care pathways are being developed worldwide to ensure sustainability of healthcare systems based on the three pillars. Transitioning to digital health solutions like DCPs has its own set of challenges for both the healthcare professionals (HCP) and patients.

In this paper, we examine research done in the context of DCPE for all age groups of patients with epilepsy in OUH.

The objective of this paper is to identify the sustainability design goals for DCPE. To achieve this, we conducted a case study on the DCPE project in collaboration with the HCPs. Based on the feedback from HCPs, we identified how the project achieves economic, social, and environmental sustainability goals. Therefore, an evidence-based study is conducted with the HCPs which can help to identify sustainability goals of DCPE.

This paper comprises of five sections. First the article discusses briefly the challenges faced by healthcare industry towards achieving the sustainability goals and reports some existing DCPs implemented around the world. Then, the methodology section describes the co-design approach followed by a team of researchers in collaboration with the HCPs on the developed template which discusses the sustainability goals for the DCPE. Afterwards, the feedback from the HCPs is given in the results and discussion section. Finally, the paper concludes with main findings on the HCP perspectives and briefly presents a future direction for further research on sustainability design goals for DCPE.

2 Background

2.1 Sustainability Challenges in Healthcare Systems

The transition of healthcare systems towards sustainability offers multifold benefits for the economy, society, and ecology of this world. The major challenge of sustainability in healthcare systems is to deal with the complexity of operations within a healthcare system [9]. The challenge is further accentuated by the uncertainty and unpredictability of innovations and changes in ICT infrastructure [15]. In this paper, we define sustainability in healthcare system with three main pillars; economic, social and environmental [16]. These pillars are interdependent and mutually reinforcing.

Economic sustainability focuses on economy-friendly practices to maximize efficient usage of resources in terms of logistics and human resources. It promises to increase prosperity and security to the healthcare system, as well as other stakeholders like professionals, staff, and patients [10]. As the costs of the healthcare are rising globally [17], it is crucial from the adoption point of view to ensure that DCP are resource efficient.

The social sustainability focuses on providing equal access to healthcare facilities for all citizens, equity, empowerment, engagement, and participation [18]. The goal of the social sustainability pillar is to consider the impacts of the DCP on social stability and capacity and capability of individuals to equally take part and benefit from healthcare.

The environmental sustainability ensures that environment-friendly practices should be promoted to help minimize the challenges of hazardous Green House Gas (GHG emissions, and utilize energy resources which are already replenishing at a rapid rate [14]. Healthcare sector global climate footprint is 4,4% [19]. In addition, healthcare sector contributes to ecotoxicity [20] and pollution, as it uses and creates variety of toxic substances. All this also causes loss of biodiversity.

There are several challenging factors which need to be addressed for the successful transition of global healthcare systems towards sustainable healthcare systems. These involve rising requirement of healthcare facilities, raising employee turnover, reduction in the number of HCPs and caregivers, expensive healthcare facilities, lack of available resources, and the overall economic crises especially in developing countries adds more burden on healthcare systems' capacities [7].

2.2 Digital Care Pathways

Digitalization in the healthcare industry offers promising alternatives like at-home or remote-treatment options [21]. The mobile applications empower the patients to self-monitor their symptoms, keep the track of their condition, share the health status with healthcare professionals, and receive treatment options while sitting at home [22]. The digitization of care pathways has multifold benefits for HCPs and patients and the overall healthcare systems [5]. Furthermore, DCPs have enabled healthcare systems to deliver more streamlined, proactive, cost-effective, and patient-centered care. Especially, patients suffering from chronic diseases like epilepsy can benefit from DCPs. According to Chronic Care Model (CCM), self-management can help the patients to get involved in better control of their symptoms and act as an equal partner along with professionals who monitor the healthcare needs of patients [23, 24].

The Health Village [3] portal is a digital health service developed by five Finnish university hospitals led by Helsinki University Hospital. My Path is a DCP tool on the Health Village website for patients to provide easy interaction with the HCPs and support their healthcare needs like self-management, guidance, appointment scheduling, and sharing health status remotely. Another model of DCP called as digital outpatient health solutions implemented in the United Kingdom (U.K.) discussed the benefits of DCP to increase the sustainability of healthcare systems and provide an evidence-base for clinicians and patients to adapt to this new model. Furthermore, ZEDOC by the Clinicians [5] provides a digital health solution platform which is developing its DCP [25] for various diseases like colorectal cancer, lung cancer, localized prostate cancer, hip and knee surgery, inflammatory arthritis, adult diabetes, cataract surgery, and general quality of life.

3 Method

In this paper a case study-based methodology is used [26, 27]. The study design is a single case of DCPE project for children, adolescents, and adult patients with epilepsy in Oulu University Hospital, Finland. We have studied DCPE to examine and explore the economic, social, and environmental sustainability goals for the project. The step-by-step methodology is illustrated in Fig. 1. We have collected qualitative data in collaboration with HCPS. We have used purposive sampling for this case study.

In the preparation phase, a group of three researchers prepared a table containing a list of factors which can contribute to achieve sustainability goals for economic, social, and environmental sustainability. The template shown in Table 1 was constructed through a literature [3–6, 10, 18, 19] survey, where similar digital healthcare solutions and their sustainability elements were discussed. The purpose of the template was to provide triggers and material for the co-design process with the HCPs.

With the help of co-authors and researchers, the table was arranged to remove repeatability of the concepts and contents to ensure maximum clarity for further discussion with HCPs. Later, the final table was shared with the HCPs for the co-design session. The purpose of the session was to collaboratively define the guiding sustainability goals for DCPE. A co-design session with two researchers and four HCPs all working as clinicians in epilepsy care at OUH (one in Neuro center, Neurology and three in Paediatric

Neurology Unit) was organized. The co-design session was organized through online Microsoft Teams. The session was recorded with the permission of HCPs and other participating researchers. The transcripts of the meeting were automatically transcribed in the Microsoft Teams and analyzed using the NVivo software.

The preliminary analysis of the data was done by a researcher leading the data collection. The preliminary results were documented and presented to HCPs participating in the co-design session and two researchers who participated in defining the data collection template. The analysis of results was collectively discussed and refined into their final format, which are the results presented in this paper. The research follows the ethical guidelines of our university. No patients were involved at this stage of the research.

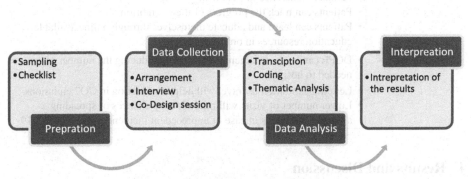

Fig. 1. Case study methodology step-by-step.

Table 1. DCPE sustainability goals

Sustainability pillar	Goals
Economic	• To reduce the treatment burden of care • To save time required for each face-to-face consultation • To be resourceful and cost-efficient for both clinicians and patients by reducing the travel costs needed to visit hospital • To reduce the energy expenditure associated with in-person visits to hospital • To reduce the number of phone calls to hospitals • To reduce the number of last-minute cancellations of scheduled appointments

(continued)

Table 1. (*continued*)

Sustainability pillar	Goals
Social	**Healthcare Professional** • Lower workload will improve job satisfaction and better work-life balance • HCPs can better utilize online consultation tools and provide personalized care to patients **Patient** • DCPE will improve patient experience and provide ease of access to consult with HCPs • Patients' adherence to treatment goes up • Patients can track the progress of their condition • Patients can learn and educate themselves through online available education resources in online portals
Environmental	• DCPE can be environmental-friendly by reducing the number of travels needed to hospital • Less transportation or travel will help in reduction in CO_2 emissions • Lower number of visits will minimize the chances of spreading airborne pathogens in case of unprecedent incidences like COVID-19

4   Results and Discussion

4.1   Economic Sustainability Goals

Based on the findings of this study, Fig. 2 shows six economic sustainability goals are identified which include (1) reduction in treatment burden, (2) reduced face-to-face consultation saves time, (3) resourceful and cost-efficient, (4) less energy expenditures due to lower hospital visits, (5) reduction in number of phone calls, and (6) reduction in last minute cancellation of appointment. In the forthcoming section, we further elaborate the feedback of HCPs about achieving these sustainability goals for the DCPE project.

Reduction in Treatment Burden of Care. Currently, the care provider struggles with having enough resources to provide care for the patient population. Therefore, HCP defined the reduction of treatment burden for the healthcare provider to be one of the leading sustainability goals of the adoption and development of the DCPE. The clinicians hoped that DCPE would reduce and optimize the workload of HCP, and at the same time, would improve the quality of care. The HCPs believed that DCPE can help to reduce the treatment burden of care. Currently, the majority of appointments take place through traditional mode of delivery by visiting the hospitals in-person. This consumes a lot of time to examine each patient and time management becomes difficult for HCPs. Consequently, HCPs get burdened with excessive workload. In future, the treatment burden of care can be by reducing the number of unnecessary face-to-face consultations and providing the facility of online appointments as per the needs of a patient with epilepsy.

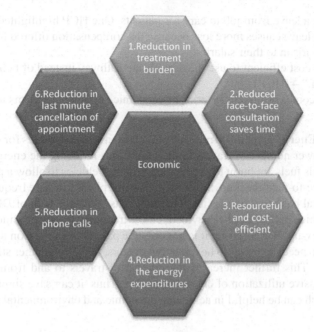

Fig. 2. Economic sustainability goals.

Time Saving for Clinicians, Patients and their Families. Treatment of epilepsy is a long journey consuming a lot of time and energy of both the clinicians and patients. According to the HCPs, a web-based version of DCPE patients is currently in place for adolescents and children. The treatment to children is planned with the help of parents. However, DCPE in a mobile version can be designed in future to provide online treatment options for younger age groups as well as adolescents and adult patients. The clinicians believed that DCPE can have an impact on changing the operational processes and routines of clinicians. Through DCPE, appointments can be made easily, and clinicians can see more patients at the same time as compared to face-to-face appointments. Furthermore, after the initial face-to-face examination, some patients can be treated remotely for follow-up checkups. It is unnecessary to come for checkup in certain cases like when the disease is stable and patient is responding well to treatment, only video conferencing might be enough for such patients to do follow-up. Thus, DCPE can save time for clinicians which can be invested towards patients who require face-to-face appointments.

Resourceful and Cost-efficient. Epilepsy is a chronic neurological disease, and it requires years of treatment. Sometimes, a major part of the life of a patient is spent receiving antiseizure medication (ASM). It is not only the patient who covers this journey alone, but the clinicians and caregivers of patients are along with him in this journey. A patient is most of the time accompanied by a caregiver, a parent, a family member, and in some cases any other person. From the parental and caregiver perspective, DCPE will be cost-efficient and save salary losses. According to the clinicians, DCPE will be cost-effective and save the economic losses incurred to patients who are working or caregivers or family members of patients who need to either compromise their professional routine or take a leave from job to care for patients. One HCP highlighted that in some cases, parental leave causes more loss because the compensation offered for such leaves is less in comparison to their salaries.

"It is more cost efficient to use the digital care pathway instead of being away from work or school." – [HCP1].

Thus, it becomes profitable in terms of economic and financial terms to use a digital care pathway.

Reduction in Energy Expenditure. The clinicians saw opportunities for saving energy costs due to lower number of travels to the clinic, thus reducing the energy needed for mobility. Fossils fuels are burnt to produce fuel for the vehicles to allow a patient to visit hospital for face-to-face checkup. Some patients with epilepsy require frequent in-person visits to hospital but some require less hospital visits. With the help of DCPE, an HCP can identify which patient can be provided remote treatment through online consultation or online follow-up. Furthermore, it is not only the patient or the person accompanying the patient who needs to travel to hospital, but doctors, nurses and other staff might also need to travel. This further increases the number of travels to and from hospital and results in excessive utilization of energy resources. Thus, it can save significant energy resources which can be helpful in achieving economic and environmental sustainability goals.

Reduction in Phone Calls. DCPE provides features which allow two-way synchronous and asynchronous communication between the patients and/or their informal carers and HCP. Patients can use these services to reach out to the HCP and inform them about their health status or seek help when needed. There are many benefits of this service. Patients do not need to wait long for phone calls. Patients can send messages to get help at any time of the day. The costs associated with phone calls are also saved. However, asynchronous communication features also have their challenges. Patients sometimes expect quick replies which cannot always be provided. It is important to design asynchronous communication features so that the patients will have realistic expectations about the response times. Moreover, if text-based communication is used, the HCPs feel that sometimes it is difficult to make the other person understand your message correctlyy.

"There is a risk of taking wrong dosing if the patient misunderstood the changes made in ASM."- [HCP2].

In this case, the patient should talk with the clinician in person to sort out their issue with regards to taking proper medication and treatment.

Reduction in Last-minute Cancellations of Appointments. According to the HCPs, the incidence of absences from scheduled appointments needs to be considered too. It happens that the patient or the person who is accompanying the appointment cannot reach and fails to inform the clinicians beforehand about cancellation. In such cases, the time and resources of the HCP and hospitals are wasted. Thus, DCPE can be fruitful in minimizing the non-attendance of patients because it will decrease the travel related occurrences of absences from appointments.

4.2 Social Sustainability Goals

The social sustainability goals can be divided into two parts as shown in Fig. 3: (1) the first part discusses the HCP perspective, which include reduction in workload, better work life balance, provide personalized care; and (2) the second part involves the patient side that consists of adherence to treatment increases, easier for patients to share epilepsy related symptoms and track progress of disease, and educate through online available education resources in DCPE.

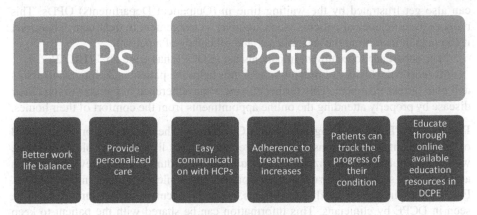

Fig. 3. Social sustainability goals.

Improvement in Work-life Balance. DCPE helps the HCPs to quicken the working processes like booking appointments for patients, taking online consultations, and prescribing medication. According to the HCPs, clinicians face the burden of treatment in face-to-face consultation, and this sometimes can lead to over-work and imbalance in personal and professional lives. Thus, DCPs need to be implemented by assigning different timing slots to invest in the in-person and online appointments.

Provide Personalized Care to Patients. The cases of patients with epilepsy vary significantly from each other. Each patient's case is unique depending upon several factors like age, gender, severity of seizures, and history of disease. The HCPs have to work to understand and make the treatment plan for every patient. DCPE can be helpful because there is a seizure diary, information about type of epilepsy seizure, aetiology, and medication taken by patients which is recorded and saved in the online portal. When a new patient is diagnosed with epilepsy for treatment then they must go through initial face to face consultation, so that doctors can make a personalized treatment plan. A personalized treatment plan can help the patient feel empowered in their treatment journey and increases overall satisfaction.

Provide Ease of Access to Consult with HCPs. DCPs like my Health village have been designed to provide people with ease of access to consult with the HCPs. The DCP of my Health Village, My Path is a DCP. Patients can access it easily by setting up a user account and providing information about their disease and ongoing treatment. Thus,

DCPE will work similarly to provide ease of access to patients with epilepsy. Patients can benefit from DCPE by making a more systematic plan of treatment and taking an active role in their treatment through collaborative approach in communicating with the doctor.

Adherence to Treatment Increases. The engagement of a patient in their treatment of epilepsy plays a significant role. The healthcare professionals believe that in-person visits are useful in building trust of patients and enhancing the patients' involvement in their journey. In some cases, the patients get exhausted from frequent trips to hospitals. Patients can also get frustrated by the waiting time in (Outpatient Departments) OPDs. This reduces the efficiency of patients' and care giver's engagement in treatment. Therefore, it can help in increasing the self-efficacy and efficiency of a patient.

"The adherence to treatment in patients using DCPE has gone up."-[HCP2].

Moreover, the history of previous check-ups helps the patient and clinician to assess and plan further treatment. This further enhances the adherence of patients to treat their disease by properly attending the online appointments from the comfort of their homes.

Patients Can Track the Progress of their Condition. The presence of previous record of appointments, medications, health related parameters like glucose, blood pressure, weight, type of epileptic seizures; the frequency, time duration, and severity of such attacks can be seen in profile created for a patient with epilepsy after an initial checkup. Furthermore, in case of paediatric patients, seizures (occurrence and duration) can be seen in DCPE by clinicians. This information can be shared with the patient to keep track of their disease and monitor the progress of their condition.

Patients Can Learn and Educate Themselves through Available Education Resources in Online Portals. According to the HCPs, education and awareness related to epilepsy can help the patient in self-care. Currently, there are different online sources of information like "Finnish Epilepsy Association", "Health Village." These provide useful resources about epilepsy for different age groups like children, adolescents, and adults, self-care advice, treatment plan, and peer-support options. Similarly, DCPE can provide educational and online resources to help patients in their journey.

4.3 Environmental Sustainability Goals

It was found that the project addresses three sustainability goals related to environmental sustainability: (1) reduces the travels needed to hospital, (2) reduction in the CO2 emissions, (3) and reduction in chances of spreading the airborne pathogens. These three goals are illustrated in Fig. 4. The HCPs perspective related to these goals are synthesized in the forthcoming subsections.

Reduction in the Travels Needed to Hospital. A bigger percentage of the population still visits hospitals in person for initial and follow-up visits. The HCPs prefer to conduct the initial evaluation of patients with epilepsy in person so that trust can be built, and a strong relationship is started for better communication between HCP and patient. Furthermore, in the initial evaluation, the clinician makes sure that they get all the required information and conducts all the required lab tests of patients.

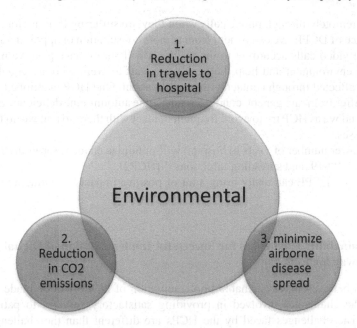

Fig. 4. Environmental sustainability goals.

However, when the follow-up visit becomes more routine, then it might not require an in-person visit. In this way, a greater number of unnecessary follow-up visits to and from hospitals can be avoided. This can reduce the carbon footprint as there is a reduced need to travel.

"Some of the patients living in the Northern Finland need to travel hundreds of kilometers to reach the clinic."-[HCP1].

This can lead to negative consequences not only from a financial perspective but also from the environmental perspective.

Reduction in CO2 Emission. Recently, there is an increased interest towards reducing healthcare activities related to carbon footprint across the globe. According to the HCPs, DCPE can certainly help in reducing the carbon footprint associated with travel to and from hospitals for clinical visits. Generally, it is believed that only patients need to travel to receive treatment. However, it is partially true, because there is a huge number of personnel in hospitals like nurses, doctors, lab specialists, and others, who are travelling for work. This sometimes accounts more for CO2 emission. An HCP expects that reduction in travels to hospital can benefit the healthcare personnel as well.

"I hope that in near future it would be possible for us doctors to work more from home, so we will have to travel less, at least not for the all the days to our workplace and back to home, so that it helps the environmental system because we will not be using all the facilities of hospital while working from home."-[HCP3].

Minimize the Chances of Spreading Airborne Pathogens. According to the healthcare experts, it is good to avoid spreading viral diseases by avoiding hospital visits when not needed. It is preferred and recommended to patients to stay at home and seek medical treatment remotely through phone calls when they are suffering from a viral illness. In the presence of DCPE, we can benefit from remote consultation or appointment through audio, and video calls according to the needs. It will surely have positive impacts on the whole environment and help the healthcare staff as well, who are equally at risk of getting affected through contact with any ill patient. One HCP mentioned that some patients suffer from rare genetic conditions and some autoimmune deficiency along with epilepsy, and we as HCP try to avoid frequent contact with them so that we do not spread viral illnesses.

"The lower number of visits to hospital will minimize chances for viral illnesses, as well as COVID-19, and spreading infections."-[HCP2].

Therefore, DCPE can really bring a lot of positive impacts on reducing the spread of viral diseases.

4.4   Sustainability Challenges for Successful Implementation of Digital Care Pathway for Epilepsy

The HCPs believed that sustainable implementation of DCPE can be made sure after meeting the challenges involved in providing satisfactory services to patients with epilepsy. The challenges faced by the HCPs are different than the challenges faced by the patients.

Sustainability Challenges for HCPs. According to the HCPs, the first challenge for them is the training required for managing the digital platforms for providing services like remote consultation through DCPE. Moreover, there is a risk of digital exclusion which can happen if a group of people do not have appropriate devices like laptop or a smart phone with working internet connection. In addition to this, there can be instances when patients are unable to access and use the digital tools or services of DCPE. Another challenge about effective communication was mentioned by an HCP which can help in proper guidelines during treatment.

"Sometimes patients expect the HCP to reply too fast because they want a quick result from the prescribed medicine, but it takes time for the medication to work."

- [HCP2].

Therefore, it can be said that careful planning and proper rescheduling pose challenges for the HCPs in successful implementation of DCPE.

Sustainability Challenges for Patients. According to the HCPs, it needs to be ensured that all the citizens are aware of the usefulness of DCPE and services like remote consultation. Particularly, the patients of epilepsy and their family members or persons involved with their treatment like friends, social workers etc. Patients can better adapt to this new mode of service after realizing its potential and advantages in their lives. Furthermore, it is important that all patients can access the digital tools and services of DCPE. For instance, it is crucial to have a laptop or PC or a smart phone to use the web or mobile application of DCPE. Besides, user satisfaction is crucial for maximizing the benefits for a patient. This can be done by implementing the principles of user centered design and verifying the developed prototypes through usability testing and user experience methods.

5 Conclusion

In this paper, we discussed and explored the sustainability goals of DCPE in collaboration with the HCPs. DCPE will offer various advantages which will contribute to the long-term goals of sustainable healthcare systems.

In terms of economic, social, and environmental factors, the project can support patients, their family members and friends, and caregivers like doctors and nurses. It is beneficial to all the stakeholders at different levels. This is done by minimizing the in-person travels needed to hospital and providing at home treatment. However, there are challenges involved in the successful implementation of a digital care pathway for smooth transitioning and delivery of online appointments. The HCPs can schedule, manage, and divide time for remote appointments and face-to-face visits as per the need of an epilepsy patient. Moreover, DCPE cannot replace every hospital visit, but it can help in reducing the unnecessary in-person visits to provide healthcare services through online portals for those with stable condition of epilepsy. Due to the nascent nature of DCPE, the HCPs perspective is highly crucial in successful and sustainable implementation of DCPE. Their firsthand experience, learning and insights will help guide the effective adoption and deployment of novel digital health solutions as well as shape its future development. Thus, we explored the subdimensions which can lead to sustainability of DCPE in collaboration with HCPs, so that an evidence-based study can help the HCPs, and patients in future.

In future, more research is required to study the sustainability goals of DCPE from an economic, social, and environmental perspective. Furthermore, we can study and examine the perspective of patients and their expectations from the sustainability perspective of DCPE. The patients can provide feedback on the usefulness and ease of use of online appointments after their first-hand experiences with DCPE. These developments and future studies can strongly support achieving the sustainability goals of DCPE.

Acknowledgments. The work has been supported by 6GESS – 6G Enabled Sustainable Society profiling program co-funded by Research Council Finland.

Disclosure of Interests. The authors have no competing interests pertaining to the content of this article to declare.

References

1. World health organization: epilepsy fact sheet. https://www.who.int/news-room/fact-sheets/detail/epilepsy

2. About epilepsy. https://www.epilepsia.fi/en/about-epilepsy/
3. Digital health village - white paper. https://www.digitalhealthvillage.com/en/white-paper
4. Tuomikoski, K., Liljamo, P., Reponen, J., Kanste, O.: Digihoitopolkujen vaikutukset ter-veydenhuollon ammattilaisten toimintaprosesseihin erikoissairaanhoidossa. Finn. J. EHealth EWelfare. 14, 326–338 (2022). https://doi.org/10.23996/fjhw.112648
5. About digital care pathways. https://theclinician.com/introduction-to-digital-care-pathways
6. Brown, M.R.D., Knight, M., Peters, C.J., Maleki, S., Motavalli, A., Nedjat-Shokouhi, B.: Digital outpatient health solutions as a vehicle to improve healthcare sustainability—a United Kingdom focused policy and practice perspective. Front. Digit. Health. 5, 1242896 (2023). https://doi.org/10.3389/fdgth.2023.1242896
7. Fischer, M.: Fit for the future? A new approach in the debate about what makes health-care systems really sustainable. Sustainability. 7, 294–312 (2015). https://doi.org/10.3390/su7010294
8. Ianculescu, M., Alexandru, A., Pop, F.: Critical analysis and evaluation of current digi-tal healthcare solutions. In: 2021 23rd International Conference on Control Systems and Computer Science (CSCS), pp. 482–488. IEEE, Bucharest, Romania (2021)
9. Faezipour, M., Ferreira, S.: Applying systems thinking to assess sustainability in healthcare system of systems. Int. J. Syst. Syst. Eng. 2, 290 (2011). https://doi.org/10.1504/IJSSE.2011.043861
10. de Preux, L., Rizmie, D.: Beyond financial efficiency to support environmental sustainability in economic evaluations. Future Healthc. J. 5, 103–107 (2018). https://doi.org/10.7861/future hosp.5-2-103
11. Thomsen, C.: Sustainability (World Commission on Environment and Development Defini-tion). Presented at the January 1 (2013)
12. Our common future world commission on environment and developement.pdf. http://ir.harambeeuniversity.edu.et/bitstream/handle/123456789/604/Our%20Common%20Future%20World%20Commission%20on%20Environment%20and%20Developement.pdf?seq uence=1&isAllowed=y
13. Chowdhury, M., Quaddus, M.A.: A multi-phased QFD based optimization approach to sus-tainable service design. Int. J. Prod. Econ. 171, 165–178 (2016). https://doi.org/10.1016/j.ijpe.2015.09.023
14. Degavre, F., et al.: Searching for sustainability in health systems: toward a multidisciplinary evaluation of mobile health innovations. Sustainability. 14, 5286 (2022). https://doi.org/10.3390/su14095286
15. Wali, S., Keshavjee, K., Demers, C.: Moving towards sustainable electronic health applica-tions. In: Heston, T.F. (ed.) eHealth - Making Health Care Smarter. In Tech (2018)
16. Choukou, M.-A.: Chapter 10 - Sustainability of mHealth solutions for healthcare system strengthening. In: Syed-Abdul, S., Zhu, X., and Fernandez-Luque, L. (eds.) Digital Health, pp. 171–189. Elsevier (2021)
17. Global spending on health: Rising to the Pandemic's Challenges. Global Spending on Health, Geneva (2022)
18. Hansmann, R., Mieg, H.A., Frischknecht, P.: Principal sustainability components: empirical analysis of synergies between the three pillars of sustainability. Int. J. Sustain. Dev. World Ecol. 19, 451–459 (2012). https://doi.org/10.1080/13504509.2012.696220
19. Karliner, J., Slotterback, S., Boyd, R., Ashby, B., Steele, K.: Health care climate footprint report (2019)
20. Hancock, T.: Beyond net-zero: toward a "One Planet" health system. Healthc. Manage. Forum 36, 184–189 (2023). https://doi.org/10.1177/08404704231162775
21. Sadegh, S.S., Khakshour Saadat, P., Sepehri, M.M., Assadi, V.: A framework for m-health service development and success evaluation. Int. J. Med. Inf. 112, 123–130 (2018). https://doi.org/10.1016/j.ijmedinf.2018.01.003

22. Heston, T.F.: eHealth: making health care smarter. BoD – books on demand (2018)
23. Austin, B., Wagner, E., Hindmarsh, M., Davis, C.: Elements of effective chronic care: a model for optimizing outcomes for the chronically Ill. Epilepsy Behav. **1**, S15–S20 (2000). https://doi.org/10.1006/ebeh.2000.0105
24. Lorig, K.: Living a healthy life with chronic conditions: self-management of heart disease, arthritis, diabetes, asthma, bronchitis, emphysema & others (2006)
25. The clinician: digital care pathway library. https://theclinician.com/care-pathways
26. Gerring, J.: What is a case study and what is it good for? Am. Polit. Sci. Rev. **98**, 341–354 (2004). https://doi.org/10.1017/S0003055404001182
27. Swanborn, P.: Case Study Research: What, Why and How? pp. 1–192 (2010)

Enhancing Independent Auditory and Speechreading Training – Two Finnish Free Mobile Applications Constructed for Deaf and Hard of Hearing Children and Adults

Kerttu Huttunen[1](✉) (iD), Jaakko Kauramäki[1,2] (iD), Kati Pajo[3] (iD), and Satu Saalasti[1,2,4] (iD)

[1] University of Oulu, 90014 Oulun yliopisto, Oulu, Finland
kerttu.huttunen@oulu.fi
[2] University of Helsinki, 00014 Helsingin yliopisto, Helsinki, Finland
[3] Helsinki University Hospital, Kasarmikatu 11–13, 00130 Helsinki, Finland
[4] University of Eastern Finland, Yliopistokatu 4, 80100 Joensuu, Finland

Abstract. The users of hearing technology often need auditory training for getting used to their hearing devices and maximally benefiting from them. Because auditory training given by professionals is only sparsely available, there is a great need for materials and applications with which self-training is possible. Moreover, deaf and hard-of-hearing persons need to improve their speechreading skills to help in speech reception and children to strengthen their reading skills. We describe the background, contents, construction and features of two Finnish free applications: Auditory Track for auditory training and Optic Track for speechreading (lip reading) training. Both can be used by children and adults, even though the Auditory Track is mainly aimed at adults and the Optic Track at primary school age children. The features of both applications include exercises carefully selected based on extensive knowledge of the acoustic and visual characteristics of speech. In addition, during the implementation of both applications, careful attention has been paid to the usability, accessibility, gamification and construction of feedback systems. The applications developed can be used in independent training, clinical use and research.

Keywords: auditory training · speechreading · lip reading

1 Introduction

Globally, almost one in five people in the world is estimated to have hearing loss, with 5% needing rehabilitation [1]. The vast majority of people with hearing problems are older adults. Especially in the elderly, impaired hearing has been found to lead to a restriction of social relations and hobbies and to loneliness [2, 3]. Hearing problems are related to anxiety and depression, particularly in males, and in some studies, increased mortality has been described as being related to impaired hearing. Of all the single risk factors, hearing loss without the use of hearing aids poses the greatest relative risk

© The Author(s) 2024
M. Särestöniemi et al. (Eds.): NCDHWS 2024, CCIS 2083, pp. 284–302, 2024.
https://doi.org/10.1007/978-3-031-59080-1_21

for dementia; those who experience hearing loss in their mid-life will be more likely to experience cognitive decline later on. However, the use of hearing aids has been suggested to decrease this risk for dementia [4].

Technical rehabilitation, that is, the use of hearing devices, forms the foundation for how problems with hearing are compensated for. Transition into a new, advanced era in hearing care took place in the 1990s when digital hearing aids and multichannel cochlear implants were implemented into clinical practice. Cochlear implants replace the severely malfunctioning or not at all functioning sensory cells in the inner ear; they transform sounds into electric signals, process them through band-pass filtering according to the encoding strategy of the sound processor device and then stimulate the hearing nerve. Additionally, a variety of assistive listening devices, such as audio induction loops (hearing loops), FM devices and infrared systems, are available to help patients at home, at work and during leisure time activities.

1.1 Auditory Training is Needed to Maximally Benefit from Technical Hearing Rehabilitation

Providing the patients with hearing devices does not suffice—they also need counselling and mental support for learning the new skills needed when starting to use their hearing devices. Additionally, their brain often needs specific training to deal with the new technically processed and, thereby, altered auditory information the hearing instruments convey or produce. Namely, hearing aids not only amplify the sounds the hearing aid user is focusing on, but they also amplify all background noises. Moreover, hearing aids also process sounds in many ways, so the outcome may sound very distorted and annoying to the device user [5]. This is why getting used to hearing aids and listening with them may take weeks or months, even up to one year. A common clinical finding verified by research (e.g., [6, 7]) is that a large share of patients prescribed with hearing aids do not actually use them at all or use them only infrequently.

Time and training are needed to get the best benefit from the hearing aids and the altered sensory input they provide. Auditory training is, indeed, frequently needed in supporting the acclimatization process, which is the improvement in auditory performance as the hearing aid user gets used to listening with their new devices [8]. Furthermore, a minority of patients have lost their hearing to the extent that cochlear implantation has been necessary. Auditory training is also often needed to maximize the benefiting from cochlear implants—devices that are expensive technology and require medical operation and lifetime care of the patients. In both patients with hearing aids and cochlear implants, auditory training is especially needed when the progress in auditory skills is slow, the expected level of speech perception is not gained, or the patient struggles with asymmetric hearing.

In many Western countries, the rapid ageing of the population has drastically increased the need for hearing rehabilitation services. Even if the technical rehabilitation with fitting of hearing devices could be arranged by public health care with patients often needing to be on the waiting list for a long time, auditory training provided by, for example, speech and language therapists, can only be offered to a fraction of those needing it [9]. This means that there is a clear need to provide patients with materials and methods that are time and cost effective. Independent auditory training (self-training) is a noteworthy option for serving that need.

Materials Constructed for Auditory Training. Auditory training as self-training in, for example, home environment has earlier been based on the use of videocassettes and CD ROM and DVD materials, such as Angel SoundTM and LACE® (Listening and Communication Enhancement) and, in Finnish, for example, Huulioluvun ja kuulonharjoituksen ohjelma [10]. Validated instruments for computer-based auditory training, such as websites or applications, are still scarce, especially when it comes to languages other than English [11]. Therefore, studies investigating the effectiveness of computer-based training in various languages typically develop new training and evaluation programs that are then aimed at being generalized into clinical use [e.g., 12-14]. Researchers have used various cloud solutions, for example, uploaded the audio files for listening onto Google Drive, and shared them with the study participants via e-mail [12] or placed the training materials onto websites, such as HEARO™, which is specifically constructed for auditory training [13, 15]. Another route for offering the participants access to the training program has been to offer them a tablet computer that has the program installed on it [16].

Today, a variety of computer-based and mobile device auditory training applications are available, though often only for English-speaking persons. Applications include, but are not limited to, the ones that Olson (2015) [17] and Völter et al. (2020) [11] have listed: AB Clix, Hear Coach, The Listening Room®, Read My Quips and LACE® (Listening and Communication Enhancement) and, for children, Angel SoundTM and i-Angel Sound and SoundScape. Examples of web-based auditory training platforms offered in languages other than English are SisTHA portal for Portuguese-speaking adults in Brazil [18] and the already mentioned HEARO™ website (Hearo.co.il) for Hebrew-speaking adults in Israel [13].

Outcomes of Auditory Training. Some earlier evidence for the effectiveness of computer-based auditory training was provided, for example, in systematic reviews by Sweetow and Palmer (2005) [8] and Henshaw and Ferguson (2013) [19]. As reported in these reviews, both analytic (identification of single sounds by using the so-called bottom-up cognitive processes) and synthetic (targeting to understand the meaning of the message delivered by using the so-called top-down cognitive processes) training methods or their combination were used in the reviewed studies. Additionally, in some studies, different noise conditions had also been included in the training. However, in the former review [8], the number of articles meeting the inclusion criteria was only six, and the number of participants in the studies was rather low. Moreover, the articles included, particularly in the latter review [19], represented very low to moderate study quality; in addition, the reported improvements in auditory skills were considered small. Furthermore, when practicing with a computer, evidence of the ability to successfully generalize the performance obtained into untrained stimuli was not robust.

Later research has shown, however, with a stronger evidence base that various forms of auditory training are beneficial for individuals with hearing loss, whether the training material includes speech [16, 20]) or music [21]. Most recently, many studies have offered even more systematic evidence, here highlighting the advantages of computer-based training (e.g., [13, 16]). Furthermore, generalizability of the skills related to word-level items has been detected; Sato et al. (2020) [22] found that independent auditory training at home by using a tablet computer increased the intelligibility of both the perceived trained and untrained words in patients who had received hearing aids or cochlear implants one year earlier. In studies reporting positive outcomes, the training dose used was at least eight hours [8], and computer-based auditory training has already been detected as effective after one month of training [13]. In addition, compliance with computer-based training was found to be high (see, e.g. [16]).

Research has suggested that auditory training in adults can improve not only auditory performance, but also working memory, attentive skills and communication [23]. In their review, Stropahl et al. (2020) [24] concluded that the use of hearing aids together with auditory training is a beneficial combination. According to common clinical experience, it is especially important to use background noise in training because the auditory signal one tries to listen to needs to be separated from the background noise for speech perception to be successful. Indeed, adding various background noises as an additional challenge while training has been detected as beneficial [15, 16]. The use of music has also been found to support the auditory training performed with speech materials. Moreover, according to a systematic review and meta-analysis [21], music used in auditory training can improve musical perception; auditory discrimination, recognition, and sound localisation skills.

1.2 Speechreading Training is Needed by Both Children and Adults with Hearing Impairment

Speech is multimodal in nature, and audiovisual information is utilized in speech reception by all people and those with impaired hearing even more so. Visual support for speech recognition is important, especially in noisy and echoic listening environments. A need to support auditorily perceived speech with visual information has drastically been shown during the COVID-19 pandemic because people with impaired hearing faced big challenges by masks covering the important visual information they need from the face [25]. In speechreading (lip reading), all available cues of the movements of lips, tongue and the face, together with head, eye and torso actions, are used to determine the intended message of a speaker. Interindividual differences in speechreading ability are large [26]. Just like with auditory training, practicing in speechreading can be done using either the analytic (use of visual patterns in articulation) or synthetic (inferring by utilizing context) methods or both [27].

Since the introduction of digital hearing aids and cochlear implants, the use of hearing technology and auditory training have been at the centre of habilitation of children with impaired hearing. The utilisation of visual information about speech seems to have largely been neglected. This situation is confusing given the research base, which suggests that, in both hearing children and those with hearing impairment, visual information is important for learning to speak, in the acquisition of phonological knowledge and even in learning to read [28, 29]. Reading skills need to be supported because they are often compromised, especially in children with more severe hearing impairment [30].

Materials Constructed for Speechreading Training. Just as with auditory training, speechreading skills take time and effort to learn. Speechreading training has traditionally been accomplished in live situations with a therapist or group, but such practice is prone to large variations. Gradually, over time, videorecorded materials have enabled more systematic training, which then advanced to the adoption of computer-aided programs and web-based applications, such as Lipreading.org. Currently, there are some speechreading computer applications available for research use [31]) and some for clinical and public use. Only a few applications can be used for free. To the best of our knowledge, some mobile applications, such as Lip Reading Academy, Seeing and Hearing Speech® and the Android application MirrorMirror [27], have thus far been developed.

Outcomes of Speechreading Training. There is a paucity of evidence on how children benefit from speechreading training. Most studies have been conducted with adults and have shown modest improvements [32–35]). Overall, research has suggested that, in adults, there is often much room to improve speechreading skills [26]. Speechreading is not an immutable skill because it has been shown that speechreading ability improves between 7 and 14 years of age [36]. Some research suggested that children [36] and adults [37] with hearing impairment may be better speechreaders than individuals with typical hearing, but contrasting evidence also exists [29, 38, 39]). In hearing children, speechreading training has been shown to improve single-word speechreading and, even more importantly, general speech sound processing skills (phonological processing) [40]. However, intensive computerized speechreading training in 5- to 7-year-old children with a hearing impairment (N = 32) led to only a small improvement in speechreading test performance but greater improvement in some other outcome measures, such as answering everyday questions presented with visual speech, vocabulary and audiovisual speech production assessment [41]. However, there was a large variation in the amount of training realized. The use of easily accessible mobile applications might increase both the usability and frequency of training.

In the present article, we describe the contents, construction and use of two Finnish free applications—Auditory Track and Optic Track—developed for persons with a hearing impairment. Both applications are suitable not only for clinical purposes (used as training material in speech therapy and in independent training at home), but also for research.

2 Methods

2.1 Contents and Construction of the Auditory Track Application

The training material included in Auditory Track [42] comprises about 3,000 audio file items consisting of one- to seven-syllable words and one- to seven-word sentences. Additionally, some 200 audio files contain the sounds of various music instruments or musical pieces. For training, there are three task types for listening to speech (Table 1) and two for listening to sounds produced with musical instruments and pieces of music (Table 2). The speech discrimination tasks were partly based on Kuulorata käyttöön [43] material, which includes exercises presented in paper form (original training material by Cochlear Corp., translated and adapted into Finnish).

Table 1. Contents of the speech discrimination tasks of the Auditory Track application.

Task Type	Task
Discrimination of Speech	Discrimination of overall sentence patterns
	Identification of sentences having different lengths
	Identification of sentences having the same length
	Identification of sounds and sentences
	Discrimination of plosives (e.g., /p, t, k/)
	Discrimination of nasals (e.g., /m, n/)
Contents of Speech	Short narratives (easy)
	Short narratives (moderate)
	Short narratives (advanced)
Games	Assembling of three- and four-word sentences
	Memory games
	Bingo game

Table 2. Contents of the music tasks of the Auditory Track application.

Task Type	Task
Instrumentals	Number of sounds produced with a musical instrument
	Pitch of sounds and pieces of music
	Tempo of sound sequences and pieces of music
	Order of sound sequences having a slow or rapid tempo
	Discrimination of pieces of music/songs
	Discrimination of musical instruments
Vocals	Only vocals or vocals with instrumental accompaniment
	Only instrumental music or vocals with instrumental accompaniment
	Solo or duet singing

Within each task type, all materials were categorized into three difficulty levels: easy, moderate and advanced. Additionally, in memory games, the difficulty level can also be further adjusted so that the user can always choose between six, eight and 12 cards (corresponding with three, four and six audio file–word pairs to be matched). At the easy level, words differ considerably from each other by phonemes and/or syllable number; at the moderate level, words are rather similar, and at the advanced level, they are very similar to each other. Within each task type and difficulty level, all target items are presented to the user in random order. Examples of some word- and sentence-level task types are illustrated in Fig. 1.

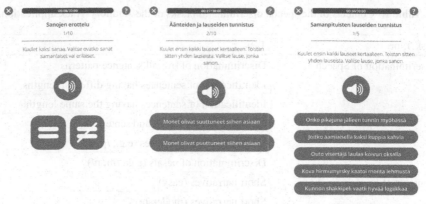

Fig. 1. Examples of the auditory training exercises (same or different word and which of the two or five sentences was heard) of the Auditory Track application.

The final task of the speech material comprises a set of 14 about two-minute narratives with five questions on the content of each narrative presented. For answering the questions after listening to cach story, four alternative choices are always given (Fig. 2). The content of the training materials has been described in Finnish in more detail by Huttunen, Vikman and Pajo (2022) [44].

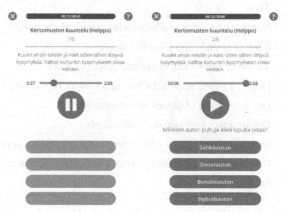

Fig. 2. After listening to a short narrative, the user of Auditory Track needs to answer five questions about the content of the story.

Both a female speech and language therapist and male professional actor spoke all the materials. Recording of the speech materials and their instructions was done using the AKG CK92 microphone and Reaper 6.14 software in a professional recording studio (the LeaF Research Infrastructure, University of Oulu, Finland). A calibration signal for the recordings was produced with a Bruel & Kjaer 4231 Sound Level Calibrator. Recording was done with a 96 kHz sampling rate and 24-bit depth, and the recordings were saved in.wav format. After this, all the materials were manually segmented using Audacity (version 2.1.3), AVS Audio Editor (version 8.0.2.501) and Praat (version 6.0.49/6.1.0) software and saved in mp3 format. When editing, all extra noises like smacks and loud, disturbing inhalations and misarticulated productions were removed. To enhance smooth streaming when using the Auditory Track application, down sampling into 48 or 44.1 kHz was done, and a variable bit rate between 170 and 210 kbps was chosen for the mp3 format. Additionally, sound level was equalized, and 1 s of silence was added to precede and to follow each single word, sentence or narrative.

Music was produced with the digital piano Kawai. The electronic sound synthesiser of the digital piano was used to produce the sounds of organs, pan flute, accordion, violin, trumpet and so forth for the tasks in which one needs to distinguish between the pitch (low/high) and tempo (slow/rapid) or the number of sounds produced with the instrument. For these same tasks and for playing the instrumental pieces of the music, acoustic guitar, violin and cello were played, in addition to the use of the digital piano. The pace of playing the songs (70 to 90 beats per minute) was determined with the help of a metronome, and 30-s musical pieces were played using the mid registers because this was seen suitable for hearing device technology and the typical features of hearing impairments.

One male adult, a trained performing musician, sang the vocal parts of the music material. For some of the songs, a female joined so that the songs were performed as a duet. All 10 musical pieces chosen to be presented were royalty free and consisted of well-known folk songs, hymns and children's songs, such as 'A Frog Went A-Courtin'' and 'Old Mac Donald Had a Farm'.

Music and sounds were mainly recorded by using Audacity software, Shure SM7B Cardoid Dynamic microphone and Focusrite iTrack Scarlett Solo external sound card. Additionally, a minor part was recorded using either Zoom H2N audio-recorder or Audacity application, AKG C 544 L microphone and Focusrite iTrack Solo external sound card.

2.2 Use of the Auditory Track Application

With its gamification features and carefully planned usability, Auditory Track aims to maximally enhance the independent training of auditory skills. These features of training materials are commonly known to be helpful in training. The gamification includes sentence-assembly tasks (Fig. 3), together with bingo and memory games.

Compliance in training with Auditory Track is supported by immediate feedback given (correctness of the answer chosen) and a reward system embedded in the software; gold, silver and bronze medals are credited after receiving a certain proportion of points (success in training) (Fig. 4).

In the task type in which short narratives are listened to, the user has, along with the option of no noise or echo (one attenuated repetition with a start delay of 0.7 s), two noise types to select from: white noise masker and speech-shaped noise masker (consisting of mixed sentence-level speech). After selecting the noise type, the user can select the noise level using a slider (see Fig. 5).

The progress bar shows the time elapsed when using the Auditory Track application. It is placed in the uppermost part of the smart device screen, with the 30-min bar automatically being reset to zero daily. According to the instructions of Auditory Track,

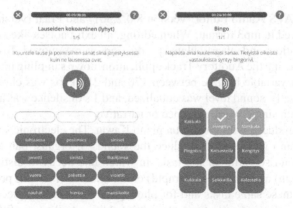

Fig. 3. Gamification examples of the Auditory Track application: assembling of three-word sentences and a bingo game.

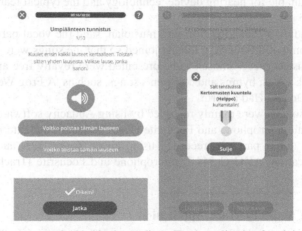

Fig. 4. Feedback system embedded in the Auditory Track application for giving visual feedback (according to the correctness of the answer and granting medals).

it is recommended that training should be done three times a week for 30 min at a time for a minimum of two months. This instruction was based on studies reporting positive outcomes in auditory training when the training dose varied from 10 to 50 h, with no difference in outcomes between training done twice or five times a week [20, 45]. In their study, Humes et al. (2014) [45] concluded that, for auditory training to be effective in older adults, practising should take place, at minimum, two or three times a week for 5–15 weeks. Streaming directly to hearing aid(s) or cochlear implant(s) is recommended [12, 16]. This also enables auditory training focusing on one ear only which is very helpful when hearing is asymmetrical or when the patient gets a new device.

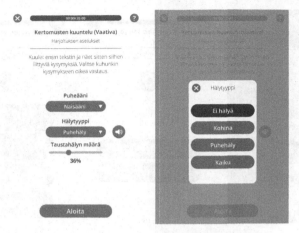

Fig. 5. Selection of the speaker (female/male) and listening mode; silence, echo and noise (including noise type and level) in the Auditory Track application.

When coding Auditory Track, an abridged pilot application, Kuulorata Pilot (available in Google Play and App Store), was used as the starting point. Technical implementation of Auditory Track was performed by a Finnish company, Outloud Ltd., by using the Unity game engine and C# language.

2.3 Contents and Construction of the Optic Track Application

The speech material included in the Optic Track application [46] comprises almost 3,800 silent videos. Most of the items are single words, having one to seven syllables, but the material also contains about 400 sentences, each having one to seven words. The frequency of words occurring in the Finnish language was also checked from some databases and other sources and considered when selecting the words. Visemes are groups of phonemes (speech sounds) having similar lip shape, articulation place or other visual cues of the articulation gestures. One of the main principles in constructing the items for the Optic Track application was to provide training material in which discrimination needs to be done between different viseme categories to separate single words from each other (e.g., *pahvi* (cardboard) – *kahvi* (coffee)). In some cases, the difference between the words to be discerned from each other is based on segment duration (e.g., *tuli* (fire) – *tuuli* (wind)) because duration is a feature affecting the meaning of words in Finnish. Both in word- and sentence-level task types, the items to be compared (same/different, which one of these two/four/five words or sentences was spoken; see Fig. 6) were allocated into easy, moderate and advanced levels. Categorization of the difficulty level was based on, for example, the viseme categories and length of words and sentences.

The tasks mainly cover word, sentence or phrase levels. In addition, a minor part of the speech material also represents connected speech level because, in one task type, the user needs to discriminate whether the three-sentence stories are identical or not.

Six speakers—three females and three males (three speech and language therapists, one teacher, one special education teacher and one layperson)—produced the speech

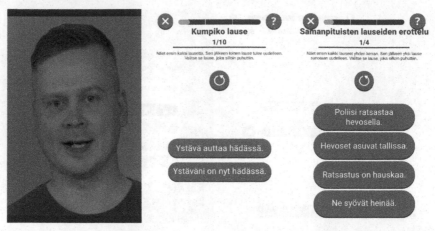

Fig. 6. Examples on the sentence-level exercises of Optic Track include discrimination between two (which one of the two sentences was spoken) or four items (which of the four sentences representing the same length was spoken).

materials at the recording studio of the Digital Pedagogics and Video Services of the University of Oulu. For recording the audiovisual materials, the Sennheiser SE 2 wireless clip-on microphone system and Panasonic AW-UE100 video camera were used, and the files were saved with Open Broadcaster Software into transport stream format (.TS with h264 codec) using a 1920 × 1080 resolution and 50 fps. A green screen was used as the background to allow for later replacement with the desired style.

Editing and cutting of the video material was done using a process with command-line tools (ffmpeg, bash) to allow precise frame-level accuracy and a unified output. The long studio sessions included several takes of words and sentences; manual editing of all samples to match the desired short clip characteristics would have been burdensome. Initially, automated subtitling was done using YuJa video platform auto-captioning. This resulted in a subtitle file in .SRT format, giving time codes within longer per-session files, despite a few auto-captioning errors. This was hand-matched to the studio session script, documenting which words and sentences were recorded. The best samples and cut points were then manually iterated at a frame-level accuracy (20 ms for 50 fps video). Special care was taken to verify that the cut points started and ended with as neutral a face as possible, with eyes open and mouth closed. These edits typically resulted in 1.5–2.0 s clips for isolated words and 2.5–4.0 s clips for longer sentences, with clear speaker-specific differences.

After the exact cut points had been defined, the original green screen was replaced with a neutral blue tint gradient background. Then, the video clips were cropped to a 3:4 aspect ratio clip containing only the facial area, with a resolution of 672 × 896. The first frame of the video was extended to 0.4 s of still face. At the end of the video clip, a symmetrical 0.4 s washout period was edited with only the background visible, so the originally cut videos were extended by 0.8 s. All the ffmpeg-based editing steps were stored in a bash shell script to allow relatively fast re-encoding from the source files in case there was a need to adjust the video clip details (start and end period durations, video format). Finally, the video files were saved without audio in an mp4 format using 50 fps and h264 codec, and the functionality of the videos was verified on a selection of mobile phones.

For alternative choices in many memory games and bingo tasks (Fig. 7), royalty-free colorful drawings or color images were selected from domestic and international image databases. In addition, about 100 colorful drawings were self-constructed when no suitable illustrations were available. Illustrations were added to the application to increase its appeal and support training motivation.

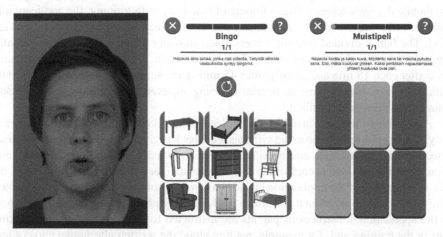

Fig. 7. Two gamification examples (bingo and memory games) of the Optic Track exercises.

Technical implementation of Optic Track was performed by a Finnish company, Outloud Ltd., by using the Unity game engine and C# language. Coding was partly based on the Auditory Track application. Special attention was paid to constructing the user interface and the graphical outlook as the main users of the application are children.

The research version of the Optic Track application, also coded by a Finnish company Outloud Ltd. and constructed for our research group, collects data on active time used for training (the application pauses after inactivity of one minute), time stamps regarding pausing and progress realised in training, that is, points and medals earned. This information is stored on the mobile device in a custom binary log file. The log file can be transferred from the device either via standard file browser and available file sharing methods (USB cable, wireless transfer) or directly from the Optic Track application via Bluetooth and computer host program written in Python. The binary log file can then be converted into a simple text CSV file for easier analysis.

2.4 Use of the Optic Track Application

The user can repeat watching the videos of the Optic Track application as many times as needed and select to play all the videos in either normal or slowed playback mode. The slowed pace is two-thirds of the pace of the normal playback pace. User interface of the application was made as clear as possible with easy-to-understand buttons helping in navigation.

The suggested amount of training with Optic Track is 45 min a week, for example, three times a week for about 15 min per training session. Practising should take place for a minimum of eight weeks, comprising a total of six hours. This recommended 'training dose' is based on research reports in which training leading to improvement of skills took place from one to five times a week and extended over a period of three to 12 weeks, with the duration of training sessions totalling from two to eight hours [31, 40, 41].

The time used for using the application is shown on a bar on the uppermost part of the mobile device's screen. After a minute of inactivity with training, the application is automatically paused with an announcement about it seen on the screen of the device used. The bar is divided into three parts, each showing 15 min. The user is verbally praised for having done the practising three times (again, a text appears on the screen), once after each 15 min and, finally, after 45 min. The user is also prompted to continue with practising, if they have an interest in doing so, even after this suggested weekly training dose has been fulfilled.

Accessibility was increased by giving feedback on correctness of the answers not only by using colors but also using symbols. Feedback is given immediately after the user selects their response and, additionally, through a reward system with gold, silver and bronze medals included in each of the 13 task types and their difficulty levels (see Fig. 8). The functionality of the application includes a summary of the number of medals earned across the whole application that can also be checked. For further improving compliance, in the application's instructions parents are instructed to support their child by taking part in the training and, for example, reading aloud the written alternative choices and feedback messages provided by the software if their child's reading skills are in an emerging phase or the child has difficulties reading.

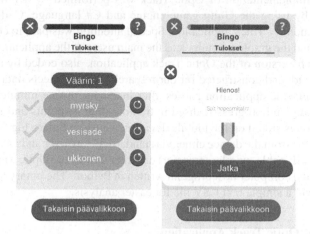

Fig. 8. Some features of the feedback system embedded in Optic Track (showing the correctness of answers and rewarding with medals according to the scores obtained).

When on the results view of the application, using the replay button (see Fig. 8), the user can look in a slow motion at the videos corresponding to the items in which they have succeeded and not in identifying the target.

3 Results

3.1 Implementation of the Auditory Track Application in the Medical Rehabilitation Field

After the Auditory Track application was completed, informing about its existence was actively taken care of. A poster presenting Auditory Track was created and sent to the 22 hearing stations and hearing centres at tertiary care Finnish hospitals in which hearing aid fittings and, in some cases, cochlear implant sound processors are also programmed. Staff members were asked to hang the poster on the wall for their patients to see. When needed, they have helped the patients download the application. Two slides giving information about the application were also created for use on digital displays of these hospitals' waiting halls. In addition, internet, social media, webinars, national seminars of hearing care professionals, patient organisation magazines and direct contact with the regional associations of the Finnish Federation for Hard of Hearing have been used as routes for reaching the potential end users of the application.

Among different digital care and rehabilitation services, independent auditory training with the help of the Auditory Track application has recently been recommended for professionals in the National Criteria for Referring People to Medical Rehabilitation 2022 Guide for Healthcare and Social Welfare Professionals and Those Working in Rehabilitation Services [47]. There is also another national route for informing about the Auditory Track: Terveyskylä (Health Village) [48] is a Finnish public 24/7 service for everyone who needs information and support in health issues. Among other advice and instructions for supporting auditory training, Auditory Track is also introduced among its materials (https://www.terveyskyla.fi/kuulotalo/ohjeita/).

About 70% of mobile phones and tablet computers in Finland have an Android operating system, and the rest have iOS. Auditory Track can be used in Android devices with an operating system of 5.1 or newer and in iOS devices 11.0 or newer. In December 2023, there were more than 2200 downloads from Google Play onto Android devices and more than 1100 downloads from the App Store onto iOS devices.

At one hospital, one cochlear implant user had realized with the help of Auditory Track that his main problem was in understanding speech in speech-shaped background noise. He found particularly valuable the possibility to train speech perception with different background noises. According to a recent MA thesis in Logopaedics [49], after an average use time of eight hours during a four-week independent training, nine adult users found Auditory Track mostly clear, convenient, and easy to use. The utility of the training application was perceived as good, the speakers were articulate, and musical parts were clear. The included gamification was appreciated, and the application helped the users become aware of their own hearing level. Some users hoped that it would be possible to change the background noise type in the middle of task execution.

3.2   Implementation of the Optic Track Application in the Medical Rehabilitation Field

A research version of Optic Track is currently used in the multidisciplinary and multiprofessional research project Gaze on lips?[1] in which, among other things, the effectiveness of Optic Track in improving the speechreading skills of hard-of-hearing children aged 8 to 11 years is studied. The aim is that the participating children use the application for 45 min a week over an eight-week period, totalling six hours of training.

After the data for the currently ongoing research project Gaze on lips?[1] have been collected, the forthcoming 'consumer version' of Optic Track will be downloadable free of charge from the application stores Google Play and App Store in the same way as Auditory Track already is. It is intended that information about the Optic Track application would also be included in the Terveyskylä (Health Village) materials.

4   Conclusions

Our aims have been obtained because we now have, for both auditory and speechreading training in Finnish, free applications that can be used by both deaf and hard-of-hearing children and adults. Additionally, research focusing on interventions can also be conducted by utilising both applications.

Since the 1980s, closed captioning has aided persons who have problems with hearing. Along with the latest huge leaps of technology based on advanced knowledge of computer linguistics, computer sciences and electrical engineering, persons with hearing loss can also get help from automatic speech recognition. With this, speech can nowadays be transformed into text practically in real time. However, the use of assisting technology does not remove the need for auditory training because of its benefits for an individuals' speech perception processes.

In addition to technology aiming to help improve the speechreading skills of human beings, automatic speech recognition technology has also been actively developed for machines and has accomplished many kinds of activities related to speechreading. According to a summary of Pu and Wang (2023) [50] and a recent systematic review based on 23 articles on deep learning by Santos, Cunha and Coelho (2023) [51], progress has been made using computerised speechreading in research projects, but at the word level, for instance, the results still remain below human performance. However, one exception—Watch, Listen, Attend and Spell—which utilises computer vision and machine learning and is based on training with immense video material, has been reported to clearly outperform at least one professional speechreader [52]. A special machine learning-based SRAVI iOS application (https://www.sravi.ai/) has been developed for, for example, staff members in hospitals in helping them understand speech produced by tracheostomy patients who cannot use their voice normally. In the future, portable speechreading technology based on artificial intelligence may also provide real-time help in real-life situations for those with hearing loss. Before reaching this situation, the aim is to help persons with impaired hearing train their skills as much as possible. This is important because most communication situations take place 'in the wild' without

---

[1] https://www.oulu.fi/en/projects/gaze-lips.

any human-technology interaction. Moreover, because speech perception is multimodal in nature, both senses need to be utilised. It is beneficial because an improvement in auditory skills can enhance speechreading improvement [53], and speechreading, in turn, is widely known to help in recognising audiovisual speech.

Acknowledgments. Coding (as a purchased service) of Auditory Track was possible with the grants received from the Finnish ORL-HNS Foundation, the Finnish Federation for Hard of Hearing and the Finnish Audiological Society. In addition, funding for the construction and coding of Optic Track has been received from the Finnish Association of Speech Therapists, the Finnish Audiological Society and the S. and A. Bovallius Foundation. Additionally, the Eudaimonia Institute of the University of Oulu has had the major role in financing the research project related to exploring the effectiveness of Optic Track.

Disclosure of Interests. The authors have no competing interests to declare that are relevant to the content of this article.

References

1. WHO: World report on hearing. World Health Organization, Geneva (2021)
2. Amieva, H., Ouvrard, C., Meillon, C., Rullier, L., Dartigues, J.-F.: Death, depression, disability, and dementia associated with self-reported hearing problems: a 25-year study. J. Gerontol. Ser. A **73**(10), 1383–1389 (2018)
3. Lawrence, B.J., Jayakody, D.M.P., Bennett, R.J., Eikelboom, R.H., Gasson, N., Friedland, P.L.: Hearing loss and depression in older adults: a systematic review and meta-analysis. Gerontologist **60**(3), e137–e154 (2020)
4. Livingston, G., Huntley, J., Sommerlad, A., et al.: Dementia prevention, intervention, and care: 2020 report of the Lancet Commission. Lancet **396**(10248), 413–446 (2020)
5. Dawes, P., Maslin, M., Munro, K.J.: 'Getting used to' hearing aids from the perspective of adult hearing-aid users. Int. J. Audiol. **53**(12), 861–870 (2014)
6. Dillon, H., Day, J., Bant, S., Munro, K.J.: Adoption, use and non-use of hearing aids: a robust estimate based on Welsh national survey statistics. Int. J. Audiol. **59**(8), 567–573 (2020)
7. Vuorialho, A., Karinen, P., Sorri, M.: Effect of hearing aids on hearing disability and quality of life in the elderly. Int. J. Audiol. **45**(7), 400–405 (2006)
8. Sweetow, R., Palmer, C.: Efficacy of individual auditory training programs in adults: a systematic review of the evidence. J. Am. Acad. Audiol. **16**(7), 494–540 (2005)
9. Huttunen, K.: Erikoissairaanhoidon tarjoamat kuulovammaisten aikuisten puheterapiapalvelut (Speech therapy services in tertiary care for adults). Puheterapeutti **2**, 16–20 (2010)
10. Lonka, E.: Huulioluvun ja kuulonharjoituksen ohjelma (Programme for speechreading and auditory training). Puheterapeuttien Kustannus, Helsinki (2003)
11. Völter, C., Schirmer, C., Stöckmann, C., Dazert, S.: Computerbasiertes Hörtraining in der Hörrehabilitation Erwachsener nach Cochleaimplantation. HNO **68**(11), 817–827 (2020)
12. Agostinelli, A., et al.: Improving auditory perception in pediatric single-sided deafness: use of cochlear implants' direct connection for remote speech perception rehabilitation. Am. J. Audiol. **32**(1), 52–58 (2023)
13. Barda, A., Shapira, Y., Fostick, L.: Individual differences in auditory training benefits for hearing aid users. Clin. Pract. **13**(5), 1196–1206 (2023)

14. Tye-Murray, N., Spehar, B., Sommers, M.S., Barcroft, J.: Auditory training with frequent communication partners. J. Speech Lang. Hear. Res. **59**(4), 871–875 (2016)
15. Barda, A., Shapira, Y., Fostick, L.: Benefits of auditory training with an open-set sentences-in-babble-noise. Appl. Sci. **13**(16), 9126 (2023)
16. Van Wilderode, M., Vermaete, E., Francart, T., Wouters, J., Van Wieringen, A.: Effectiveness of auditory training in experienced hearing-aid users, and an exploration of their health-related quality of life and coping strategies. Trends Hearing **27**, 1–14 (2023)
17. Olson, A.D.: Options for auditory training for adults with hearing loss. Semin. Hear. **36**(4), 284–295 (2015)
18. Vitti, S.V., Blasca, W.Q., Sigulem, D., Torres Pisa, I.: Web-based auditory self-training system for adult and elderly users of hearing aids. In: Studies in Health Technology and Informatics, MEDINFO 2015: eHealth-enabled Health, vol. 216, pp. 168–172 (2015)
19. Henshaw, H., Ferguson, M.A.: Efficacy of individual computer-based auditory training for people with hearing loss: a systematic review of the evidence. PLoS ONE **8**(5), e62836 (2013)
20. Tye-Murray, N., Spehar, B., Barcroft, J., Sommers, M.: Auditory training for adults who have hearing loss: a comparison of spaced versus massed practice schedules. J. Speech Lang. Hear. Res. **60**(8), 2337–2345 (2017)
21. Ab Shukor, N.F., Lee, J., Seo, Y.J., Han, W.: Efficacy of music training in hearing aid and cochlear implant users: a systematic review and meta-analysis. Clin. Exp. Otorhinolaryngology **14**(1), 15–28 (2021)
22. Sato, T., Yabushita, T., Sakamoto, S., Katori, Y., Kawase, T.: In-home auditory training using audiovisual stimuli on a tablet computer: feasibility and preliminary results. Auris Nasus Larynx **47**(3), 348–352 (2020)
23. Ferguson, M.A., Henshaw, H.: Auditory training can improve working memory, attention, and communication in adverse conditions for adults with hearing loss. Front. Psychol. **6**, 556 (2015)
24. Stropahl, M., Besser, J., Launer, S.: Auditory training supports auditory rehabilitation: a state-of-the-art review. Ear Hear. **41**(4), 697–704 (2020)
25. Mendel, L.L., Larson, B., Pousson, M.A., Shukla, B., Sander, K.: Listening effort and speech perception performance using different facemasks. J. Speech Lang. Hear. Res. **6**(11), 4354–4368 (2022)
26. Altieri, N.A., Pisoni, D.B., Townsend, J.T.: Some normative data on lip-reading skills. J. Acoust. Soc. Am. **130**(1), 1–4 (2011)
27. Gorman, B.R., Flatla, D.R.: MirrorMirror: a mobile application to improve speechreading acquisition. In: CHI '18: Proceedings of the 2018 CHI Conference on Human Factors in Computing Systems, Paper No. 26, pp. 1–12. Association for Computing Machinery, New York (2018)
28. Buchanan-Worster, E., et al.: Speechreading ability is related to phonological awareness and single-word reading in both deaf and hearing children. J. Speech Lang. Hear. Res. **63**(11), 3775–3785 (2020)
29. Kyle, F., Campbell, R., MacSweeney, M.: The relative contributions of speechreading and vocabulary to deaf and hearing children's reading ability. Res. Dev. Disabil. **48**, 13–24 (2016)
30. Trezek, B., Mayer, C.: Reading and deafness: state of the evidence and implications for research and practice. Educ. Sci. **9**(3), 216 (2019)
31. Tye-Murray, N., Spehar, B., Sommers, M., Mauzé, E., Barcroft, J., Grantham, H.: Teaching children with hearing loss to recognize speech: gains made with computer-based auditory and/or speechreading training. Ear Hear. **43**(1), 181–191 (2022)
32. Bernstein, L.E., Auer, E.T., Tucker, P.E.: Enhanced speechreading in deaf adults: can short-term training/practice close the gap for hearing adults? J. Speech Lang. Hear. Res. **44**(1), 5–18 (2001)

33. Blumsack, J.T., Bower, C.R., Ross, M.E.: Comparison of speechreading training regimens. Percept. Mot. Skills **105**(3), 988–996 (2007)
34. Bothe, H-H.: Training of speechreading for severely hearing-impaired persons by human and computer. In: Seventh IEEE International Conference on Advanced Learning Technologies (ICALT 2007), Niigata, Japan, vol. 2007, pp. 913–924. IEEE, Piscataway, NJ (2007)
35. Lonka, E.: Speechreading instruction for hard-of-hearing adults. Effects of training face-to-face and with a video programme. Scandinavian Audiology **24**(3), 193–198 (1995)
36. Tye-Murray, N., Hale, S., Spehar, B., Myerson, J., Sommers, M.S.: Lipreading in school-age children: the roles of age, hearing status, and cognitive ability. J. Speech Lang. Hear. Res. **57**(2), 556–565 (2014)
37. Pimperton, H., Ralph-Lewis, A., MacSweeney, M.: Speechreading in deaf adults with cochlear implants: evidence for perceptual compensation. Front. Psychol. **8**, 106 (2017)
38. Conrad, R.: Lip-reading by deaf and hearing children. Br. J. Educ. Psychol. **47**(1), 60–65 (1977)
39. Kyle, F.E., Campbell, R., Mohammed, T., Coleman, M., MacSweeney, M.: Speechreading development in deaf and hearing children: introducing the test of child speechreading. J. Speech Lang. Hear. Res. **56**(2), 416–426 (2013)
40. Buchanan-Worster, E., Hulme, C., Dennan, R., MacSweeney, M.: Speechreading in hearing children can be improved by training. Dev. Sci. **24**, e13124 (2021)
41. Pimperton, H., et al.: Computerized speechreading training for deaf children: a randomized controlled trial. J. Speech Lang. Hear. Res. **62**(8), 2882–2894 (2019)
42. Huttunen, K., Vikman, S., Pajo, K.: Kuulorata. Kuulonharjoitussovellus (Auditory Track. Application for auditory training). Coding: Outloud Ltd. Available for free at Google Play and App Store (2021)
43. Lonka, E., Aulanko, R.: Kuulorata käyttöön. Puheterapeuttien Kustannus, Helsinki (1999)
44. Huttunen, K., Vikman, S., Pajo, K.: Kuulorata-sovellus avuksi kuulonharjoitusten oma-toimiseen tekemiseen (The Auditory Track application for helping independent auditory training). In: Laitakari, J. & Yliaska, M. (eds.), XLII Valtakunnalliset audiologian päivät ja tekninen audiologia Oulussa 7.–8.4.2022, pp. 59–71. Suomen audiologian yhdistys, Helsinki (2022)
45. Humes, L.E., Kinney, D.L, Brown, S.E, Kiener, A.L., Quigley, T.M.: The effects of dosage and duration of auditory training for older adults with hearing impairment. J. Acoust. Soc. Am. **136**(3), EL224 (2014)
46. Huttunen, K., Saalasti, S.: Näkörata. Huulioluvun harjoitussovellus (Optic Track. Application for speechreading training). Yet unpublished, research version of the application currently being in research use. Coding: Outloud Ltd. Consumer version will be available for free at Google Play and App Store
47. Aarnisalo, A., et al.: Kuulon kuntoutus. In Valtakunnalliset lääkinnälliseen kuntoutukseen ohjaamisen perusteet. Opas terveyden- ja sosiaalihuollon ammattilaisille ja kuntoutuksen parissa työskenteleville (National Criteria for Referring People to Medical Rehabilitation 2022 Guide for Healthcare and Social Welfare Professionals and Those Working in Rehabil-itation Services), pp. 215–225. Sosiaali- ja terveysministeriön julkaisuja 2022:17. Sosiaali-ja terveysministeriö, Helsinki (2022)
48. Terveyskylä (Health Village). https://www.terveyskyla.fi/kuulotalo/ohjeita/ Accessed 10 Jan 2024
49. Hulkkonen, E.: Puheen vastaanoton omatoiminen harjoittelu – Muutokset Kuulorata-sovellusta kokeilleiden aikuisten elämänlaadussa ja käyttökokemuksia sovelluksesta (Inde-pendent training of speech reception – Changes in the quality of life and user experiences of adults who have tried the Auditory Track application). MA thesis in Logopaedics. Faculty of Humanities, University of Oulu, Oulu (2023)

50. Pu, G., Wang, H.: Review on research progress of machine lip reading. Vis. Comput. **39**, 3041–3057 (2023). https://doi.org/10.1007/s00371-022-02511-4
51. Santos, C., Cunha, A., Coelho, P.: A review on deep learning-based automatic lipreading. In: Cunha, A., M. Garcia, N., Marx Gómez, J., Pereira, S. (eds.) Wireless Mobile Communication and Healthcare. MobiHealth 2022, LNICS, Social Informatics and Telecommunications Engineering, vol. 484, pp 180–195. Springer, Cham (2023). https://doi.org/10.1007/978-3-031-32029-3_17
52. Chung, J.S., Senior, A., Vinyals, O., Zisserman, A.: Lip reading sentences in the wild. In: 2017 IEEE Conference on Computer Vision and Pattern Recognition (CVPR), pp. 3444–3453. IEEE Computer Society, Washington, DC (2017)
53. Strelnikov, K., Rouger, J., Lagleyre, S., Fraysse, B., Deguine, O., Barone, P.: Improvement in speech-reading ability by auditory training: evidence from gender differences in normally hearing, deaf and cochlear implanted subjects. Neuropsychologia **47**(4), 972–979 (2009)

Visual Modeling of Multiple Sclerosis Patient Pathways: The Healthcare Workers' Perspectives

Binyam Bogale[1]([✉]) [iD], Ingrid Konstanse Ledel Solem[2], Elisabeth Gulowsen Celius[1,3], and Ragnhild Halvorsrud[4]

[1] Institute of Clinical Medicine, Department of Neurology, University of Oslo, Oslo, Norway
b.b.bungudo@medisin.uio.no
[2] Department of Health, SINTEF Digital, Oslo, Norway
[3] Oslo University Hospital, Ullevål, Norway
[4] Sustainable Communication Technologies, SINTEF Digital, Oslo, Norway

Abstract. Multiple Sclerosis (MS) necessitates tailored care along intricate pathways throughout a patient's lifetime. Visualizing these pathways enhances the collective understanding of care processes and fosters collaboration among stakeholders. This study employed a qualitative study to map and the Customer Journey Modeling Language (CJML) to model MS patient pathways. A total of six purposefully selected healthcare professionals working in specialized healthcare, at a hospital and separate rehabilitation center, contributed to the care process mapping, participating in both pre- and post-modeling in-depth interviews. CJML, designed to capture planned and actual journeys from the service users' perspective was adapted in this study to showcase the service provider's viewpoints, revealing insights into the existing organization of MS care. Involving more than one service provision level in mapping and modeling care processes requires dealing with handovers and its associated challenges. The final visualizations illustrate potential areas for improvement, including the need for more standardized procedures, potentially leading to variations in the quality of care and/or inefficient processes. However, the mapping process highlighted the difficulties in visualizing the MS care pathway due to its highly personalized nature, including challenges with creating personas or case groups that would allow for a unified service model. Participants' feedback on the visualizations was essential, illustrating the importance of member checking when dealing with complex concepts such as patient pathways and organization of care.

Keywords: Visual modeling · Customer Journey Modeling Language (CJML) · Patient Pathways · Multiple Sclerosis

1 Introduction

Multiple Sclerosis (MS) is an inflammatory demyelinating condition resulting from an autoimmune attack of the myeline sheath of the neurons in the central nervous system [1, 2]. It is a severe neurological disorder with varying presentations and disease progression

© The Author(s) 2024
M. Särestöniemi et al. (Eds.): NCDHWS 2024, CCIS 2083, pp. 303–317, 2024.
https://doi.org/10.1007/978-3-031-59080-1_22

from person to person [1–3]. The global prevalence of MS is increasing, disproportionately affecting productive age groups and females [4]. Highly effective disease modifying treatments are increasingly utilized for this lifelong condition with the ultimate aim of reducing the frequency and severity of relapses, slowing the disease progression, and managing symptoms [5]. Along with non-pharmacological [6] and rehabilitation services [7], the overall goal is to improve quality of life. Time plays a crucial role to achieve the best outcome in MS care [8]. One of the factors delaying the timely intervention is the organization of care processes. There are international clinical guidelines and national efforts to streamline the MS patient pathways [8–10], however, these are recommendations prone to limitations in actual implementation. The care processes are described in a text and flowchart formats in many situations. Managing complex conditions such as MS further complicates the already complex organization of healthcare system. When a business processes for non-linear and less predictable processes, such as managing MS, presented in a narrative form, comprehending the complexity becomes difficult.

Visual models are useful in enabling easy understanding of processes, which improves communication and mutual understanding among stakeholders [11]. Several visual modeling languages exist, broadly classified into domain specific (i.e., health or clinical oriented in this case) or general purpose [12]. In this case study, we employed the Customer Journey Modeling Language (CJML), which is designed to visually model both the planned and executed journeys [13]. CJML has previously been used in the healthcare domain and shown to model both the planned journey (or the patient pathway) and the actual journey from the perspective of the patients [14]. With the increasing use of patient centric pathway implementations, CJML is well suited to model patient pathways. In this case study, we explored the potential of CJML in modeling more personalized care pathways from the perspective of service providers.

The healthcare in Norway is organized into municipal and specialized care services [15]. The mandate of establishing diagnoses and initiating treatment for MS resides at the specialist care, usually at the public hospital level, in the department of neurology where MS specialized neurologists are available. Long-term rehabilitation services are mainly provided by a specialized centers for neurological disorders, which is organized independently under the specialist care. Integration of services such as MS along multiple levels of care requires efficient organization of processes. In this study, we emphasize on visualizing the handovers and challenges that follow in the integration of services in the MS patient pathways.

This study is part of larger research project working towards creating a comprehensive toolkit for managing and communicating patient pathways. The aim of this study was to map and visually model the current MS patient pathways within specialized healthcare, including diagnosis, treatment, and follow-up at the hospital level and rehabilitation services at the neurology specialized rehabilitation center from the healthcare workers' perspectives.

Specific objectives were to:

- Assess the existing MS care delivery processes at the hospital and the rehabilitation center
- Identify and map actors and touchpoints in the MS patient pathways

- Identify practices and procedures related to handovers within and across healthcare levels
- Assess the feasibility of Customer Journey Modeling Language (CJML) to visually represent the MS patient pathways from healthcare workers' perspectives

2 Methods

2.1 Study Design, Area and Participants

The study utilized a qualitative study design, using semi-structured interviews to systematically collect insights on the MS patient pathways as seen from the perspectives of healthcare providers' working within the specialized healthcare (a department of neurology and outpatient clinic and a MS rehabilitation center). This study was conducted in Oslo University Hospital, which serves the largest number of MS patients in the country. The hospital has several specialists and allied professionals dedicated to MS research and clinical care provision. The MS rehabilitation service is situated in one of the neurology related specialized rehabilitation centers close to the city of Oslo. The center provides rehabilitation services to patients with other neurological disorders. The center accepts patients from all over the county for inpatient rehabilitation services. To gain a comprehensive understanding of the MS care delivery process, participants were purposively selected, representing different disciplines, roles, and services within MS care. The final six participants included two neurologists, one health secretary and one nurse working at the hospital MS clinic and a leader and a coordinator (both are health professionals) at the MS rehabilitation center. Half of the participants were females. All participants had several years of experiences in their respective role. All approached healthcare providers agreed to participate in the study. The data collection spanned from June – November 2023.

2.2 Data Collection

The material was collected in two phases; In the first phase, a semi-structed interview guide was used to gather detailed information about the touchpoints and interactions the participant (e.g., the nurse) was involved in during the MS patient pathway. The interview guide aimed at exploring step-by-step organizational and clinical processes undertaken by the participants and their colleagues in their respective roles. These spanned from the very first contact with the patient (e.g., receiving a referral from the general practitioner) throughout the entire treatment/care provision up to patients' exit. The interview guide was semi-structured with open-ended questions to facilitate the free narration of the care processes. It was developed by the researchers and iteratively improved throughout the two phases of the interviews.

Based on the insights from the first interview, the first author (BB) visualized the MS patient pathways using Customer Journey Modeling Language (CJML). The visualizations were then used as discussion points in the following round of interviews (second phase). The aims of these post-modeling interviews were to present the visualizations and get feedback on 1) potential gaps from the initial round of interviews, 2) errors and needs for adjustment, 3) understandability of the visualizations and 4) the usefulness of these kinds of visualizations. The final visual models were based on iterative improvements in addition to the feedbacks from the participants.

Except one virtual meeting, the data collections were conducted physically, at the premises of the institutions. The interviews were conducted by two of the authors (BB and IKLS) who are not associated to the MS patient care, and while one lead the interview the other took notes. Each interview lasted for around 1,5–2 h in each phase. Since this is for process mapping and modeling, we did not aim for information saturation to determine the adequacy of number of participants, rather diversity of participants. Most of the interviews were conducted in English. However, two of the interviews were conducted in local language with notes later being translated into English. All interviews were recorded and later transcribed.

The study was approved by regional and institutional ethics committee and collected in accordance with the Helsinki Declaration [16]. All participants signed informed consent before participation. Data was stored in a secure directory and results presented anonymously, by observing the personal data protection rules [17].

2.3 Data Analysis

In the first step of analysis, two of the authors (BB and IKLS; both external researchers) listened to the recordings and took notes, supplementing the original notes taken at the time of the interviews. Then the entire MS patient pathways in both institutions were divided into sub-processes for the sake of simplicity during modeling procedure and presentation of the CJML models. The notes were then sorted based on these sub-processes for further analysis of the interview materials. The next step in the analysis process was that the first author (BB) identified and mapped actors (patients, individual healthcare professionals, or a unit in healthcare system) and touchpoints (i.e., actions, medium, and instances of communications between the patient and the healthcare institution actors), and further visualized these using CJML. The visualizations were then used in the follow-up interview with each participant to get feedback, ensuring that the insights and details were understood correctly, while also providing an opportunity for additional data and details left out from first interview. The interview material from second phase interviews also were sorted into sub-processes in the same manner as the first phase interviews.

The data material was revisited to identify common themes discussed during the two phased interviews. Using the sorted data under each sub-process, the first author grouped and labelled the major themes discussed by the participants. Main themes are presented together with illustrating quotes, ensuring transparency in the interpretation of results. Thus, several rounds of revisiting the material were required to iteratively improve the final version of the model. The output of the process, visual models of selected sub-processes using CJML is presented to illustrate parts of the current MS patient pathways in these institutions.

3   Results

The result section is structed into sub-processes in the MS patient pathway and are hence divided into the following sections: 1) referrals, 2) internal handovers, 3) admission processing, 4) diagnosis, 4) treatment and symptom management, and 5) follow-up. As most sub-processes apply to both institutions (i.e., the hospital and the rehabilitation center), findings are presented together to allow for comparisons.

3.1   Referral Processing

There are two main routes of referrals to the hospital for a MS specialist care: 1) directly from primary care, mainly from the general practitioner's office presenting with mild or moderate symptoms, or 2) referred from the same hospital or other healthcare outlets after receiving emergency management. Figure 1 shows the CJML model of the referral processing sub-process using a swimlane diagram. Similarly, the rehabilitation center also receives referrals from a MS specialist at the hospital or general practitioner through regional approving authority (Fig. 2). For both facilities, the models in Fig. 1 and 2 show the first referral routes to illustrate the involved actors and touchpoints. The other route is not shown due to space restrictions.

Assumptions: Referral is from GP for a mild or moderate symptoms.

All the requests from the communicator are accepted; or not declined by the receiver of the request or information.

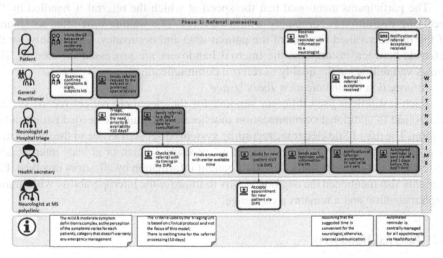

Fig. 1. CJML model of MS patient pathway sub-process at hospital specialist care

Major themes discussed by the participants regarding this sub-process are as follows.
Communication Between Institutions
The participants discussed the ways in which the referring professionals communicate to their institutions. Some made a call before processing the referral requests,

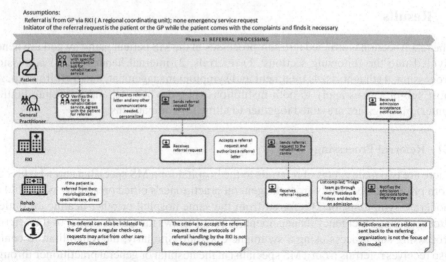

Fig. 2. CJML model of MS patient pathway sub-process at the specialist rehabilitation center

while others only referred the patients through the digital communication channels. The content of the referral letter also varied. The participant from rehabilitation center stated that "*some time the referral letter says, 'this patient needs rehabilitation'. Others (mentioned a professional by name) detail what specifically the patient needs the rehabilitation service.*"

The participants mentioned that the speed at which the referral is handled by the receiving institution is commonly within 10 days. The waiting time after acceptance of the referrals varied because of the patient load and occupancy. This is only for the referrals between institutions; the internal handovers are processed differently. This shows variabilities in the quality of referral communication.

Information Communication Tools Usage

Each institutions used different vendors for the electronic patient record system, which lead to additional communication touchpoint to obtain the needed patient information. The use of Silo electronic recording systems discussed as one of the information flow hinderers between facilities. The effect of using similar, or at least interoperable systems, would mean real time access of patient information by all actors involved. Participants also mentioned the ongoing efforts to improve the interoperability with limited implementation and it remains a challenge.

3.2 Internal Handovers

In addition to the referrals between institutions tasked with different care provisions, there is internal handovers for semi-independent actors in the MS pathways at the hospital specialist care. The neurologist who diagnosed the patient hands over to the MS nurse at the out-patient clinic to administer the treatment and manage the patient (Fig. 5). There are differences following the type of medication to be administered, however, the majority who take intravenous infusions are managed, both clinically and organization-ally, by the MS nurses at the out-patient clinic with limited or no involvement from the diagnosing MS specialist neurologist.

Informal Communication Works Best Internally

The actor who is handing over the care internally communicates to the other party, often in person despite the presence of internal electronic communications channel. The digital communication is also used but informal communications believed to be feasible in small institutions. Any communication that transcends a department, for example, to a laboratory department, however, follows standard operating procedure of the hospital.

Information Communication Tools Usage

Internally, the same electronic tool is being used. This allowed a real time information exchange (including yellow notes for urgent attention) between the neurologists and MS nurses. The electronic health record under use required some expertise to locate the information a given professional may need, which might have hindered the effective use of the digital tool for internal communication. The administrative information is easier for the health secretary to obtain and process but maybe challenging for the clinicians. Health secretary said that "*you have to click several places to retrieve information, which is easier for us since we use the system a lot.*"

3.3 Admission

This sub-process applies to the rehabilitation services. However, the information needs, and retrieval applies to the hospital services to some extent, except that majority of the patient data about the MS is generated at the hospital level. Coupled with the less detailed description in the referral letter, the retrieval of information during and after admission became very laborious, which can also lead to inaccuracies. The participants stated that the rehabilitation center conducts a lot of communications via different channels to obtain patient specific information needed to commence the service. One of the participants said, "*we do a lot of calls…does not matter who makes the calls as long as the information is obtained*". Figure 3 shows the CJML model of the communication needs that arise although it is not possible to list all the actors as it depends on the individual cases.

Flexible to Accommodate More Patients and Operate More Quickly

Both the health secretaries who manage the appointment scheduling and the physi-cians cooperate to help the patients get appointments faster. The patients are also given options to get the diagnosis at private specialist practitioners if there is no possibility of finding appointments shortly. The health secretary said that "*We also collaborate with the private sector to give the patients options to get timely diagnosis if we could not find free spots with our specialists*". Clinicians also use their spare time and adjust their schedules to accommodate patients. One of the physicians said that "*We try to exploit the system or adjust somethings…and I think we are actually quite good at adapting.*"

3.4 Establishing Diagnosis

The diagnosis for MS is established by the neurologist at the hospital specialist care. The process involves imaging and diagnostic lumbar puncture, which involves other

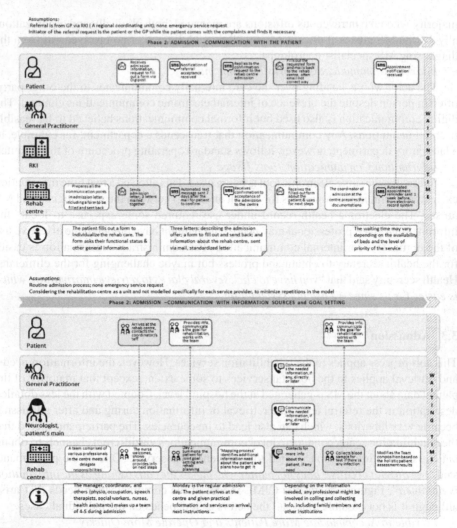

Fig. 3. CJML model of patient and stakeholder communication to retrieve patient information at the rehabilitation center.

actors in the pathway. All the internal communications between actors were made via the same EHR system, in addition, in person consultation of senior physicians. Figure 4 demonstrates the actors involved with the communication touchpoints.

Variable Approaches Among Clinicians

Some clinicians take the initiative to contact their patients to notify the results. One participant stated *"I think there might be a difference there. I usually call the patients after the MRI because I know that they are very anxiously waiting"*.

Uncertain Waiting Time for Diagnostic Results

Due to waiting time for the laboratory and imaging services, the diagnostic results might not come in the duration the neurologist hopes to receive. This affects the next

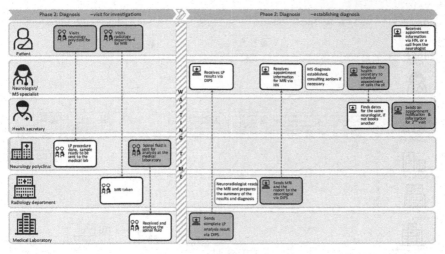

Fig. 4. CJML model of MS patient pathway diagnosis sub-process at the hospital

scheduling and patients are anxiously waiting for the result. For emergency cases, however, the neurologist can put a flag in the electronic order so that the result turnover is quicker.

3.5 Treatment and Symptoms Monitoring

This sub-process at the hospital and at the rehabilitation center aimed at different focus, but the actors' involvement at the team level makes the organization of care somehow similar. First, the treatment is administered by the out-patient clinic (polyclinic) which operate semi-independently. The patient communication, internal communication between departments and the diagnosing neurologist, and the monitoring of treatment progress is planned and managed after the handover is completed.

3.6 Follow-Ups

Since the MS management is a lifelong process, the follow up at the different service outlets is warranted. Specially, patients are scheduled for a follow up with preferably the diagnosing neurologist at least after 6 months of diagnosis, unless there was no other indication for more frequent visits. The neurologists promise their patient an estimated time for the follow up visit but are not in control because of the long waiting list. The scheduling is also monitored by the health secretary who has to follow the queue in the waiting list. Sometimes, the patient has to be scheduled with another neurologist than the one who diagnosed them first, which is not welcomed by the neurologists.

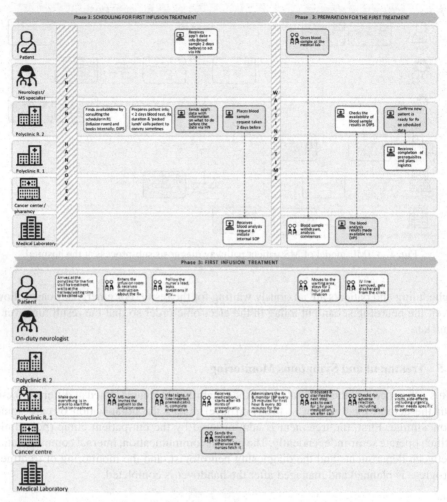

Fig. 5. CJML model for infusion treatment at the neurology out-patient clinic

4 Discussion

Employing an iterative approach, we visually modeled the MS patient pathways at the hospital specialist care and a rehabilitation center using CJML. The three main contributions of this study were identifying and dealing with the challenges and opportunities of visually illustrating care processes with highly personalized care, as in the case of MS patient pathways; applying CJML to model from the perspective of the healthcare service providers; and the complexities of modeling handovers by including more than one care level. In the following paragraphs, we discuss these points selectively to share our approaches. The process of visually modeling a care process presents opportunities to bottleneck analysis for the future improvements of services. This study contributed to the first stages of bottleneck analysis and process optimization [18]. Assessing and modeling an existing care process, the 'as-is', is a step in developing a 'to-be', or future ideal organization of care by addressing the bottlenecks or even optimizing a functioning pathways [19, 20]. The studied MS patient pathways is based on international guidelines and national care process organization recommendations [8, 9]. Assessments like this, along with insights from studies such as [21] on care variations among patients, offer valuable input to develop integrated MS patient pathways, centered around a life-course approach, based on a proactive, multidisciplinary, and patient pathways concept.

Visually modeling every scenario for health condition with a variable presentation and disease course is a difficult task [11]. As to the first contribution, we understood the necessary variations arising from individualization or other clinical factors that can be modeled separately. However, we only modeled the commonest pathways while recognizing individual variations within. For example, there are several treatment options for MS tailored to individual factors [22]. In the study area, however, majority of the patients are using highly effective disease modifying therapy, which is modeled as a common treatment pathway on a higher level of abstraction. Our modeling does not go into the clinical decisions where further individualization of the therapy is made [22]. Therefore, the abstraction of a visual model is at a higher or group level. This may have reduced the usual trap of a complex visual models of a process that is hard to understand and often not used [11]. Modeling should always allow individual variations because of unpredictable factors in the care delivery process [23]. Such complexity calls for a more adaptive modeling that has a flexibility to present the individualization process in a planned pathway.

Since patient care for conditions such as MS spans over lifetime and involves several stakeholders, considering the integration of care throughout multiple levels of healthcare is vital [24, 25]. Where there is inter-institutional communication, the flow of patient information is affected by several factors. We identified challenges encountered during referral processing. One of the challenges emanates from the usage of a silo electronic health record (EHR) systems, placing additional workflow issues, where providers spend time in collecting information about the patient, otherwise would have been automatically retrieved [26]. In addition to the logistics it requires, the quality of patient information is compromised when other ways of communications were employed. During modeling, we also run into an overwhelming number of actors and touchpoints, which was also different for individual cases. Pertaining to modeling the handovers contribution of this study, the work around in the modeling was to provide assumptions (Fig. 3). The within institution handovers where the same EMR is used have not encountered as much difficulty in finding patient information as in the case of referrals between institutions (Fig. 5). One important aspect discussed in the process of handovers and management of follow-ups was expressed by the physicians, concerning the long waiting time, which is against the very idea of 'time matters in MS'[8].

Visual modeling of a process works best for predictable and linear processes [27, 28]. Most business process modeling languages work well when a process meets those criteria. The healthcare domain, due to its complex nature (e.g., dealing with human health, not a production line), has been a challenging area to easily adapt process modeling languages and apply [12]. Therefore, several studies demonstrated that the domain requirements are being met by different approaches, including adapting a modeling language to the domain needs [29]. Push factors such as using a patient-centered approach in a care delivery model, with the growing literature on patient journey studies pave the way for opting for a customer-oriented modeling languages over process modeling languages with a focus on beyond line of visibility for customers (service blueprints) [14]. One such example is CJML [13]. In this study, we demonstrated how information gathered from healthcare works with multidisciplinary background and roles can also be used to model. The CJML provides two diagram types, where swimlane is one of them. We used swimlane diagram type where all the actors, including the patient can be depicted (as presented in the models in Fig. 1, 2, 3, 4 and 5) in a model. Processes happening beyond the line of visibility for the patient can be modeled and used as a service blueprint best using other modeling languages. Approaching from the client perspective provides opportunity to model the individual pathways whereas modeling from the perspective of the service providers presents a holistic process of the organization of a given care. The advantage of approaching from both providers' and patients' perspectives for a more standardized patient pathways is underway within the umbrella project this study is a part of.

This study has strength and limitations as any research projects. We worked with the same participant twice –before and after the modeling exercise. This approach, we believe, allowed us to refine the modeling process. There were several questions that we identified in the process of modeling the first iteration based on the first interview, which we used to get clarification in the post-modeling interview. Without such a process, there would have been incomplete or misleading visualization of the process. The inclusion of professionals with different roles and responsibilities in the patient pathway also provided a comprehensive mapping of the processes.

Using the patient-centered modeling language helps to put the patient at the center of the process modeling even though the data is from the providers' perspectives. Commonly used visual models present the service blueprints, dealing with the hidden part of the process from the users, missing the crucial touchpoints with the patients along with the end-users' feelings that affects the overall effect of care delivery process [13].

Since creating personas or grouping cases is a challenging task as the care provision is highly personalized and the touchpoints are dependent on the care providers' innovative approach and dedication, we presented the models with assumptions by only modeling the commonest, yet without going into low level of abstractions. Such categorization cannot be exhaustive enough to include all the different variations. During the interview, we explored ways of categorizing and creating personas with the participants. The lesson learned from the process was that it is challenging and probably needs a refined methodology for future studies of similar kinds.

Future similar studies may consider a hands-on modeling of the process with the participants. We only involved them in the refinement process to some extent but co-creating the models could give them more agency in presenting the process even more accurately. It has been demonstrated earlier that non-modelers can easily adopt CJML and make precise models of a process [30]. Especially when there is an attempt to create a 'to-be' type of patient pathways, hands-on approach might be even more relevant. We also did not carry out a thorough feasibility study by involving more stakeholders than the participants in the interview. This can be improved by including other healthcare workers to thoroughly assess the understandability, usability, and feasibility of CJML models.

5 Conclusions

The process of modeling a care system allows for reflection on care delivery organization. Mapping the actors and touchpoints in MS patient pathways at a hospital and specialized rehabilitation center, involving healthcare workers in various roles, helps comprehend the current organization of care processes. Visualizing highly individualized patient pathways for chronic conditions managed across multiple care levels with numerous stakeholders is inherently complex. While modeling languages like CJML can aid in visually representing patient pathways, further studies are needed to enhance methods and address all domain needs comprehensively.

Acknowledgments. We acknowledge the participants for their invaluable contribution and dedication. This work was funded by The Research Council of Norway, under the Pathway project (no. 316342).

Disclosure of Interests. The authors have no competing interests to declare that are relevant to the content of this article.

References

1. Compston, A., Coles, A.: Multiple sclerosis. Lancet Lond. Engl. **372**(9648), 1502–1517 (2008). https://doi.org/10.1016/S0140-6736(08)61620-7
2. Multiple sclerosis [Internet]. https://www.who.int/news-room/fact-sheets/detail/multiple-sclerosis. Accessed 23 Jan 2024
3. Goura, K., Harsoor, A.: A systematic review on multiple sclerosis. In: Kumar, A., Ghinea, G., Merugu, S. (eds.) ICCIC 2022, pp. 685–90. Springer, Singapore (2023). (Cognitive Science and Technology). https://doi.org/10.1007/978-981-99-2746-3_67
4. Walton, C., et al.: Rising prevalence of multiple sclerosis worldwide: insights from the Atlas of MS, third edition. Mult Scler Houndmills Basingstoke Engl. **26**(14), 1816–1821 (2020)
5. Rae-Grant, A., et al.: Comprehensive systematic review summary: disease-modifying therapies for adults with multiple sclerosis. Neurology **90**(17), 789–800 (2018)
6. Gitman, V., Moss, K., Hodgson, D.: A systematic review and meta-analysis of the effects of non-pharmacological interventions on quality of life in adults with multiple sclerosis. Eur. J. Med. Res. **28**(1), 294 (2023)
7. Khan, F., Amatya, B.: Rehabilitation in multiple sclerosis: a systematic review of systematic reviews. Arch. Phys. Med. Rehabil. **98**(2), 353–367 (2017)
8. Hobart, J., et al.: International consensus on quality standards for brain health-focused care in multiple sclerosis. Mult Scler Houndmills Basingstoke Engl. **25**(13), 1809–1818 (2019)
9. Nasjonal standard [Internet]. https://www.helse-bergen.no/nasjonal-kompetansetjeneste-for-multippel-sklerose-ms/nasjonal-standard. Accessed 23 Jan 2024

10. Multippel sklerose - nasjonal faglig retningslinje [Internet]. Helsebiblioteket. https://www.hel sebiblioteket.no/innhold/nasjonal-faglig-retningslinje/multippel-sklerose. Accessed 23 Jan 2024
11. Figl, K.: Comprehension of procedural visual business process models. Bus. Inf. Syst. Eng. **59**(1), 41–67 (2017)
12. Ruiz, F., et al.: Business process modeling in healthcare. Stud. Health Technol. Inform. **179**, 75–87 (2012)
13. Halvorsrud, R., Sanchez, O.R., Boletsis, C., Skjuve, M.: Involving users in the development of a modeling language for customer journeys. Softw. Syst. Model. **22**(5), 1589–1618 (2023)
14. Halvorsrud, R., Lillegaard, A.L., Røhne, M., Jensen, A.M.: Managing complex patient journeys in healthcare. In: Pfannstiel, M.A., Rasche, C. (eds.) Service Design and Service Thinking in Healthcare and Hospital Management. Springer, Cham (2019). https://doi.org/10.1007/978-3-030-00749-2_19
15. European Observatory on Health Systems and Policies (2022), Norway: Health System Summary. WHO Regional Office for Europe on behalf of the European Observatory on Health Systems and Policies, Copenhagen. ISBN 9789289059053 [Internet]. https://iris.who.int/bit stream/handle/10665/356963/9789289059053-eng.pdf?sequence=3. Accessed 23 Jan 2024
16. WMA - The World Medical Association-WMA Declaration of Helsinki – Ethical Principles for Medical Research Involving Human Subjects [Internet]. https://www.wma.net/pol icies-post/wma-declaration-of-helsinki-ethical-principles-for-medical-research-involving-human-subjects/. Accessed 23 Jan 2024
17. General Data Protection Regulation (GDPR) – Official Legal Text [Internet]. General Data Protection Regulation (GDPR). https://gdpr-info.eu/. Accessed 7 Feb 2024
18. Bottleneck Analysis Explained - Steps, Benefits & Tools – Workfellow [Internet]. https://www.workfellow.ai/learn/bottleneck-analysis-simply-explained. Accessed 23 Jan 2024
19. Seys, D., et al.: Care pathways are complex interventions in complex systems: New European Pathway Association framework. Int. J. Care Coord. **22**(1), 5–9 (2019)
20. Gartner, J.B., Abasse, K.S., Bergeron, F., Landa, P., Lemaire, C., Côté, A.: Definition and conceptualization of the patient-centered care pathway, a proposed integrative framework for consensus: a concept analysis and systematic review. BMC Health Serv. Res. **22**(1), 558 (2022)
21. Flemmen, H.Ø., Simonsen, C.S., Broch, L., Brunborg, C., Berg-Hansen, P., Moen, S.M., et al.: The influence of socioeconomic factors on access to disease modifying treatment in a Norwegian multiple sclerosis cohort. Mult Scler Relat Disord. **61**, 103759 (2022)
22. Holmøy, T., Nygaard, G.O., Myhr, K.M., Bø, L.: Disease-modifying therapy for multiple sclerosis. Tidsskr Den Nor Legeforening [Internet]. 2021 May 10. https://tidsskriftet.no/en/2021/05/kronikk/disease-modifying-therapy-multiple-sclerosis. Accessed 23 Jan 2024
23. Guizani, K., Ghannouchi, S.A.: An approach for selecting a business process modeling language that best meets the requirements of a modeler. Procedia Comput Sci. **1**(181), 843–851 (2021)
24. Ardito, C., Caivano, D., Colizzi, L., Dimauro, G., Verardi, L.: Design and execution of integrated clinical pathway: a simplified meta-model and associated methodology. Inf Switz [Internet] **11**(7) (2020). https://www.scopus.com/inward/record.uri?eid=2-s2.0-850 89949950&doi=10.3390%2finfo11070362&partnerID=40&md5=bede563f9ce5d1dd1d1e1 7a240502a26
25. Bowles, J., Caminati, M.B., Cha, S.: An integrated framework for verifying multiple care pathways, pp. 1–8 (2018). https://www.scopus.com/inward/record.uri?eid=2-s2.0-850506 87720&doi=10.1109%2fTASE.2017.8285628&partnerID=40&md5=9a4ff774e32826b263 1a346da46b6faa
26. Shah, B., Allen, J.L.Y., Chaudhury, H., O'Shaughnessy, J., Tyrrell, C.S.B.: The role of digital health in the future of integrated care. Clin Integr Care. **1**(15), 100131 (2022)

27. Moody, D.: The, "Physics" of notations: toward a scientific basis for constructing visual notations in software engineering. IEEE Trans. Softw. Eng. **35**(6), 756–779 (2009)
28. Farshidi, S., Kwantes, I.B., Jansen, S.: Business process modeling language selection for research modelers. Softw Syst Model [Internet]. 2023 May 29. https://doi.org/10.1007/s10 270-023-01110-8. Accessed 31 Oct 2023
29. Zarour, K., Benmerzoug, D., Guermouche, N., Drira, K.: A systematic literature review on BPMN extensions. Bus. Process. Manag. J. **26**(6), 1473–1503 (2019)
30. Halvorsrud, R., Haugstveit, I.M., Pultier, A.: Evaluation of a modelling language for customer journeys. In: 2016 IEEE Symposium Visual Lang Human-Centric Computing VLHCC, 40–8 (2016)

The Viewpoint of Informal Carers of People with Multiple Sclerosis in Digital Health Research: A Scoping Review

Tiia Yrttiaho[1][(✉)] , Vasiliki Mylonopoulou[2] , Guido Giunti[1] ,
and Minna Isomursu[1,3]

[1] Faculty of Medicine, University of Oulu, Oulu, Finland
tiia.yrttiaho@oulu.fi
[2] Applied IT, University of Gothenburg, Gothenburg, Sweden
[3] Faculty of Information Technology and Electrical Engineering, University of Oulu, Oulu, Finland

Abstract. Multiple sclerosis (MS) is a common neurological disease that can impact not only individuals diagnosed with the condition but also their informal carers, i.e. family members and friends. This scoping review aimed to map the role that family members and friends of people with multiple sclerosis have had in digital health research. The scoping review was reported according to PRISMA-ScR. The search was done in Scopus, CINAHL, Pubmed, and Web of Science. A total of 14 studies met the inclusion criteria. These studies were about telemedicine, rehabilitative video games, online education, user research, and development. Usually, family members and friends had a side part in the research. One study focused exclusively on them, and in total, in eight studies family and friends were participants in the study. Otherwise, they were accompanying the person with multiple sclerosis, were seen as possible users of the digital solution or they appeared in results by someone else. In this scoping review, it was seen that informal carers can get support and information from digital sources, they are able to act as informal carers in digital environments, healthcare professionals can receive information from them and family and friends can help in remote assessments, and digital solutions can help informal carers and people with MS to connect in a new or better way. Our results highlight that digital health can bring benefits to family members, people with multiple sclerosis, and healthcare.

Keywords: Digital Health · Digital rehabilitation · Informal carers · Multiple sclerosis · Patient Education · Telehealth · Telemedicine · Telerehabilitation

1 Introduction

There are more than 1,8 million people with multiple sclerosis (pwMS) in the world. Multiple sclerosis (MS) is usually diagnosed in young adulthood, and it is more common in women. It can cause various symptoms that can be disabling [1]. Informal carers, including family and friends (F&F) provide care for their loved ones with long-term

M. Särestöniemi et al. (Eds.): NCDHWS 2024, CCIS 2083, pp. 318–330, 2024.
https://doi.org/10.1007/978-3-031-59080-1_23

conditions. Informal care is care that is provided by non-professionals. Some of the informal carers get financial compensation for their effort. Among older people informal carers are often the only ones that provide care [2]. About half of the pwMS receive informal care from their F&F [3, 4], on average 10,5 h per week [4]. People with a severe form of MS need most help from F&F, as much as 8 h a day throughout the day. The amount of support pwMS receive from formal care affects how much they need help from their F&F [3].

MS also causes costs for informal carers as a form of absenteeism, presenteeism, early retirement, and productivity loss in volunteer work. In the United States alone this is estimated to cost 4 182 million dollars annually [5]. Informal carers are less likely to work full-time [6] and they have lower socioeconomic status [7]. Informal caregiving can lead to the society receiving less taxes and the informal carers earning smaller pensions [6]. Informal carers of pwMS may also experience carer burden, anxiety, depression, poor quality of life, and poor sleep [8].

Family members and loved ones of a person with a long-term condition do not always see themselves as carers and are concerned that labeling themselves as carers could lead to more responsibilities. People receiving care also might have difficulties accepting their need for support, which is also a reason for avoiding being called a carer. Without a carer identity, people do not necessarily feel that getting support is for them. They might also avoid recognizing how the disease affects them. Sometimes informal carers need outsiders, like healthcare professionals (HCP), to validate them as carers and encourage them to accept support. Responsibilities also can limit carers' opportunities to look for support for themselves [9].

Digital health is a broad umbrella term that covers the use of digital technologies to improve health [10]. Digital health includes for example telehealth, big data, artificial intelligence, and mobile health devices [11]. Through the application of digital health technologies, for example to consumers, there is a possibility to strengthen the health system [10]. Digital health solutions enable sustainable health systems, but to reach this they must respond to health needs [11]. Digital solutions could provide opportunities for family and friends to participate or ease their burden. Digitalization can bring healthcare to home and the daily life of pwMS that they share with their family and friends.

To our knowledge, any kind of review of the role of informal carers of pwMS in digital health research has not been made before. This scoping review was made to map the research that has been done on this topic. Results can guide future research and be used to create more appropriate digital health solutions.

2 Methods

This scoping review was conducted to systematically map the research and to identify possible gaps in knowledge in the literature about the role of informal carers of pwMS in digital health research. This report was written according to the Preferred Reporting Items for Systematics Reviews and Meta-Analyses: Extension for Scoping Reviews (PRISMA-ScR) [12]. This research aimed to explore and summarize how this concept has been studied over time and secondarily to identify knowledge gaps, which makes scoping review a suitable method [13].

Research questions:

1. What roles informal carers of pwMS have had in digital health research?
2. What was the digital health aspect of the included studies?
3. What results do the included studies report related to informal carers of pwMS in digital health?

Inclusion criteria for this scoping review were: the research explored aspects about family or friends of pwMS, is about digital health, is original research, research is peer-reviewed and the full text is in English. Exclusion criteria were: no family or friends of pwMS, not about digital health, or the article was protocol, editorial, comment, or review.

The search was done in four databases: Pubmed, Web of Science, Scopus, and CINAHL in November 2022. No time limit or other limitations were set. Search words used in databases are presented in Table 1. Words in each search word group were combined with the Boolean operator "OR" and groups were attached with the Boolean operator "AND".

Table 1. Words used in the search

Search word 1	Search word 2	Search word 3
digital*	"multiple sclerosis"	informal
ehealth	"ms-disease"	famil*
"e-health"		spous*
mhealth		partner*
"mobile health"		couple*
telemedicine		child*
telemedicine		parent*
telerehabilitation		friend*
"health informatics"		relative*
		caregiv*

One researcher (TY) executed the title, abstract, and full-text screening based on the inclusion and exclusion criteria. The identification of included studies is represented in Fig. 1. Included full texts were then discussed by two researchers (TY, VM). Two researchers (TY, VM) independently read the included articles, wrote information about the included studies to the Google Sheets file, and then discussed the findings and synthesized the results.

3 Results

The search in the databases resulted in a total of 723 results. Search results were uploaded to Covidence [14]. Covidence identified 189 duplicates, which were removed. A total of 534 search results ended in title and abstract screening. 45 of them continued to full-text screening, but one full-text was not available. A total of 14 articles were included in this review. The study identification process is described in Fig. 1.

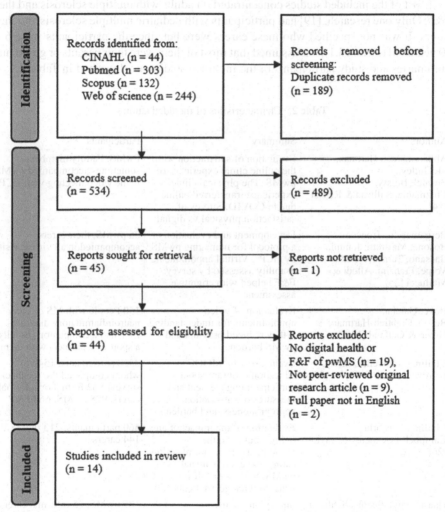

Fig. 1. Preferred Reporting Items for Systematics Reviews and Meta-Analyses Flow diagram of identification of studies

3.1   Characteristics of Included Studies

One article was published in 2014 [15], two in 2016 [16, 17], one in 2018 [18], three in 2020 [19–21], four in 2021 [22–25] and three in 2022 [26–28]. Six of the included studies were conducted in the United States [18–21, 24, 27], two in Australia with international participants (the educational intervention was in English) [23, 26], two in Italy [25, 28], one in Spain [16], one in Germany [22], one in Belgium [15] and one in the United Kingdom [17].

Most of the included studies concentrated on adults with multiple sclerosis and their F&F. Only one research, [19] had participants with pediatric multiple sclerosis and their carers. It was not specified who these carers were but since the participants were 6 to 20 years old (mean 13.1), it is assumed that most of them were their parents or guardians. Summaries and study participants of the included studies are described in Table 2.

Table 2.   Characteristics of included studies

Authors	Summary	Participants
Abbatemarco., Hartman, McGinley, Bermel, Boissy, Chizmadia, Sullivan & Rensel [24]	Evaluation of satisfaction with the online clinic experience of pwMS. The physical clinic experience transferred online due to COVID. Survey of satisfaction physical vs digital	PwMS. Family members sometimes accompanied pwMS in the video meeting with HCP[a]
Bergamaschi, Tronconi, Bosone, Mastretti, Jommi, Bassano, Turrini, Benati, Volpe, Franzini, Allodi & Mallucci [25]	Development and evaluation of a protocol for managing pwMS by HCP[a]. Virtual appointment, usability assessed by survey. F&F helped with cognitive assessment	25 pwMS, their carers accompanied in all virtual visits
Bove, Garcha, Bevan, Crabtree-Hartman, Green & Gelfand [18]	Evaluation of video appointments for understanding if they reduced provider and pwMS burden	150 People with MS or other neuroinflammatory disorders. 27% had a companion (usually a spouse or partner) with them
Claflin, Campbell, Doherty, Farrow, Bessing & Taylor [23]	Evaluation of a MOOC[b] education program about participant engagement and measures of satisfaction, appropriateness, and burden	3518 participants, 1549 of whom completed the feedback survey: 862 formal or informal carers, 928 pwMS, 664 F&F
Claflin, Mainsbridge, Campbell, Klekociuk & Taylor [26]	Evaluation of the impact of an online course on the participants' behavior regarding eating and exercising habits of pwMS. Survey of self-reported behavior change after education	560 participants: 213 pwMS, 144 carers
Haase, Voigt, Scholz, Schlieter, Benedict, Susky, Dillenseger & Ziemssen [22]	Survey on the use of information technology, barriers, needs, requirements, and adopting technology solutions for MS	185 pwMS, 25 informal carers, 24 Healthcare professionals

(*continued*)

Table 2. (*continued*)

Authors	Summary	Participants
Halstead, Leavitt, Fiore & Mueser [21]	A feasibility study of an online resilience education program for pwMS and their family	62 participants, 31 dyads: 28 pwMS and partners, 3 parent-child dyads
Harder, Hernandez, Hague, Neumann, McCreary, Cullum & Greenberg [19]	Comparison between the home-based pediatric videoconference and in-person neuropsychology assessment. Evaluation of user satisfaction and validity	95 participants, ages 9–20 years, and their carers. 24% have MS or clinically isolated syndrome
Octavia & Coninx [15]	Evaluation of the impact of adaptive, personalized, collaborative games for rehabilitation	9 pwMS and therapist. A game was designed to play with for example family members, but it was not studied with family members
Palacios-Ceña, Ortiz-Gutiérrez, Buesa-Estellez, Galán-Del-Río, Cachón-Pérez, Martínez-Piedrola, Velarde-García & Cano-De-La-Cuerda [16]	Exploring the experience of pwMS on the virtual home exercise program and its impact. Video games were used as a rehabilitation tool	24pwMS received treatment using Kinect, control group (25pwMS) received physiotherapy twice a week. Family and friends had joined Kinect games with pwMS
Roth, Minden, Maloni, Miles & Wallin [27]	Interviewing participants to understand their perspectives about telemedicine for provision of MS care	20pwMS, 15 HCP[a], 15 payers and policy experts (from health insurance companies)
Schleimer, Pearce, Barnecut, Rowles, Lizee, Klein, Block, Santaniello, Renschen, Gomez, Keshavan, Gelfand, Henry, Hauser & Bove [20]	Expanding the design of a medical digital platform to have an interface for pwMS, where they can monitor and understand their health condition to make meaningful decisions. Designing and testing the solution	Phase I: 6 clinicians, 12 pwMS (with family, friend, carer), industry and advocacy experts. Phase II: 10 pwMS, MS support group. Phase III: MS support group, 15 pwMS advocacy group for feedback & 24 pwMS for testing
Sillence, Hardy, Briggs & Harris [17]	Study of F&F impressions and needs of online support and information forums	20 F&F of pwMS. In all but one case pwMS was their spouse
Toscano, Patti, Grazia Chisari, Arena, Finocchiaro, Schillaci & Zappia [28]	Evaluation of reliability and satisfaction of televisits	76 pwMS, 23 F&F

[a] HCP: healthcare professional, [b] MOOC: Massive open online course

3.2   Role of Family and Friends of PwMS in Included Studies

Role of family members and friends varied greatly in the included studies. One of the 14 included studies had their main focus solely on the F&F of pwMS [17] and two had them in a significant role [19, 21]. Harder et al. were the only ones studying pediatric pwMS and their informal carers. In their study carers made the necessary arrangements but they were not allowed to be in the room with the child patient during testing. Informal carers also filled out the satisfaction survey [19]. Figure 2 represents how centric roles informal carers had in different studies.

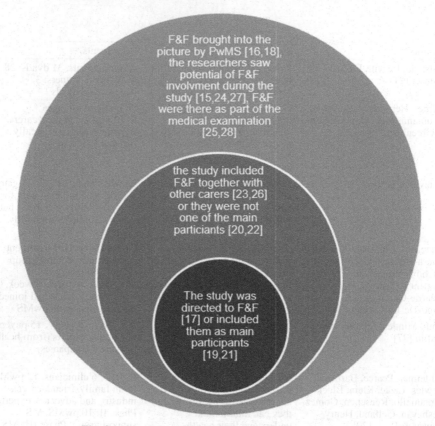

Fig. 2. The role of informal carers in the included studies

In two studies F&F had been mentioned as possible users in the methods section but they were not part of the study, and they were not separately discussed in the results [15, 20]. In one study, it was planned that family members would be using the solution with pwMS, but they ended up testing it with HCP only [15] and in one study it was recognized that the user could finally be the patient's informal carer [20]. Some studies had not written about F&F participating in their methods, but F&F had appeared in the study [16, 18, 27]. In Claflin et al. [23, 26] studies, they did not define any group specifically as participants. They invited all people who had registered for their multiple sclerosis course or completed it. Table 3. Represents in what part of the research article informal carers were mentioned.

Table 3. Informal carers in included studies

	Yes	No
F&F were mentioned in the methods section of the research	7 studies [15, 17, 20–25, 28]	6 studies [16, 18, 19, 26, 27]
F&F were participants in the study	8 studies [17, 19, 21–23, 26, 28]	6 studies [15, 16, 18, 20, 24, 25, 27]
F&F accompanied pwMS during the research	8 studies [16, 18, 20, 21, 24, 25, 27, 28]	6studies [15, 17, 19, 22, 23, 26]
F&F appeared in the results or discussion section of the research	11 studies [16–19, 21–28]	2 studies [15, 20]

3.3 The Digital Health Aspect of the Included Studies

Telemedicine. Six out of 14 included studies were about telemedicine, meaning they arranged video appointments instead or in addition to in-person appointments at the clinic [18, 19, 24, 25, 27, 28]. Video appointment was organized with Zoom [18], VSee [19], Express Care Online telemedicine platform [24], or Skype [25, 28]. In one study software that was used in telemedicine was not mentioned [27]. Telemedicine made it possible for F&F to attend appointments from a third location [18, 27] and in some cases, pwMS did not need to leave the workplace to attend the appointment[18]. F&F often accompanied their cared ones with multiple sclerosis during their video appointment [18, 24, 25, 27, 28]. F&F also helped in arrangements or health assessments [19, 25, 28].

Online Education Course. Three of the included studies were about online education targeted to increase awareness or knowledge about MS [21, 23, 26]. In Claflin et al. studies [23, 26] they arranged it by Massive open online course (MOOC). Halstead et al. [21] had a web-based portal called MS hub, that was developed for their study. It was used for resilience intervention for pwMS and their partners.

Telerehabilitation with Video Games. In the included studies, there were two that studied telerehabilitation, in these cases digital rehabilitative games. Neither of them had F&F as participants in their study [15, 16]. Octavia et al. [15] had created a rehabilitative game that pwMS could play together with their family members but tested it in their research with HCP. They used individualized technology-supported and robot-assisted virtual learning environments (I-TRAVALE) and MOOG HapticMaster, a haptic robot, while the healthy co-player uses a WiiMote. They had developed games for individual and collaborative use. They thought that collaborative rehabilitation would have a positive effect on pwMS motivation, and it could provide social support, sympathy, and empathy [15]. Palacios-Ceña et al. [16] used for rehabilitative purposes pre-existing games for Xbox360 with Microsoft Kinect that were monitored with videoconference. They used the Kinect Virtual Home-Exercise Programme and the games they used were Kinect Joy Ride, Kinect Adventures, and Kinect Sports. During testing, F&F had joined a game with their loved one with MS [16].

User research and Software Development. In Sillence et al. [17] study F&F selected and used websites of their interest from a list. Websites contained information and experiences of MS and carers. Haase et al. [22] studied the use of information technology, barriers, needs, and requirements for eHealth solutions for a user-centered development process for a care portal for MS. Schleimer et al. [20] developed and studied the development of an app version of a data infrastructure platform called MS BioScreen that gathers data from various sources and visualizes the disease course.

3.4 Family- and Friend-Related Results of Included Studies

Two of the included studies did report F&F-related results [15, 20]. In one article family and friends' answers were combined with pwMS answers [22] and in two articles participants without MS were divided into two groups based on whether they identified themselves as carers. Informal and formal carers were combined in one group and another group was people who did not identify as carers [23, 26]. These results were not included in this section as F&F-related results could not be specified. Nine of the included articles reported F&F-related results.

Support and Information from Digital Sources. Especially those F&F whose loved ones had been recently diagnosed with MS wanted to find information about the condition. Those who had lived with the condition for a longer time were also interested in carers' experiences, especially in ideas on how to tackle everyday problems. People share their difficult experiences online more openly than in face-to-face support groups, but not all want to be reminded of difficulties [17].

Family Members and Friends as Carers. Some pwMS rely on their carer being with them in the appointment taking notes and asking questions. Telemedicine can make it easier for F&F to attend [27]. Telemedicine can also reduce carer burden as F&F can avoid taking time off from work [18]. F&F did not always see themselves as carers. Instead, some considered that they were going through things together with pwMS [17]. It can also happen that the person who usually drives pwMS to appointments does not attend remote appointments [27]. In Bove [18] et al. study, they also found that F&F attended not so often remote appointments than in-person appointments at the clinic. In Harder et al. [19] pediatric patients' carers arranged the remote appointments and 94% of them were satisfied with the videoconference health testing session and most of them considered it as acceptable as in-person health testing. 21% would rather choose an in-person assessment and 16% would rather use videoconference [19].

Family Members and Friends as a Source of Information for Healthcare Professionals. Telemedicine gives HCPs the possibility to meet informal carers of pwMS who maybe would not come to in-person appointments. This provides HCPs an opportunity to see who at home provides support for pwMS [27]. Meeting with the members of the household sometimes gave a different perspective of pwMS needs and status [24]. Toscano et al. [28] compared remote and in-person appointments' inter-rater agreement and in most health tests, it was better when informal carers accompanied patients. In visual assessment, carers made it possible to do the assessment properly. In

Bergamaschi et al. [25] research F&F's presence was considered important, especially in remote cognitive assessment.

Connecting People. Playing the Xbox Kinect game gave pwMS a new type of opportunity to connect with their family members as it was something that they could do together even though pwMS had limitations with their mobility. Instead of suffering treatments, pwMS were able to have fun with F&F by playing with them with Kinect [16]. Online education intervention was found to increase family members' satisfaction with their relationship with pwMS and improve their communication [21].

4 Discussion

In this scoping review, we identified 14 studies that had some information about family members and friends of pwMS in digital health research. Even though there was no time limit, the oldest research was from the year 2014 [15]. Most of the included articles, 10 out of 14 were from this decade, from the years 2020–2022 [19–28]. Only one of the 14 included studies had their main focus on the informal carers of pwMS [17] and two had them as one of the main participants [19, 21]. In Harder et al. [19] study patients were children and the research could not have happened without their guardians. All the other studies had adult participants.

Digital health aspects of the research were telemedicine, online education, telerehabilitation with video games, user research, and development. Telemedicine was the most common type of digital health, and it was examined in six out of 14 included studies. In most of these F&F were accompanying pwMS during their remote appointment with HCP [18, 24, 25, 27, 28]. In one study F&F arranged a remote appointment for a child but were not in the same room during the appointment [19].

11 out of 14 included studies had outcomes related to F&F [16–19, 21–23, 25–28]. Overall, in the included studies, there were not many outcomes considering F&F, but the results related to F&F were positive toward digital health. In this scoping review was seen that F&F can get support and information from digital sources, they are able to act as a carer in digital environments, HCP can receive information from them, and with their help and digital solutions can help F&F and pwMS to connect in a new or better way. In some studies, results related to F&F were reported by an HCP [24, 25, 27] or pwMS [16, 18, 27]. In one of the included studies, one reason for adding mental health services to telemedicine was that HCPs had noticed an increase in domestic violence during the COVID-19 epidemic [24]. It is good to keep in mind that families can also have interactions that can have a negative impact.

52 million people take care of their loved ones with disabilities in the EU weekly. In addition to taking their time and causing a financial burden, it affects their mental health [6]. Digital health has the potential to ease carers' burden. For example, transportation is one of the most common things F&F helps pwMS with [8]. One of the benefits of telemedicine is that pwMS and F&F can avoid traveling to a clinic that can be far away. Sometimes pwMS could travel by themselves but they need their F&F to accompany them at the appointment and for example to ask necessary questions [27]. In earlier studies, web-based interventions have decreased the stress, anxiety, and depression of informal carers [29, 30].

There were possible limitations in this study. Due to the resources, only one researcher did the screening, it would have been more reliable if it had been made independently by two researchers. It is a limitation that studies were only sought and included studies reported in English. Most of the included studies were from English-speaking countries and it might be explained by language limitation. Also, two articles were excluded in the full-text stage because they were not in English.

Currently, there is a limited body of evidence addressing the F&F of pwMS in digital health research. F&F may be often overlooked when designing digital health and its research. As populations in numerous countries age and health challenges become more prevalent, healthcare resources are becoming increasingly scarce. The rise of informal caregiving is anticipated across various health conditions, including multiple sclerosis. There is significant potential for digital health to aid informal carers in effectively caring for both their loved ones and themselves, thereby saving time and resources for everyone involved. This research shows that there is a lack of research on the inclusion of F&F of pwMS in digital health. Further research is imperative to fully understand and harness the benefits of digital health.

Disclosure of Interests. The authors have no competing interests to declare that are relevant to the content of this article.

References

1. World Health Organization: Multiple sclerosis (2023). https://www.who.int/news-room/fact-sheets/detail/multiple-sclerosis. Accessed 13 Dec 2023
2. Rocard, E., Llena-Nozal, A.: OECD Health Working Papers No. 140. Supporting informal carers of older people: Policies to leave no carer behind (2022). https://doi.org/10.1787/0f0c0d52-en
3. Kobelt, G., Thompson, A., Berg, J., Gannedahl, M., Eriksson, J.: New insights into the burden and costs of multiple sclerosis in Europe. Mult. Scler. **23**, 1123–1136 (2017). https://doi.org/10.1177/1352458517694432
4. Ruutiainen, J., Viita, A.M., Hahl, J., Sundell, J., Nissinen, H.: Burden of illness in multiple sclerosis (DEFENSE) study: the costs and quality-of-life of Finnish patients with multiple sclerosis. J. Med. Econ. **19**, 21–33 (2016). https://doi.org/10.3111/13696998.2015.1086362
5. Bebo, B., et al.: The economic burden of multiple sclerosis in the United States: estimate of direct and indirect costs. Neurology **98**, E1810–E1817 (2022). https://doi.org/10.1212/WNL.0000000000200150
6. European Commission, D.-G. for E.S.A. and I.: Study on exploring the incidence and costs of informal long-term care in the EU (2021)
7. Quashie, N.T., Wagner, M., Verbakel, E., Deindl, C.: Socioeconomic differences in informal caregiving in Europe. Eur. J. Ageing **19**, 621–632 (2022). https://doi.org/10.1007/s10433-021-00666-y
8. Rajachandrakumar, R., Finlayson, M.: Multiple sclerosis caregiving: a systematic scoping review to map current state of knowledge (2022). https://doi.org/10.1111/hsc.13687
9. Knowles, S., Combs, R., Kirk, S., Griffiths, M., Patel, N., Sanders, C.: Hidden caring, hidden carers? Exploring the experience of carers for people with long-term conditions. Health Soc. Care Community **24**, 203–213 (2016). https://doi.org/10.1111/hsc.12207
10. World Health Organization: Global strategy on digital health 2020–2025 (2021)

11. World Health Organization: The ongoing journey to commitment and transformation Digital health in the WHO European Region 2023 (2023)
12. Tricco, A.C., et al.: PRISMA extension for scoping reviews (PRISMA-ScR): checklist and explanation. Ann. Intern. Med. **169**, 467–473 (2018). https://doi.org/10.7326/M18-0850
13. Peters, M.D.J., Godfrey, C.M., Khalil, H., McInerney, P., Parker, D., Soares, C.B.: Guidance for conducting systematic scoping reviews. Int. J. Evid. Based Healthc. **13**, 141–146 (2015). https://doi.org/10.1097/XEB.0000000000000050
14. Covidence: Covidence Systematic Review Tool (2023). https://www.covidence.org/. Accessed 13 Nov 2023
15. Octavia, J.R., Coninx, K.: Adaptive personalized training games for individual and collaborative rehabilitation of people with multiple sclerosis. Biomed. Res. Int. 2014 (2014). https://doi.org/10.1155/2014/345728
16. Palacios-Ceña, D., et al.: Multiple sclerosis patients' experiences in relation to the impact of the kinect virtual home-exercise programme: a qualitative study. Eur. J. Phys. Rehabil. Med. **52**, 347–355 (2016)
17. Sillence, E., Hardy, C., Briggs, P., Harris, P.R.: How do carers of people with multiple sclerosis engage with websites containing the personal experiences of other carers and patients? Health Informatics J. **22**, 1045–1054 (2016). https://doi.org/10.1177/1460458215607938
18. Bove, R., Garcha, P., Bevan, C.J., Crabtree-Hartman, E., Green, A.J., Gelfand, J.M.: Clinic to in-home telemedicine reduces barriers to care for patients with MS or other neuroimmunologic conditions. Neurol Neuroimmunol Neuroinflamm. **5** (2018). https://doi.org/10.1212/NXI.0000000000000505
19. Harder, L., et al.: Home-based pediatric teleneuropsychology: a validation study. Arch. Clin. Neuropsychol. **35**, 1266–1275 (2020). https://doi.org/10.1093/arclin/acaa070
20. Schleimer, E., et al.: A precision medicine tool for patients with multiple sclerosis (the open ms bioscreen): human-centered design and development. J. Med. Internet Res. **22** (2020). https://doi.org/10.2196/15605
21. Halstead, E.J., Leavitt, V.M., Fiore, D., Mueser, K.T.: A feasibility study of a manualized resilience-based telehealth program for persons with multiple sclerosis and their support partners. Mult Scler. J. Exp. Transl. Clin. **6** (2020). https://doi.org/10.1177/2055217320941250
22. Haase, R., et al.: Profiles of ehealth adoption in persons with multiple sclerosis and their caregivers. Brain Sci. **11** (2021). https://doi.org/10.3390/brainsci11081087
23. Claflin, S.B., Campbell, J.A., Doherty, K., Farrow, M., Bessing, B., Taylor, B.V.: Evaluating course completion, appropriateness, and burden in the understanding multiple sclerosis massive open online course: cohort study. J. Med. Internet Res. **23** (2021). https://doi.org/10.2196/21681
24. Abbatemarco, J.R., et al.: Providing person-centered care via telemedicine in the era of COVID-19 in multiple sclerosis. J. Patient Exp. 8, (2021). https://doi.org/10.1177/23743735209814 74
25. Bergamaschi, R., et al.: Description and preliminary experience with Virtual Visit Assessment (ViVA) during the COVID-19 pandemic, a structured virtual management protocol for patients with multiple sclerosis. Neurol. Sci. **43**, 1207–1214 (2022). https://doi.org/10.1007/s10072-021-05371-3
26. Claflin, S.B., Mainsbridge, C., Campbell, J., Klekociuk, S., Taylor, B.V.: Self-reported behaviour change among multiple sclerosis community members and interested laypeople following participation in a free online course about multiple sclerosis. Health Promot. J. Austr. **33**, 768–778 (2022). https://doi.org/10.1002/hpja.559
27. Roth, E.G., Minden, S.L., Maloni, H.W., Miles, Z.J., Wallin, M.T.: A qualitative, multiperspective inquiry of multiple sclerosis telemedicine in the United States. Int. J. MS Care. (2022). https://doi.org/10.7224/1537-2073.2021-117

28. Toscano, S., et al.: Reliability of televisits for patients with mild relapsing–remitting multiple sclerosis in the COVID-19 era. Neurol. Sci. **43**, 2253–2261 (2022). https://doi.org/10.1007/s10072-022-05868-5
29. Graven, L.J., Glueckauf, R.L., Regal, R.A., Merbitz, N.K., Lustria, M.L.A., James, B.A.: Telehealth interventions for family caregivers of persons with chronic health conditions: a systematic review of randomized controlled trials (2021). https://doi.org/10.1155/2021/3518050
30. Zhai, S., Chu, F., Tan, M., Chi, N.C., Ward, T., Yuwen, W.: Digital health interventions to support family caregivers: an updated systematic review (2023). https://doi.org/10.1177/20552076231171967

Intelligent Mental Workload Mobile Application in Personalized Digital Care Pathway for Lifestyle Chronic Disease

Pantea Keikhosrokiani[1,2]([✉]) [iD], Minna Isomursu[1,2] [iD], Olli Korhonen[1] [iD], and Tan Teik Sean[3]

[1] Faculty of Information Technology and Electrical Engineering, University of Oulu, Oulu, Finland
Pantea.keikhosrokiani@oulu.fi
[2] Faculty of Medicine, University of Oulu, Oulu, Finland
[3] School of Computer Sciences, Universiti Sains Malaysia, 11800 Gelugor, Penang, Malaysia

Abstract. In the new healthcare paradigm, personalized digital care pathway enables the provision of tailored information and empowers patients. In healthcare, it is crucial to attend to patients' physical and emotional requirements. Stress and heavy mental workload can be detrimental to managing chronic lifestyle disorders. However, a reliable, standardized, and widely used paradigm for incorporating mental workload into the digital care pathway for providing long-term personalized care is missing from the current care pathway. Therefore, this study aims to investigate the use of mental workload tools and mobile applications in personalized digital care pathways for managing lifestyle chronic diseases. The study was focused on determining and characterizing the variables that determine mental workload; and then, investigating the ways in which these variables might function as supplementary data sources to enhance the personalization of care pathway. Based on the proposed mental workload tool, data was collected from 304 employees in the manufacturing industry, software development department. An intelligent mobile application was developed to manage and classify mental workload. Ensemble learning algorithms were used for mental workload classification, among which Hard Voting Ensemble Model outperforms the other techniques with 0.97 accuracy. Based on the findings, the most variable factor of mental workload is psychological factors with a median of 3.25, suggesting that individual differences or specific psychological conditions can significantly affect mental workload. Regarding personalization for managing chronic diseases, the mental workload variables may be utilized to individually adjust digital treatments to the specific requirements of every patient in a person-centered care.

Keywords: mHealth · Mental workload · Digital care pathway · Machine learning · Lifestyle chronic disease

© The Author(s) 2024
M. Särestöniemi et al. (Eds.): NCDHWS 2024, CCIS 2083, pp. 331–349, 2024.
https://doi.org/10.1007/978-3-031-59080-1_24

1 Introduction

1.1 Background and the Aim of the Study

Healthcare is changing from a paternalistic healthcare model to a more proactive care, and finally predictive care. It this new paradigm, the patient is at the center of care, surrounded by various technological solutions that empower them, supporting awareness of factors influencing their health and well-being [1]. This change aligns with the World Health Organization's (WHO) digital health strategy (2021) [2], advocating for putting people at the center of care through the adaptation and utilization of digital health technologies. This patient-centered approach is also referred to as person-centered care (PCC), emphasizing the ongoing interaction in healthcare between the individual and their healthcare team, with support from digital health technologies [3].

Care pathways (also known as clinical pathways or care maps) are treatment plans describing all desired diagnostic and treatment steps to guide and ensure standardized and evidence-based healthcare [4]. By adapting and utilizing digital health technologies, there are opportunities to personalize care pathways more according to the individual patient's needs. The development of tools, such as a personalized healthcare pathway (PHP) [5], an eHealth care pathway that is tailored to the needs of patients with lifestyle chronic diseases [6] and a personalized digital care pathway (PDCP) tool that facilitates tailored information provision [7], are examples of how care pathways can be personalized through the adoption and utilization of digital health technologies.

There is some evidence suggesting that patients can be positive towards the use of different digital health technologies at all stages of their care pathway [8]. These technologies can offer support in personalizing care pathways by providing data to support individuals in adopting healthier lifestyles [6]. In addition, digital health can serve as an additional data source, complementing clinical data. Integrating digital narrative elements from patients into clinical data has shown promising results in conditions like epilepsy, where connecting the clinical perspective with the personal experience of patients has traditionally been challenging [9].

In healthcare, there is an increasing need to address both the mental and physical needs of individuals [10]. Especially in the case of chronic lifestyle diseases, the high mental workload and stress may impact on handling the condition. However, there is still a lack of a consistent, trustworthy, and broadly applicable framework for integrating mental workload into the care pathway for providing sustainable care [11, 12].

This study aims to explore how intelligent mental workload management mobile applications can be integrated to personalized digital care pathways for lifestyle chronic diseases. Specifically, our focus had two primary aspects: firstly, in identifying and establishing factors to assess mental workload, and secondly, exploring how these factors can serve as a complementary data source to contribute to personalization of care pathways. Our research question is: What are the factors related to mental workload, and in what ways can they support the personalization of care pathways?

The rest of the paper reviewed the connection between mental workload and personalization for digital care pathways related to lifestyle chronic diseases. Then the proposed method including the details for system design, multidimensional personalized tool, and the classification of mental workload are presented. Afterwards, the results and analysis section, which consists of multidimensional personalization tool, the effects of different factors on mental workload, mental workload classification using machine learning, and system implementation and interface are reported. Finally, the paper is wrapped up with discussion and conclusion.

1.2 Mental Workload Assessment and Lifestyle Chronic Diseases

The Belgian Health Interview Survey (BHIS) examined the relationship between a healthy lifestyle and mental health outcomes [13]. Assessing and predicting mental health aspects, including psychological distress, vitality, life satisfaction, self-perceived health, depressive and generalized anxiety disorders, and suicidal ideation have significant impacts on the management of lifestyle chronic diseases. Healthy lifestyle habits are positively associated with mental health and well-being [13–20].

High mental workload in employees may potentially affect the onset and management of lifestyle chronic diseases [21]. Chronic mental stress can lead to unhealthy behaviors like poor diet, physical inactivity, smoking, and alcohol use, which are risk factors for diseases like heart disease, diabetes, cancer, obesity, and hypertension [16, 21, 22]. Prolonged stress may also directly impact physiological processes, exacerbating these conditions. Moreover, mental workload can affect sleep patterns and recovery, further influencing the development and management of chronic diseases [22]. Employers should consider these factors in their workplace health strategies.

1.3 Personalization and Digital Care Pathways

Personalization is a key component in PCC, emphasizing the empowerment of individuals to acquire the knowledge, skills and confidence they need for managing and making informed decisions about their health. It promotes the concept of active individual in managing their health, surrounded by healthcare professionals who use digital health technologies to complement the individual's resources, fostering the creation and exchange of health-related knowledge between the individual and the healthcare professional [23]. The development of digital health technologies provides new opportunities to enhance individual awareness of factors influencing their health and wellbeing [1]. Various technologies such as sensors and wearables can continuously provide real-time data about the individual, contributing to personalization related decision-making in care [24].

Digital health technologies have the potential to serve as a data source for supporting the personalization of care pathways [6, 9]. This support can vary from technology-driven automated assistance to a more collaborative approach involving data-driven decision-making [25]. There is a growing interest in developing tools and solutions for personalized care pathways. A personalized digital care pathway (PDCP) was introduced by [7], serving as a digital tool offering healthcare professionals and patients an overview of a personal care pathway, displaying adequate and dosed information gradually as the care pathway progressed. The information tailored to the individual serves as the foundation for collaborative decision making in care, fostering a more person-centered approach throughout the care process. In [9] narrative medicine methodologies were integrated into clinical practices using a digital platform. Patient narratives collected digitally were integrated with the clinical data to personalize the care pathway for individual patients. Both healthcare professionals and patients could benefit from these data as digital interactions allowed patients to share important aspects of treatment plans, such as more personal and emotional experiences of their condition, which may be challenging to express in the traditional healthcare setting. Furthermore, a personalized eHealth care pathway specifically tailored for patients with lifestyle related chronic diseases, supporting patients in making psychological and lifestyle adjustments was introduced by [6]. This care pathway tool automatically detected increased risk profiles but also provided personalized support to help patients to actively adopt a healthy lifestyle with a focus on psychological and lifestyle-related assistance.

Integrating mental workload management into personalized digital care pathways can significantly enhance healthcare delivery by tailoring treatments to individual patient needs while also ensuring that healthcare providers operate efficiently and without extreme cognitive burden. By incorporating mental workload management, digital care pathways can provide decision support that is tailored not just to the patient's needs, but also to the specific context and capabilities of the healthcare provider. For instance, a system might offer more focused guidance to a patient under high workload conditions, thus ensuring that patient care and well-being are optimized [26–28].

2 Method

2.1 System Design and Modules

The proposed mobile application two-tier architecture diagram is illustrated in Fig. 1. The first layer is the presentation tier where it corresponds to the client-side of the mobile application built with React Native. It handles the user interface, user interactions, and rendering of the application on the mobile device. The second layer is a data tier which consists of the backend components that interact with data and external services. The proposed AI-Mental application utilizes Flask as the web framework hosting the machine learning model, Firebase as the database for storing and managing data, and integration with the ChatGPT API for incorporating conversational AI capabilities. The main users for this application are employees and employers in the manufacturing workplace. The main input of the mobile application is the mental workload assessment provided by the users, which is used to predict employee mental workload. The employee mental workload record, results of the mental workload assessment and classification will be displayed on the dashboard as the main output of the system.

AI-mental consists of four main modules including: (1) account management module, (2) assessment module for data collection, (3) ensemble learning module for data analytics, and (4) dashboard or visualization module. The account management module is responsible for registering new accounts, login, updating profiles, and managing employee accounts whereas assessment module main task is collecting mental workload data from the users. Ensemble learning module is designed to classify mental workload, generate advice and suggestions based on the use status. Dashboard module, as the main output of the system, displays user profile, visualizes the mental workload prediction results and advice, and generates a summary for the employers. AI-mental mobile application provides user interface for all modules, which allows user to understand and interact with the system.

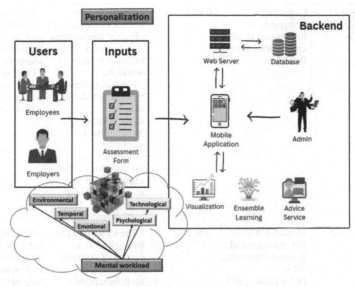

Fig. 1. Overall Architecture Diagram for Mental Workload Mobile Application.

2.2 Process to Design a Multidimensional Personalization Tool for Assessing Mental Workload

In order to classify mental workload, different types of data can be utilized. In this study, we have decided not to use the mental workload classification method based on physiological and performance-based techniques. The physiological technique, which requires specialized EEG measurement devices and experienced professionals to conduct the EEG test, is not preferred due to its high cost and complexity. Similarly, the performance-based technique is not ideal as it is not sufficiently sensitive to workload changes, and the measurement of secondary tasks may compromise the accuracy of the results. Therefore, this study will solely implement the subjective technique, specifically the self-assessment method.

This study aims to integrate mental workload related factors from patients into digital care pathways to provide personalized care specially for lifestyle chronic diseases. Therefore, a multidimensional personalization tool is designed in this study to improve mental well-being in digital care pathway. Furthermore, the study goal is to classify mental workload using machine learning techniques based on the data collected from multidimensional personalization tool or questionnaire. For this reason, the proposed questionnaire was distributed to individuals with employee roles. The existing self-assessment tools are compared in terms of dimensions, rating scale, strengths, and weaknesses as shown in Table 1.

Table 1. Comparison of Existing self-assessment tools.

Self-assessment Technique	Dimensions	Rating Scale	Strengths	Weaknesses
Carga Mental Questionnaire (CarMen-Q)	Cognitive, Temporal, Emotional, Health, and Performance Demands	0 to 3	- The technique does not include physical demands as it is not practical in measure mental workload - Identifies areas where individuals may be experiencing high levels of mental workload - Allows interventions to be implemented to reduce stress and improve performance	- Relies on self-report, which may be influenced by individual biases and perceptions - Does not measure all aspects of mental workload such as social demand
NASA task load index (NASA-TLX)	Mental demand, Physical demand, Temporal demand, Effort, Performance, and Frustration level	0 to 20	- The technique can be applied to a variety of domains due to its multidimensional and generic measurement property - It is relatively easy to administer and can be completed in a short amount of time	- Requires the participants to complete during their work which may not be feasible in certain situation such as high-stress environment - Result might be influenced by personal factor such as stress, fatigue, and motivation - Not be sensitive enough to capture small changes in workload over time, or to distinguish between different levels of workload within a single task
Subjective Workload Assessment Technique (SWAT)	Time Load, Mental Effort Load, and Psychological Stress Load	1 to 3	- Identifies potential areas for improvement or delegating tasks to better distribute workload - Provides a more personalized and accurate assessment of workload for individual employees	- Not very sensitive for low workload conditions - Requires a time-consuming pre-task card sorting procedure

Different existing tools or questionnaires were considered to propose the multidimensional personalization tool for this study. Some of the existing self-assessment techniques that used by the previous research papers including Depression Anxiety and Stress Scale 21 (DASS-21) [29], Carga Mental Questionnaire (CarMen-Q) [30], NASA Task Load Index (NASA-TLX) [31], Subjective Workload Assessment Technique (SWAT) [32], Cooper-Harper Rating Scale [33] and more. Among those questionnaires used for assessing mental workload, the most popular subjective techniques used are the Carga Mental Questionnaire (Carmen-Q), NASA Task Load Index (NASA-TLX), and Subjective Workload Assessment Technique (SWAT).

After the comparison of existing tools, the proposed multidimensional personalization tool was designed, and the dimensions were selected. The proposed tool was reviewed and verified by an expert in psychoanalysis from the School of Humanities. Then the questionnaire was used for data collection and the pilot study. 304 responses were received from the employees in the manufacturing industry, the software development unit, providing valuable data for the analysis and classification of mental workload levels.

2.3   The Process Flow of Mental Workload Classification

The main objective of ensemble module was the classification of mental workload using machine learning techniques based on the data collected from multidimensional personalization tool or questionnaire. Figure 2 illustrates the step-by-step process of training the machine learning model. First, several preprocessing techniques have been applied to the dataset to ensure its quality and suitability for analysis such as checking missing values, verifying the presence of any invalid responses for both inputs and output. Next, the inputs and outputs of the dataset were converted to integer format to facilitate their utilization in training machine learning models. The pre-processed dataset is then divided into 80% train data and 20% test data. Since the dataset contains imbalanced classes, the Synthetic Minority Oversampling Technique (SMOTE) was implemented for classification. It is important to note that SMOTE was applied only to the training data and not the test data to prevent overfitting. By applying SMOTE to the training data, the minority class instances are oversampled to balance the class distribution. This helps to mitigate the impact of class imbalance and ensures that the machine learning model is trained on a more representative dataset.

Furthermore, the machine learning models are trained and evaluated using various classification algorithms. The models selected for evaluation include K-Nearest Neighbors (KNN), Decision Tree, Support Vector Machine (SVM), Logistic Regression, and Naive Bayes. Each model is fitted to the training data using their respective algorithms. The evaluation results for each model are calculated, showcasing their precision, recall, F-1 score, and accuracy scores. Logistic regression model shows a relatively poor performance based on the evaluation results. After that, hyperparameter tuning using GridSearchCV is performed to optimize the models' performance by finding the hyperparameter settings that yield the highest accuracy or other evaluation metrics such as precision, recall, or F-1 score. This helps to fine-tune the models and improve their predictive capabilities on the given dataset. The best hyperparameters are shown in the figure below. The machine learning models are then trained and evaluated using the hyperparameters.

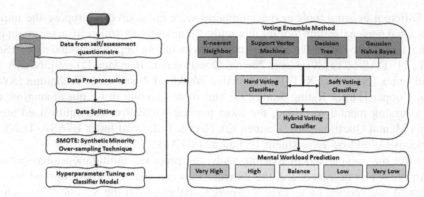

Fig. 2. Process Flow of the Proposed Mental Workload Classification Model using Ensemble Learning.

3   Results and Analysis

3.1   Multidimensional Personalization Tool

This study aims to design a personalized digital care pathway by integrating mental workload related factors for patients with lifestyle chronic diseases. Therefore, a multidimensional personalization tool is designed in this study (Fig. 3) to improve mental well-being in digital care pathway. The proposed multidimensional personalization tool illustrates various dimensions of overall mental workload, which is defined as the total cognitive burden placed on an individual at a given time, encompassing all cognitive processes required to perform tasks. Assessing overall mental workload involves considering both the demands imposed by the task and the individual's capacity to handle these demands, taking into account their skills, experience, and current psychological state.

Incorporating factors like Environmental, Psychological, Technical, Emotional, and Temporal into understanding and managing mental workload can significantly enhance the personalization of care pathways. A clinical understanding of the impact of physical and social environments on an individual's mental workload can lead to personalized interventions. This might include modifying lighting, noise levels, or even the arrangement of living or working spaces. Tailoring work of living environments to reduce unnecessary stressors or distractions. For example, providing a quiet and comfortable space for someone who is easily overstimulated by noise or crowding.

Recognizing personal psychological traits such as resilience, anxiety levels, or coping mechanisms can help predict how individuals handle mental workload. Developing stress management or resilience training programs tailored to the individual's psychological profile. For example, providing cognitive-behavioral therapy for someone prone to anxiety or stress. Identifying how comfortable and efficient individuals are with the technology and tools they use daily can influence their mental workload. Offering training or tools better suited to an individual's technical skills and preferences or redesigning workflows to reduce technical burdens. Considering the emotional states and variability in how individuals emotionally respond to stressors can inform care pathways. Integrating emotional support structures, counseling, or techniques like mindfulness and emotional regulation strategies tailored to how the individual experiences and processes emotions.

Recognizing the effects of time pressure, deadlines, and the pacing of activities on mental workload is crucial. Adjusting schedules, setting realistic deadlines, or creating time management plans that accommodate an individual's pace and workload capacity is useful for mental workload management. Continuously assessing mental workload allows for dynamic adjustments in care and support strategies, ensuring they match the individual's current needs. Implementing adaptive interventions that respond to real-time assessments of mental workload, perhaps using wearable tech or self-reporting tools for immediate feedback.

Combining insights from all factors of mental workload assists us to understand the multifaceted nature of an individual's experience, which involves creating a comprehensive profile that considers all dimensions. Regularly monitoring each factor's impact and adjusting the care pathway is needed to include routine assessments and the flexibility to change strategies as the individual's situation or responses evolve. Engaging the individual in understanding the mental workload factors and incorporating their preferences and feedback into the care pathway design is suggested to enhance the current digital care pathways. This ensures the solutions are not only personalized but also embraced by the individual. By considering these factors as parameters of personalization, care pathways can be more effectively tailored to each individual, enhancing the likelihood of successful outcomes, improving engagement, and reducing the overall mental workload. This holistic and nuanced approach ensures that interventions are not only technically sound but also resonate with the individual's unique circumstances, preferences, and needs.

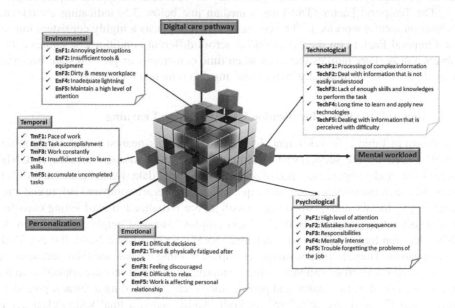

Fig. 3. Multidimensional Personalization Tool to Improve Mental Well-being in Lifestyle Chronic Diseases Digital Care Pathway.

3.2 The Effects of Different Factors on Mental Workload

Figure 4 shows the data distribution of the factors based on the collected data. For the Environmental Factors (EnF), the median is at 3.5, suggesting a moderate impact on mental workload. The narrow interquartile range (IQR) implies that the Environmental Factor's impact on mental workload is relatively consistent among the subjects or conditions tested. The absence of outliers indicates that extreme conditions of the environmental factor are either not present or do not significantly deviate from the typical impact on mental workload. However, the median for Psychological Factor (PsF) is slightly lower than EnF at 3.25, suggesting a slightly less overall impact on mental workload. The wide IQR, however, indicates that the impact of PsF on mental workload varies more significantly among individuals or situations than the Environmental Factor does. The presence of an outlier at a low value indicates that there may be certain psychological conditions or events that can extremely reduce mental workload.

With a median above 3.5, Technological Factor (TechF) might have a slightly higher impact on mental workload compared to Environmental and Psychological Factors. The moderate IQR suggests some variability in how different technological factors influence mental workload but less so than Psychological Factors. No outliers suggest that extreme technological factors are not significantly different in terms of their impact on mental workload. The median for Emotional Factor (EmF) is around 3.25, which is similar to the Psychological Factor, suggesting a comparable level of impact on mental workload. The IQR is not as wide as for PsF, which indicates that while Emotional Factors affect mental workload, the degree of this impact may be more predictable and less variable than Psychological Factors. The lack of outliers suggests that extreme emotional conditions do not commonly occur or do not significantly deviate from the typical impact range.

The Temporal Factor (TmF) has a median just below 3.5, indicating a moderate impact on mental workload. The very narrow IQR suggests a highly consistent impact of Temporal Factors on mental workload across different conditions or subjects. The absence of outliers implies that even when time constraints or pressures are irregular, they do not have an unusually high or low impact on mental workload.

3.3 Mental Workload Classification Using Machine Learning

As shown in Table 2, four different algorithms including k-nearest neighbors algorithm (k-NN), decision tree, support vector machine (SVM), and Gaussian Naive Bayes (GNB) are selected and compared in terms of performance. Since data was imbalanced, SMOTE was utilized as the oversampling technique and the results are compared before and after applying it. In this study, two voting classifiers are initialized: a hard voting classifier and a soft voting classifier. Both classifiers employ k-nearest neighbors algorithm (k-NN), decision tree, support vector machine (SVM), and Gaussian Naive Bayes (GNB) as estimators. They are trained on the resampled training dataset and their performance is evaluated using cross-validation. Subsequently, these classifiers are applied to make predictions on the test dataset, and performance metrics including accuracy, precision, recall, and F1 score are calculated for both. Additionally, a final voting classifier is created by combining the hard and soft voting classifiers. This final classifier is then used for predictions on the test dataset.

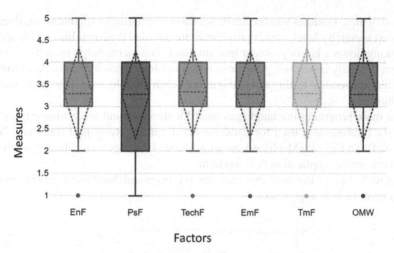

Fig. 4. Data Distribution for Mental Workload Variables.

Table 2. Performance Comparison of Different Machine Learning Techniques.

Machine Learning Model	Precision		Recall		F-1		Accuracy	
	Before	After	Before	After	Before	After	Before	After
KNN	0.86	0.96	0.80	0.87	0.87	0.93	0.87	0.93
Decision Tree	0.94	0.94	0.81	0.81	0.89	0.89	0.90	0.90
Support Vector Machine	0.94	0.97	0.87	0.82	0.92	0.91	0.92	0.91
Naive Bayes	0.90	0.90	0.80	0.80	0.84	0.87	0.89	0.89
Hard Voting Ensemble Model	0.93		0.92		0.91		0.97	
Soft Voting Ensemble Model	0.93		0.92		0.91		0.96	
Hybrid							0.92	

3.4 System Implementation and User Interface

Agile development methodology is selected for this study as it allows developers to deliver high-quality products faster, with greater flexibility and collaboration. It enables the developers to adapt quickly and to respond to new or changing features during development. Furthermore, it mainly concentrates on the deliverables and involves less planning than other traditional methodologies [15, 34, 35]. Therefore, it is suitable for AI-mental application due to the short timescale.

The proposed employee mental workload management application has adopted a top-down approach as its implementation strategy. This choice was made because the system was developed from scratch, requiring a generalized system model during the initial stages of design and implementation. To achieve this, the system was divided into four main modules: (1) Employee Management Module, (2) Assessment Module, (3) Ensemble Learning Model Analytics Module, and (4) Result Visualization Module.

Each of these modules was further broken down into smaller fragments until reaching the lowest hierarchy level, which provides more detailed functionalities. This approach of breaking down a larger problem into smaller components helps to reduce complexities that typically arise during the design and implementation phases. Additionally, it facilitates independent testing and debugging of each module since they can be evaluated individually.

The main programming languages used for development were Javascript, Python, and SQL. Firebase was used for database development. React.js (Front-end), Node.js (Back-end), and Flask (Machine Learning Model Hosting) were utilized as the main framework for the application development.

Figure 5 depicts the user interface for the proposed intelligent mental workload management mobile application.

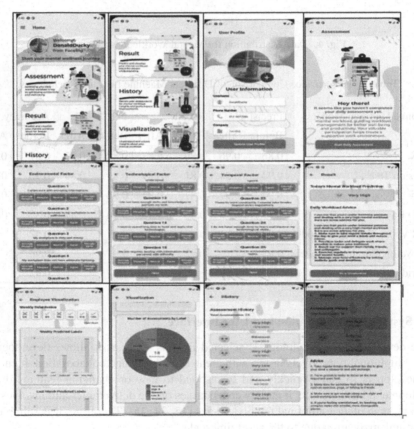

Fig. 5. User Interface for The Developed Personalized Mobile Application.

The login screen serves as the landing page. Users without an account can register via the Sign-Up Screen. After logging in, employees are directed to the Home Screen, which offers access to various screens through the navigation bar and users can update their profile. As for the assessment screen, users who haven't completed their daily assessment will see the screen. Those who have completed it will see another screen. The assessment consists of six screens, each with five questions. Assessment results will be shown in the Result Screen, and past results can be accessed on the History Screen and the history of mental workload assessment for the last week or month will be displayed in the history screen.

Furthermore, a visualization presenting assessment data in graphs and statistics will be depicted in the visualization screen. Employers are presented with a home screen and can manage employees using the Management Screen. This screen allows access to employee information, and the ability to delete or add employees. The Add New User Screen for adding new employees is part of the management screen. To monitor the mental workload of employees, employers use the Tracker Screen. They also have access to employee assessment results, visualizations, and assessment history. For an overview of employees' mental workload, the overall visualization screen will be displayed.

3.5 The Proposed Personalized Process for Lifestyle Chronic Disease Care Pathway

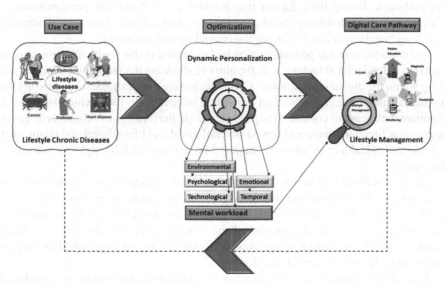

Fig. 6. The Proposed Iterative Process for Personalized Care Pathway for Lifestyle Chronic Disease.

Based on the results illustrated in Fig. 4, we can infer that while each factor has a moderate and consistent impact on mental workload, there are some differences. For instance, Psychological Factors show the most variability, indicating that individual differences or specific psychological conditions can significantly affect mental workload. Technological Factors show a slightly higher median impact, which could be due to the challenges of using new or complex technologies. Temporal Factors have the least variability, suggesting that time-related pressures are a consistent and predictable source of mental workload. Environmental and Emotional Factors appear to have a moderate and consistent impact on mental workload.

We propose that these mental workload related factors can serve as a complementary data source, enhancing the personalization of care pathways. They take into account various aspects of an individual's mental workload, emphasizing the importance of understanding the person as a whole. In Fig. 6 an iterative process for personalized care pathway for lifestyle chronic diseases is proposed. In the use case of lifestyle chronic diseases, the personalization process is dynamic, considering the factors that all contribute to an individual's lifestyle management within the care pathways, aiming to improve the mental well-being of an individual.

4 Discussion and Conclusion

This study investigated the factors related to mental workload, and the way they can support the personalization of care pathways specially for lifestyle chronic diseases. It proposes five factors: Environmental, Psychological, Technical, Emotional, and Temporal and examines how these factors can serve as parameters of personalization in care pathways. Taking these factors into account may enhance the personalization of care pathways for individuals, thereby increasing the likelihood of successful outcomes, improving engagement, and reducing the overall mental workload.

The multidimensional personalization tool presented in this study offers insights into mental workload related factors, with the aim of enhancing the individual's mental well-being within the digital care pathway. Given the growing importance of addressing both the mental and physical needs of an individual in healthcare [36], which is especially important in the case of chronic lifestyle diseases [6] the findings of this study align with the previous literature that considers on psychological and lifestyle-related factors in the personalized eHealth care pathways, targeted for patients with lifestyle-related chronic diseases [6].

The results illustrated in Fig. 4 suggest that when considering interventions to manage mental workload, attention should be given to the variability within Psychological Factors, as this is where individual differences are the most noticeable. Technological Factors may need to be closely monitored and managed to prevent an increase in mental workload. Temporal Factors, while consistent, should not be overlooked as they still contribute to the overall mental workload.

Since the environmental factor has a consistent but moderate impact on mental workload, digital care pathways can be personalized by considering the patient's environment. For example, the interface and notifications can be tailored to be less intrusive if a patient is in a stressful environment.

The high variability and the presence of outliers in psychological factors suggest that mental workload is significantly influenced by personal psychological conditions. Personalization in this aspect could mean incorporating cognitive-behavioral strategies, stress management, and coping mechanisms into the digital care pathway. This can help in providing a more tailored approach to managing psychological stressors that affect chronic disease management.

With technology having a slightly higher median impact on mental workload, digital care pathways need to be intuitive and user-friendly. Personalization could involve adapting the technology to the user's proficiency, providing training modules, or simplifying the user interface to reduce cognitive load.

Emotional factors affect mental workload to a degree like psychological factors but with less variability. Digital care pathways can incorporate features that monitor mood and provide emotional support, such as through motivational messages or alerts to seek human support when needed.

Temporal factors show a consistent impact on mental workload, indicating the importance of time management in chronic disease care. Personalization could involve scheduling medication reminders, appointments, and activities at times when the patient is less likely to be stressed.

Finally, digital care pathways should aim to distribute the mental workload evenly, avoiding overwhelming the patient. This can be achieved by decreasing the information overload on patient or reducing the tasks at once and by providing a personalized schedule that considers the patient's daily routine and capacity.

In relation to personalization for chronic disease management, these factors can be used to tailor digital interventions to each patient's unique needs in a person-centered manner. For instance, the platform can have *adaptive content*. It could adjust the information complexity based on the user's current cognitive load and emotional state. Furthermore, *user-centered design* can be considered. Interfaces can be designed considering the user's technological proficiency to avoid additional stress or workload. *Behavioral tracking* is another feature that can be incorporated into the care pathway to track psychological and emotional status to adjust the care plan. *Context-aware notifications* and reminders could be sent considering the patient's environment and time constraints to avoid adding stress. Integrating *stress management tools* for relaxation and stress relief can manage emotional and psychological factors that contribute to mental workload. *Support systems* facilitate access to support groups or counseling through the digital pathway that can address emotional and psychological needs. Finally, personalizing digital care pathways in these ways can help in managing the overall burden on patients with chronic diseases, leading to better engagement, adherence, and potentially better health outcomes.

Moreover, based on the results of this paper, we suggest conceptualizing an iterative personalized digital care pathway for lifestyle chronic diseases, as illustrated in Fig. 7. The iterative personalized digital care pathway emphasizes a holistic approach to care. This involves addressing diagnosis and treatment aspects, but also incorporating patient education and lifestyle management. Mental workload related factors play an important role, particularly in the lifestyle management of individuals. This aligns with the research from [6] where personalized support was provided to patients to actively adopt healthier lifestyles. By incorporating data on mental workload assessment, we believe there is an opportunity to increase individuals' awareness of the factors that can influence their health and well-being [1]. Also, the adoption and integration of digital health technologies offers possibilities to empower the patient. When combined with other data sources and care collaboration with healthcare professionals, these aspects can enhance the personalization of care pathways for individuals.

If employees' mental workload is managed effectively, it can contribute to lifestyle behaviors and conditions that elevate the risk of chronic diseases. Therefore, workplace health promotion programs are vital in mitigating these risks and fostering a healthier, more productive workforce.

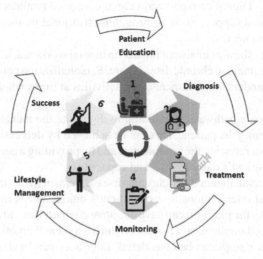

Fig. 7. Conceptualizing an Iterative Personalized Digital Care Pathway for Lifestyle Chronic Diseases.

Limitations. This study has some limitations. An expert in psychoanalysis reviewed and verified the suggested multidimensional personalization tool. However, integrating the tool with the clinical data was beyond the scope of this paper. Previous literature provides examples of incorporating data generated by digital health solutions into clinical data to personalize care pathways [9]. In this paper, we believe that the introduction of a multidimensional personalization tool and established factors for assessing mental workload can serve as a starting point for exploring the integration of this tool with clinical data in the future.

References

1. Sharma, D., Singh Aujla, G., Bajaj, R.: Evolution from ancient medication to human-centered Healthcare 4.0: a review on health care recommender systems. Int. J. Commun. Syst. **36**, e4058 (2023). https://doi.org/10.1002/dac.4058
2. Cancer. World Health Organization (WHO). https://www.who.int/health-topics/cancer#tab=tab_1. Accessed 11 Jan 2024
3. Morton, R.L., Sellars, M.: From patient-centered to person-centered care for kidney diseases. Clin. J. Am. Soc. Nephrol. **14**, 623–625 (2019)
4. Kinsman, L., Rotter, T., James, E., et al.: What is a clinical pathway? Development of a definition to inform the debate. BMC Med. **8**, 31 (2010). https://doi.org/10.1186/1741-7015-8-31
5. Fico, G., Fioravanti, A., Arredondo, M.T., et al.: Integration of personalized healthcare pathways in an ICT platform for diabetes managements: a small-scale exploratory study. IEEE J. Biomed. Health Inform. **20**, 29–38 (2016). https://doi.org/10.1109/JBHI.2014.2367863
6. Cardol, C.K., Tommel, J., van Middendorp, H., et al.: Detecting and treating psychosocial and lifestyle-related difficulties in chronic disease: development and treatment protocol of the E-GOAL eHealth care pathway. Int. J. Environ. Res. Public Health **18**, 3292 (2021). https://doi.org/10.3390/ijerph18063292
7. Heijsters, F., Santema, J., Mullender, M., et al.: Stakeholders barriers and facilitators for the implementation of a personalised digital care pathway: a qualitative study. BMJ Open **12**, e065778 (2022). https://doi.org/10.1136/bmjopen-2022-065778
8. Van der Ven, J., et al.: Preferences of patients with musculoskeletal disorders regarding the timing and channel of eHealth and factors influencing its use: mixed methods study. JMIR Hum. Factors **10**, e44885 (2023). https://doi.org/10.2196/44885
9. Cenci, C., Mecarelli, O.: Digital narrative medicine for the personalization of epilepsy care pathways. Epilepsy Behav. **111**, 107143 (2020). https://doi.org/10.1016/j.yebeh.2020.107143
10. Hudson, J.L., Moss-Morris, R.: Treating illness distress in chronic illness: integrating mental health approaches with illness self-management. Eur. Psychol. **24**, 26–37 (2019). https://doi.org/10.1027/1016-9040/a000352
11. Sather, E.W., Iversen, V.C., Svindseth, M.F., et al.: Exploring sustainable care pathways - a scoping review. BMC Health Serv. Res. **22**, 1595 (2022). https://doi.org/10.1186/s12913-022-08863-w
12. Longo, L., Wickens, C.D., Hancock, G., Hancock, P.A.: Human mental workload: a survey and a novel inclusive definition. Front. Psychol. **13**, 883321 (2022). https://doi.org/10.3389/fpsyg.2022.883321
13. Hautekiet, P., Saenen, N.D., Martens, D.S., et al.: A healthy lifestyle is positively associated with mental health and well-being and core markers in ageing. BMC Med. **20**, 328 (2022). https://doi.org/10.1186/s12916-022-02524-9
14. Hu, G., Qin, H., Su, B., et al.: Composite healthy lifestyle, socioeconomic deprivation, and mental well-being during the COVID-19 pandemic: a prospective analysis. Mol. Psychiatry (2023). https://doi.org/10.1038/s41380-023-02338-y
15. Mei, A.W.S., Keikhosrokiani, P., Isomursu, M.: LiveHeart: AI-augmented lifestyle habit monitoring system for decision making in digital care pathway. In: Kasurinen, J., Päivärinta, T. (eds.) CEUR Workshop Proceedings, Oulu, pp. 1–12 (2023)
16. Xuan, W.C., Keikhosrokiani, P.: Habitpad: a habit-change person-centric healthcare mobile application with machine leaning and gamification features for obesity. In: Barsocchi, P., Parvathaneni, N.S., Garg, A., Bhoi, A.K., Palumbo, F. (eds.) Enabling Person-Centric Healthcare Using Ambient Assistive Technology. Studies in Computational Intelligence, vol. 1108, pp. 27–56. Springer, Cham (2023). https://doi.org/10.1007/978-3-031-38281-9_2

17. Yee, L.S., Keikhosrokiani, P.: Hospital data analytics system for tracking and predicting obese patients' lifestyle habits. In: Keikhosrokiani, P. (ed.) Big Data Analytics for Healthcare, chap. 14, pp. 165–178. Academic Press (2022)

18. Augustine, C.A., Keikhosrokiani, P.: A hospital information management system with habit-change features and medial analytical support for decision making. Int. J. Inf. Technol. Syst. Approach (IJITSA) **15**, 1–24 (2022). https://doi.org/10.4018/IJITSA.307019

19. Ravichandran, B.D., Keikhosrokiani, P.: An emotional-persuasive habit-change support mobile application for heart disease patients (BeHabit). In: Saeed, F., Mohammed, F., Al-Nahari, A. (eds.) IRICT 2020. LNDECT, vol. 72, pp. 252–262. Springer, Cham (2021). https://doi.org/10.1007/978-3-030-70713-2_25

20. Augustine, C.A., Keikhosrokiani, P.: A habit-change support web-based system with big data analytical features for hospitals (doctive). In: Saeed, F., Mohammed, F., Al-Nahari, A. (eds.) IRICT 2020. LNDECT, vol. 72, pp. 91–101. Springer, Cham (2021). https://doi.org/10.1007/978-3-030-70713-2_10

21. Chen, B., Wang, L., Li, B., Liu, W.: Work stress, mental health, and employee performance. Front. Psychol. **13**, 1006580 (2022)

22. Shiri, R., Väänänen, A., Mattila-Holappa, P., et al.: The effect of healthy lifestyle changes on work ability and mental health symptoms: a randomized controlled trial. Int. J. Environ. Res. Public Health **19**, 13206 (2022). https://doi.org/10.3390/ijerph192013206

23. von Thiele Schwarz, U.: Co-care: producing better health outcome through interactions between patients, care providers and information and communication technology. Health Serv. Manage. Res. **29**, 10–15 (2016). https://doi.org/10.1177/0951484816637746

24. Awad, A., Trenfield, S.J., Pollard, T.D., et al.: Connected healthcare: improving patient care using digital health technologies. Adv. Drug Deliv. Rev. **178**, 113958 (2021). https://doi.org/10.1016/j.addr.2021.113958

25. Korhonen, O., Isomursu, M.: Identifying personalization in a care pathway: a single-case study of a Finnish healthcare service provider. In: Proceedings of the 25th European Conference on Information Systems (ECIS), Guimarães, Portugal, 5–10 June 2017. Research Papers. Association for Information Systems (2017)

26. Alshyyab, M.A., FitzGerald, G., Dingle, K., et al.: Developing a conceptual framework for patient safety culture in emergency department: a review of the literature. Int. J. Health Plann. Manage. **34**, 42–55 (2019). https://doi.org/10.1002/hpm.2640

27. Delbanco, T., Walker, J., Bell, S.K., et al.: Inviting patients to read their doctors' notes: a quasi-experimental study and a look ahead. Ann. Intern. Med. **157**, 461–470 (2012). https://doi.org/10.7326/0003-4819-157-7-201210020-00002

28. Van Nunen, K., Reniers, G., Ponnet, K.: Measuring safety culture using an integrative approach: the development of a comprehensive conceptual framework and an applied safety culture assessment instrument. Int. J. Environ. Res. Public Health **19**, 13602 (2022). https://doi.org/10.3390/ijerph192013602

29. Luximon, A., Goonetilleke, R.S.: Simplified subjective workload assessment technique. Ergonomics **44**, 229–243 (2001). https://doi.org/10.1080/00140130010000901

30. Rubio Valdehita, S., López Núñez, M.I., López-Higes Sánchez, R., Díaz Ramiro, E.M.: Development of the CarMen-Q questionnaire for mental workload assessment. Psicothema (2017). https://doi.org/10.7334/psicothema2017.151

31. Hart, S.G.: NASA-task load index (NASA-TLX); 20 years later. In: Proceedings of the Human Factors and Ergonomics Society Annual Meeting, vol. 50, pp. 904–908 (2006). https://doi.org/10.1177/154193120605000909

32. Reid, G.B., Nygren, T.E.: The subjective workload assessment technique: a scaling procedure for measuring mental workload. In: Hancock, P.A., Meshkati, N. (eds.) Advances in Psychology, pp. 185–218. North-Holland, Amsterdam (1988)

33. Mansikka, H., Virtanen, K., Harris, D.: Comparison of NASA-TLX scale, modified Cooper-Harper scale and mean inter-beat interval as measures of pilot mental workload during simulated flight tasks. Ergonomics **62**, 246–254 (2019). https://doi.org/10.1080/00140139.2018.1471159
34. Keikhosrokiani, P.: Perspectives in the development of mobile medical information systems: life cycle, management, methodological approach and application (2019)
35. Dybå, T., Dingsøyr, T.: Empirical studies of agile software development: a systematic review. Inf. Softw. Technol. **50**, 833–859 (2008). https://doi.org/10.1016/j.infsof.2008.01.006
36. Hudson, J.L., Moss-Morris, R.: Treating illness distress in chronic illness. Eur. Psychol. (2019)

Digitalization in Health Education

Factors Affecting Marginalized Older Peoples' Digital Exclusion Evaluated by Gerontological Social Work Professionals

Virpi Paananen[1], Susanna Rivinen[2] (iD), Anniina Tohmola[3] (iD), and Satu Elo[4](✉) (iD)

[1] The Wellbeing Services County of East Uusimaa, Mannerheiminkatu 20K, 06100 Porvoo, Finland
[2] Faculty of Education, University of Lapland, Media Education Hub, P.O. box 122, 96101 Rovaniemi, Finland
[3] Lapland University of Applied Sciences, Future Health Services, Tietokatu 1, 98400 Kemi, Finland
[4] Oulu University of Applied Sciences, Wellbeing and Cultural Field of Expertise, Kiviharjuntie 4, 90220 Oulu, Finland
satu.elo@oamk.fi

Abstract. Digitalization is one of today's megatrends, and the increased development and use of various digital services emphasize the importance of sufficient guidance, support, and digital skills. The purpose of this study was to describe factors that can lead to an increased possibility of digital exclusion of marginalized older people evaluated by gerontological social work professionals. The aim was to obtain knowledge for developing age-friendly digital literacy education for older people. The research was qualitative: data was collected from gerontological social work professionals (n = 23) through an open-ended electronic survey and analyzed by using inductive content analysis. Professionals considered that marginalized older people had personal difficulties reaching or adopting digital services with deteriorating cognitive and physical abilities, such as impaired functioning, a lack of motivation or fears, and missing equipment. The possibility of digital exclusion of older people can also be increased by external factors, such as a lack of support and counseling resources, and competence from professionals. Therefore, to be able to utilize digital services, marginalized older people need plenty of support from care workers which should be considered in the service time. In addition, the digitalization of services prevents marginalized older people from managing their own lives unnecessarily early. There is a need to develop facilitating services, and support for acquiring digital skills and advocacy.

Keywords: Digitalization · Digital exclusion · Marginalized older people · Older people · Social work professionals

1 Introduction

Digitalization is one of today's megatrends [1], which challenges and offers opportunities for developers and producers of services and their users. Global societal challenges, such as COVID-19, have further increased the need to rapidly develop digital service

M. Särestöniemi et al. (Eds.): NCDHWS 2024, CCIS 2083, pp. 353–362, 2024.
https://doi.org/10.1007/978-3-031-59080-1_25

channels, the use of which has also increased during the COVID-19 pandemic [2, 3]. After the pandemic, the use of various digital services has continued to be used, which at the same time emphasizes the importance of developing service guidance and support. For instance, a survey conducted by Kyytsönen et al. (2021) suggests that one in five Finns needs guidance in the use of online social and healthcare services and that there is a significant need for supported use of the internet and digital services in Finland [4]. In addition, 15% of those who responded to the survey felt that digital services were not barrier-free and the ability to use the internet was felt to weaken with higher age groups [4]. According to Pirhonen and his colleagues (2020), digitalization can increase inequality between older people, especially between those with different social, cognitive, and physical resources, and different social and financial standing. Therefore, one of the disadvantages of digitalization can be considered to be that it can increase inequality in the availability of services, especially between older people and generations [5].

The use of digital services requires citizens to have digital skills. In the present research, digital skills are understood, according to the DigComp 2.2 framework created by the European Commission [6], to mean a wide-ranging ability to use, understand, and evaluate digital information; communicate, collaborate, promote health, and safety in digital environments; and produce digital content [7–9]. Advanced digital skills also include the ability to help and guide others with questions related to digital skills [6].

Currently, not everyone has the necessary digital skills, and the concern is particularly accentuated in the older age group. According to Digital and Population Data Services Agency (2023) up to 78 percent of 75–89-year-olds have no digital skills and only half of those aged 65–74 have at least basic digital skills. [10] A lack of digital skills can potentially cause digital exclusion and increasing inequality as a full member of society, which means, in other words, that part of the population still has unequal access and capacity as well as willingness to use digital technologies and media that are necessary for participation in society [11]. However, digital exclusion does not directly mean the exclusion of an individual in other ways as well, but rather focuses specifically on the themes of exclusion from digitalization and services [12], although international literature suggests that it has a strong connection with social exclusion [11, 13, 14]. Yet, the phenomenon also works the other way, because individuals who are in poor health, socially isolated, or in a socioeconomically weaker position are more vulnerable to digital exclusion [13].

Previous studies find that there are mutual and digital exclusion connections between age, education level, the urbanity of the place of residence as well as poor health status and social isolation [12, 15–17]. For example, on average, older age groups are less educated than younger generations, and advanced age is also seen to be significantly related to the risk of digital exclusion compared to younger adults, due to increased functional impairments [5]. However, advanced age alone does not explain digital exclusion or the level of digital skills in general, although differences can be found between older and younger age groups, for example, what digital technologies and media are used and how they are used [18, 19]. Older people in this study refers to the population aged 65 or older who are entitled to an old-age pension according to Finnish law [20]. They form a heterogeneous, large, and growing population group nationally and globally, that are less experienced users of digital technologies and media compared to younger adults [17, 21]. For instance, older people use social media less than younger generations, although it should still be remembered that older people are a heterogeneous group of people and there are differences within a large group [22].

The purpose of the present study is to describe factors that can lead to an increased possibility of digital exclusion of marginalized older people evaluated by gerontological social work professionals. Marginalized older people in this study are defined as gerontological social work clients in a vulnerable position and having one or more risks related to health, livelihood, social relationships, or living conditions, which, if realized, may lead to a socially weak position. To achieve the set goal, the qualitative research answers the following question: What factors challenge the marginalized older people's digital service adoption and usage?

2 Materials and Methods

The present study was conducted using a qualitative approach. The data was collected through an open-ended electronic survey from gerontological social workers (n = 23), such as special social workers, social workers, social counselors, and home care assistants, from one large city in Finland. The target group of the survey was selected on the basis that they work closely with older people with special needs and their views and experiences were perceived as valuable information. Daily, these gerontological social workers meet marginalized older people because gerontological social work clients need special support, and most of them have a reduced ability to apply services, and often they do not have helpful relatives to support them.

The open-ended electronic survey included a total of six open questions, which focused on the situations of digital service deployment and the support needed from professionals (Table 1). Three social and health professionals tested the open-ended questions and based on the feedback, minor changes were made to the questions and the format, such as harmonizing the terms used and improving the layout of the questions.

The survey was sent through the organization's liaison to the respondents by email and the response time was three weeks. The basic information of the study was given to the respondents before the data collection. The respondents answered voluntarily and by answering, gave informed consent to participate in the study. One reminder of the questionnaire was sent, extending the response time by four days. The data consists of descriptions of 23 respondents to the six open-ended questions.

Using the approach of Elo & Kyngäs (2008), the data were analyzed by qualitative inductive content analysis [23]. When using content analysis, the aim is to describe the phenomenon in a conceptual form. During the preparation phase of the analysis, an analysis unit was decided, which can be a unit of meaning, a sentence, or a word. Here, the unit of meaning was used. The analysis is guided by a research question and was started by reducing the responses to a meaning unit and subdividing similar responses into subcategories. The classification was continued by combining the same content into the upper categories. Eventually, the categories were named according to the unifying factor into the main categories, resulting in five main categories. The main categories were used to describe situations in which professionals became concerned about the increased possibility of digital exclusion of marginalized older people.

Table 1. Open-ended questions.

	Open-ended question
1	Describe briefly how your customers are able to adopt and use the digital services
2	What kind of challenges have you faced that have prevented or made it difficult for your customers to adopt and use digital services?
3	What kind of support do your customers need in order to adopt and use digital services?
4	What is your biggest concern regarding your customers' digital service adoption and usage?
5	Related to the previous question: How do you think your concern should be answered?
6	Is there something else you would like to tell?

3   Results

Based on content analysis of social work professionals' descriptions, the challenging factors which can lead to an increased possibility of digital exclusion of marginalized older people are divided into factors related to marginalized older people themselves and factors related to the competence and resources of social work professionals.

3.1   Factors Related to Marginalized Older People Itself

Factors that can lead to an increased possibility of digital exclusion of marginalized older people based on gerontological social work professionals' descriptions are 1. impaired cognitive or physical functioning, 2. a lack of knowledge, low motivation or fears, and 3. missing or outdated equipment. Professionals evaluated that marginalized older peoples' impaired cognitive and physical functioning prevented and hindered the use of digital services. Impairment of cognitive functioning was manifested as difficulties in learning, understanding the service, adopting the use of the digital service, and following the guidelines. Social work professionals pointed out that the use of digital services requires strong cognitive abilities, and e.g. online banking authentication alone could be very challenging for older people. In addition, the use of complex, changing, and multi-location digital services with impaired cognition further complicates the use of digital services.

"We practiced using online banking with the client's smartphone at home. The assignments were successful when I was involved in mentoring, but the 65-year-old client was not able to work independently. However, the client has an academic degree and had a career as a special education teacher." Professional #12

Professionals evaluated that impaired sensory and fine motor skills also made it more difficult for older people to use digital services, even if they otherwise had the ability to function. Due to poor eyesight, it was difficult to see the small screen clearly, and the clumsiness of the fingers and the trembling of the hands prevented the right keys from being hit.

The gerontological social work professionals pointed out that older people's lack of previous experience with digital solutions and weak digital skills often led to difficulties in learning how to use digital services. Even if older people had some experience, information technology would have changed since the last time they had used it actively, and older people also have difficulties understanding the vocabulary used.

"If everything, starting with the use of devices and the language used in the digital services, is completely foreign, then there is not much of a basis on which to build a new way of operating in the world." Professional #4

Low motivation and fears against technology were also identified as key issues regarding the adoption and use of digital services by older people. Several professionals highlighted older peoples' fears and prejudices about devices, machines, and their reluctance to use digital services. Moreover, the desire to use traditional, not digitalized services was strong. In addition, the informants described that the fear of being overwhelmed or feeling of unsafety in the digital world limited the activity when it was not understood how the digital service works. The inexperience of older people in digital services also increased the professionals' concerns about the possibility of being abused.

Missing or outdated equipment was mentioned by gerontological social work professionals as one factor increasing the risk of digital exhaustion. The lack of a computer, a mobile device, digital identification, an internet connection, or outdated equipment was seen as a significant hindering factor for marginalized older people in using digital services. This was usually the result of weak health status as well as a reduced ability to function: due to reduced cognitive and physical functioning, marginalized older people are often unable to acquire equipment. Consequently, professionals pointed out that if older people do not have sufficient devices due to their economic situation there was a high possibility of digital exclusion. Outdated equipment such as traditional phones also made it difficult to receive guidance from customer service.

"When calling client support, it is impossible for the younger generation to realize that an older person has an old-fashioned telephone, for example. Explaining it to them is sometimes even comical when they ask them to enter identification codes or try hard to tell a customer to send a text message or online banking ID to complete authentication." Professional #10

3.2 Factors Related to Competences and Resources of Social Work Professionals

In the present study, social work professionals pointed out that their competencies are also related to their customers' digital exclusion of marginalized older people. These factors are 1. a lack of digital competence of professionals for supporting older people, and 2. insufficient counseling resources and competence of professionals.

First of all, professionals described that a lack of digital competence of professionals can lead to a risk of older people being marginalized: unless professionals have insufficient know-how and digital skills, clients are at risk of being excluded from digital services because they do not receive adequate support. Some professionals felt that in addition to older people, they needed digital support. Indeed, professionals needed information and support on how to use the services and how to deal with problems. They needed information about easy-to-use and age-friendly services. Furthermore, professionals needed information on where to get reliable digital support for themselves and their clients. The perceived experience of telephone digital support had seemed necessary, and the answers suggested the profession of a digital counselor as a solution.

"... for example, a digital counselor who also provides support by phone to professionals." Professional #17

Professionals evaluated that the insufficient resources for the time required to support the use of digital services made it difficult to support the marginalized older peoples' use of digital services and might lead to digital exhaustion. To take up the digital service, the marginalized older people needed a lot of guidance, which also involved a lot of work time. Commonly, the need for guidance was not transient. Instead, older people needed constant guidance and support. In their responses to the research questions, the professionals indicated that the employer should consider the time taken to introduce and support the use of digital services by marginalized older people.

"Guidance is not always enough, but the customer needs constant support in using the services, for example, due to a memory disorder." Professional #7

According to professionals, good counseling skills and resources were the key elements for supporting digital skills and encouraging older people to develop them. Counseling requires the professional's competence to adapt to the needs of older people. Social care professionals mentioned that a letter sent home from a remote service does not encourage seniors to try the service, but instead requires an encouraging conversation with a professional, which in turn takes time. There was a need for both face-to-face and remote counseling. Professionals pointed out that it is important to have room for attendance just when older people need it; this requires practice together and encouragement. Introducing the digital service and the support of the digital skills consists of side-to-side counseling, for example just practicing together how to attend remote meetings. The importance of repetition was emphasized: older people needed counseling and practice many times over in a calm atmosphere. Indeed, older people might be insecure about their skills, and a professional's calm and encouraging guidance would lead to the safer use of digital services.

"The customer has his computer and basic digital skills. Together, we went through the steps of making a digital application of benefits and finally, I wrote the instructions step by step. These instructions will enable the customer to use the digital service." Professional #12

4 Discussion

The results of the present study showed that the factors that can lead to an increased possibility of digital exclusion of marginalized older people evaluated by gerontological social work professionals are related to 1. marginalized older people themselves and 2. social work professionals' competencies and resources. More specifically, the factors include impaired cognitive or physical functioning lack of knowledge, low motivation or fears; missing or outdated equipment; a lack of digital competence of professionals for supporting older people; and insufficient counselling resources and competence of professionals.

Impaired cognitive or physical functioning increases the possibility of using digital services. Older people have difficulties reaching or using digital service tools when their cognitive and physical functioning ability has weakened, which confirmed the results of previous studies [26]. To use digital services, there must be a cognitive and physical ability to function, basic information technology skills, motivation, guidance, and an internet connection [27]. Moreover, using digital services requires a sufficient cognitive ability including the ability to learn and adopt new things. The use of digital services requires, for example, a moderate ability to see and hear and fine motor skills to hit the right choice on the keyboard. There is therefore a need to develop the accessibility of digital services so that they can be used by adults with poor vision, poor hearing, and clumsy fingers. To achieve the accessibility of digital services, it is important not only to look at the individual's characteristics but also to consider issues at a social level, such as guidelines and regulations on age-friendly design (e.g. size of screens and buttons) and intuitive software [5]. As an example, so far, the market economy has still poorly identified older people alongside the young, and if the situation remains like this, older peoples' needs will not be fully supported, and they will be discriminated against [22].

Older peoples' lack of knowledge, low motivation, or fears lead to digital exclusion. The results of the research also showed that the digitization of services and the difficulty of using services in other ways displaced adults from managing their own lives unnecessarily early. Not only did the negative experiences cause concern, but the inability to use services pushed the aging adults beyond the control of their lives. Further, the digitalization of social and health services can increase inequality [4], and negative experiences cause concern about losing control of one's life and facing alienation from society [5]. Deficiencies in digital services must not affect the loss of a sense of control over life or a deterioration in the quality of life. There is a risk that the inaccessibility of digital services leads to new forms of disadvantage. Overall, this can be seen as contradicting the equality laws of Finnish society and the assumption that everyone has equal opportunities to use digital services, which is not true [22]. Although previous studies have demonstrated the positive impact of technology, there are still barriers to using it because of psychological issues in motivation, attitudes, privacy, and trust, and social issues involving learning to use the technology [28].

Digital exclusion can result from the lack of social work professional's digital competence for supporting older people. In the present study, the results showed that professionals assessed whether the aging person could use digital services at all or whether they needed encouragement and support. One important division is to evaluate who cannot and those who do not want to use digital technologies in later life, which might also call for different approaches when trying to reach these target groups [16]. To achieve these professionals should have warm and social skills that will help clarify the needs of older people about the use of digital services and technologies through discussion and questions. When necessary, such professionals also know how to create a friendly atmosphere and choose pedagogically appropriate approaches, where the use of digital services and technologies is encouraged and supported, considering the changes brought about by the heterogeneity and age of the target group [27].

Insufficient counseling resources and the competence of professionals prevent older peoples' use of digital technology. The results of the present study highlighted the fact that professionals should have enough time to guide them in using digital services, as social support is important in learning digital skills [27, 29]. In learning digital skills and services, it is especially important to provide long-lasting learning sessions and systematic support where things can be repeated and practiced [27]. Recent research also shows that learning to use, in particular, eHealth services for older people in the learning and care ecosystem is a long-term process that is not just a one-time experience only when it is initially introduced [29]. In this sense, employees play a significant role in the implementation of services, and they will offer the opportunity and resources to support the customer [30]. Insufficient resources for the time required to support the use of digital services and the tools required for use have hindered and prevented older people from using digital services. Sufficient resources for professionals are particularly important because older people are outside formal education and working life where skills can otherwise be developed [27].

For the broad target groups of the aging population, it is necessary to plan versatile interventions and approaches for different ages. It would be important to take a closer look at this group from an age point of view because in this heterogeneous group digital skills are already various and will become more diverse with age, so it may matter whether we look at 65-year-olds or, for example, over 75-year-olds (Digital and Population Information Agency, 2023). Another important division might lie between those who cannot and those who do not want to use digital technologies in later life, which might also call for different approaches when trying to reach these target groups. This also suggests that gerontology should not only put the non-use of digital technologies on its research agenda, but also technology reluctance, resistance, neglect, or taste, and that policies should take these constructs more closely into account when designing interventions.

5 Conclusions

The results show that marginalized older people had personal difficulties reaching or adopting digital services with deteriorating cognitive and physical abilities, such as impaired functioning, a lack of motivation or fears, and missing equipment. The possibility of digital exclusion of older people can also be increased by external factors, such as a lack of support and counseling resources, and competence from professionals. Therefore, to be able to utilize digital services, marginalized older people need plenty of support from care workers which should be considered in the service time. In conclusion, we can state that the insufficiency of resources supporting the use time of services or systems makes it difficult and prevents older people from using digital services. Thus, sufficient resources are required to identify these obstacles and to support and guide users.

Ethics. This study was held to the principles of research ethics [24, 25] and a research permit was obtained from the city of Helsinki (diary number HEL 2021-002864). The study did not need a prior ethical review, because the respondents were not under-aged or it did not collect sensitive information, such as respondents' identification information. A covering letter attached to the front page of the electronic survey included information about the aim of the study, voluntary participation, anonymity, and confidentiality. By giving a response to the survey, the respondent gave their informed consent to participate in the study and to the processing of the data. The cover letter stated that the respondent has the right to refuse to participate, to interrupt their participation or to withdraw their consent.

References

1. Dufta, M.: Megatrendit 2020. Sitra, Helsinki (2020)
2. Almeida, F., Duarte Santos, J., Augusto Monteiro, J.: The challenges and opportunities in the digitalization of companies in a post-COVID-19 world. IEEE Eng. Manag. Rev. 48 (2020). https://doi.org/10.1109/EMR.2020.3013206
3. De', R., Pandey, N., Pal, A.: Impact of digital surge during Covid-19 pandemic: a viewpoint on research and practice. Int. J. Inf. Manag. 55 (2020). https://doi.org/10.1016/j.ijinfomgt.2020.102171
4. Kyytsönen, M., Aalto, A.-M., Vehko, T.: Sosiaali- ja terveydenhuollon sähköinen asiointi 2020–2021: Väestön kokemukset. THL, Helsinki (2021)
5. Pirhonen, J., Lolich, L., Tuominen, K., Jolanki, O., Timonen, V.: "These devices have not been made for older people's needs" – Older adults' perceptions of digital technologies in Finland and Ireland. Technol. Soc. 62 (2020). https://doi.org/10.1016/j.techsoc.2020.101287
6. Vuorikari, R., Kluzer, S., Punie, Y.: DigComp 2.2. the digital competence framework for citizens. With new examples of knowledge, skills and attitudes. Publications Office of the European Union, Luxembourg (2022)
7. Forsman, M.: Digital competence and the future media citizen: a preliminary conceptual analysis. J. Media Literacy 65, 24–29 (2018)
8. Ilomäki, L., Paavola, S., Lakkala, M., Kantosalo, A.: Digital competence – an emergent boundary concept for policy and educational research. Educ. Inf. Technol. (Dordr) 21 (2016). https://doi.org/10.1007/s10639-014-9346-4
9. Vuorikari, R., Punie, Y., Carretero, S., Van Den Brande, L.: DigComp 2.0: The Digital Competence Framework for Citizens. Publications Office of the European Union, Luxembourg (2016)
10. Digital and Population Data Services Agency: Digital skills report 2023 (2023). https://urly.fi/3rS5. Accessed 26 Feb 2024
11. Martin, C., Hope, S., Zubiri, S., Ipsos MORI Scotland: the role of digital exclusion in social exclusion. Carnegie UK Trust (2016)
12. Ahola, N., Hirvonen, J.: Digitalisaation huipulla ja reunalla. Verkkopalvelujen käyttö ja digisyrjäytyminen Helsingissä ja Suomessa. Kaupunkitieto, Helsinki (2021)
13. Heponiemi, T., Jormanainen, V., Leemann, L., Manderbacka, K., Aalto, A.M., Hyppönen, H.: Digital divide in perceived benefits of online health care and social welfare services: national cross-sectional survey study. J. Med. Internet Res. 22, (2020). https://doi.org/10.2196/17616
14. Seifert, A., Cotten, S.R., Xie, B.: A double burden of exclusion? Digital and social exclusion of older adults in times of COVID-19. J. Gerontol. – Ser. B Psychol. Sci. Soc. Sci. 76 (2021). https://doi.org/10.1093/geronb/gbaa098
15. Formosa, M.: Digital exclusion in later life: a Maltese case study. Human. Soc. Sci. 1 (2013). https://doi.org/10.11648/j.hss.20130101.14
16. Gallistl, V., Rohner, R., Seifert, A., Wanka, A.: Configuring the older non-user: between research, policy and practice of digital exclusion. Soc. Incl. 8 (2020). https://doi.org/10.17645/si.v8i2.2607
17. Olson, K.E., O'Brien, M.A., Rogers, W.A., Charness, N.: Diffusion of technology: frequency of use for younger and older adults. Ageing Int. 36 (2011). https://doi.org/10.1007/s12126-010-9077-9
18. Official Statistics of Finland (OSF): Use of information and communications technology by individuals (2022)
19. Rasi, P., Vuojärvi, H., Hyvönen, P.: Aikuisten ja ikääntyneiden mediakasvatus. In: Pekkala, L., Salomaa, S., Spisak, S. (eds.) Monimuotoinen mediakasvatus, pp. 198–212 (2016)

20. Lee, S.B., Oh, J.H., Park, J.H., Choi, S.P., Wee, J.H.: Differences in youngest-old, middle-old, and oldest-old patients who visit the emergency department. Clin. Exp. Emerg. Med. **5** (2018). https://doi.org/10.15441/ceem.17.261

21. Van Volkom, M., Stapley, J.C., Amaturo, V.: Revisiting the digital divide: generational differences in technology use in everyday life. N. Am. J. Psychol. **16** (2014)

22. Rasi, P., Vuojärvi, H., Rivinen, S.: Promoting media literacy among older people: a systematic review. Adult Educ. Q. **71**, 37–54 (2021). https://doi.org/10.1177/0741713620923755

23. Elo, S., Kyngäs, H.: The qualitative content analysis process. J. Adv. Nurs. **62** (2008). https://doi.org/10.1111/j.1365-2648.2007.04569.x

24. Finnish National Board on Research Integrity: The Finnish Code of Conduct for Research Integrity and Procedures for Handling Alleged Violations of Research Integrity in Finland. TENK, Helsinki (2023)

25. All European Academies: The European Code of Conduct for Research Integrity. Revised Edition 2023 (2023)

26. Haase, K.R., Cosco, T., Kervin, L., Riadi, I., O'Connell, M.E.: Older adults' experiences with using technology for socialization during the COVID-19 pandemic: cross-sectional survey study. JMIR Aging **23:4**(2), e28010 (2021). https://doi.org/10.2196/28010

27. Tilles-Tirkkonen, T., Lappi, J., Karhunen, L., Harjumaa, M., Absetz, P., Pihlajamäki, J.: Sosioekonomisesti heikommassa asemassa olevien kiinnostus ja mahdollisuudet digitaalisten terveyspalveluiden käyttöön. Yhteiskuntapolitiikka **83**, 317–323 (2018)

28. Marston, H.R., Musselwhite, C.B.A.: Improving older people's lives through digital technology and practices. Gerontol Geriatr Med **7**, 23337214211036256 (2021). https://doi.org/10.1177/23337214211036255

29. Airola, E.: Older adults, and eHealth service use. An exploration of a complex learning and care ecosystem in the rural areas of Finnish Lapland, University of Lapland, Lauda (2022)

30. Karisalmi, N., Kaipio, J., Kujala, S.: Hoitohenkilökunnan rooli potilaiden motivoinnissa ja ohjaamisessa terveydenhuollon sähköisten palveluiden käyttöön. Fin. J. eHealth eWelfare **10** (2018). https://doi.org/10.23996/fjhw.69145

Social and Health Care Teachers' Experiences of Implementing Multidisciplinary Specialisation Studies in a Digital Learning Environment

Hanna Naakka[1](✉) , Jarmo Heinonen[2] , Merja Männistö[3] , Sami Perälä[4] ,
Anna Rauha[4] , Mika Paldanius[5] , Outi Ahonen[2] , and Päivi Sanerma[1]

[1] Häme University of Applied Sciences, Hameenlinna, Finland
hanna.naakka@hamk.fi
[2] Laurea, University of Applied Sciences, Vantaa, Finland
[3] Diaconia University of Applied Sciences, Helsinki, Finland
[4] Seinäjoki University of Applied Sciences, Seinajoki, Finland
[5] Oulu University of Applied Sciences, Oulu, Finland

Abstract. The aim of the study was to find out how teachers and project actors experienced the implementation of the specialisation education in a digital learning environment. The methods were triangulation with paired t-test, ANOVA and content analysis of qualitative data. The results showed a statistical difference between the responses after the first and second implementation of specialisation education. The overall results show that teachers and project actors demonstrate a strong commitment to producing and developing student-centred and work-life-centred online specialisation education.

Keywords: specialisation education · multiprofessional cooperation · digitalisation

1 Background

The constant changes of the social and health sector require teachers to update and specialise their competences. The rise of digital learning environments offers a unique opportunity to expand teaching methods and support teachers' multidisciplinary specialisation [1].

Social and health care is a field where rapid technological developments and changing practices pose constant challenges for teachers. Providing multidisciplinary specialisation education is one way of meeting this challenge, and digital learning environments offer an effective means of supporting such training [2] Digitalisation enables diversification of teaching, increased flexibility, and different ways of engaging students. The digital learning environment opens new opportunities for multidisciplinary specialisation studies. It allows students to participate at any time and from any place, making it easier to combine work and study [3].

M. Särestöniemi et al. (Eds.): NCDHWS 2024, CCIS 2083, pp. 363–370, 2024.
https://doi.org/10.1007/978-3-031-59080-1_26

Digital learning environments allow teachers to create a variety of learning tasks and e-learning environments, which promote multi-faceted learning [4] Teachers are critical of the successful use of digital learning environments in the delivery of multidisciplinary specialisation studies. Their experiences range from enthusiasm and success to challenges and uncertainty [5].

Student learning in Europe is defined based on European Credit Transfer and accumulation systems (ECTS). One ECTS credit equals 27 h of student work. This system is important because it provides a framework for studying in different countries and in different higher education institutions across Europe [6] In Finland, specialisation education is defined at levels 6–7 of the European Qualification Framework (EQF) in the social and health care sector, specialisation education is defined at level 6, which is equivalent to bachelor level education. Specialisation education is strongly connected to working life [7, 8] and is one form of lifelong learning. It complements and updates the competencies needed in an evolving working life. Lifelong learning relevant to the work life is now often offered online in the form of short courses. The advantage of online studies is in their affordability, flexibility of learning independent of time and location, and accessibility [9, 10].

A national UUDO project, implemented by 14 different universities of applied sciences (UAS), designed, and implemented a fully web-based specialisation education on digital health and social care service. Both students and teachers in the education came from all over Finland. Students of the specialisation education mostly had more than ten years of work experience and they evaluated the content of the studies important [11, 12] The teachers may have had different roles during the project: some as course teachers, others as tutors, but some also as project managers or in other project management roles. In Finland, UAS are independent institutions. They can cooperate with other UAS, and they support regional cooperation [13]. The multidisciplinary digitalised specialisation education is driven by the objectives of the national Digivision project, which aims to increase common digital studies and the possibility for students to study seamlessly across different UAS [14].

This article explores teachers' and project actors' perceptions of teaching and learning and how to further improve the multidisciplinary specialisation education. The aim of the study was to find out how teachers and project actors experienced the implementation of the specialisation education. **The research question** is how teachers and project actors describe the implementation of the specialisation education and multiprofessional cooperation.

2 Materials and Methods

The respondents in the study were all the experts in social and health care and other professional fields who either taught in the first, second or both implementations of the specialisation education or acted as project actors without teaching responsibilities.

Quantitative and qualitative research methods and data triangulation were used. Samples were collected from teachers after both specialisation educations (5/2022 and 8–10/2023) using an electronic form. The instrument for data collection was a structured survey. The themes of the survey were: 1. Content and requirements (3 questions), 2. Implementation of the education (10), 3. Resourcing of work (5), 4. Cooperation with students (8), 5. Learning outcomes (5) and 6. The development of professional competence (6). Each thematic category included the above number of Likert-scale questions (1–4) and open-ended questions that allowed the respondents to share their reflections on each theme.

The research data consisted of teachers´ and project actors´ answers and statements related to the research question in the two consecutive specialisation educations. The anonymized qualitative data consisted 52 answers to 6 open ended questions. In the first education (2021–2022) the total number of responses was 22. In the second education (2022–2023), the total number of responses was 11. Thus, a total of 33 participants responded to the survey, some of whom taught in both specialisation educations.

SPSS 28.0 with t-test was used for statistical analysis to find the relationship between the first implementation answers and the second implementation answers. Paired t-test is an arithmetic mean test between two variables means, to check any differences [15, 16]. The significance level was 5%. Significant test ($p < 0,05$) shows that only one question (242) shows differences between the first implementation answers and the second implementation answers.

Answers to open-ended questions were analysed by using qualitative content analysis [17]. This data was compiled, tabulated, and analysed by using inductive content analysis [18]. At the end of the analysis, triangulation of the results was used. Triangulation is a research method in which different methods are used to collect data on the same phenomenon [18]. In this study, triangulation was used to view qualitative results with quantitative results and the aim was to understand them by reviewing the different results. The qualitative research data was copied from the tables separately and transferred to separate files. The research data was analysed by two researchers who reviewed the result categories and results obtained. Meaningful expressions were separated into their own groups and result categories were created. The categories were compared and refined. Finally, the results were viewed with quantitative and qualitative results and conclusions and findings were drawn.

3 Results

The statistical results are only indicative, because the sample is small. Out of these 37 questions only one shows statistical significancy ($p < 0,05$). Question "Student cooperation: 24.2 The common instructions given to the tutors have been clear" (p 0,02) showed a statistical difference between the first and the second responses. The questions "Student collaboration: 24.4 student collaboration between higher education institutions (0.08) and "Development of professional's own skills: 26.1 Collaboration between higher education institutions has increased knowledge of different learning environments" (0,06) showed slight significance, indicating only uncertain results. There were no statistical differences between the years 2021–2023 answers except the answers mentioned above.

The qualitative results have been divided into two main categories based on the analysis. The categories are: 1) Teachers' experiences of the implementation and 2) Teachers' experiences of learning in educational development. The main categories were further divided into subcategories, which are described in Table 1. Teachers´ experiences of implementation and development of specialisation education.

3.1   Teachers' Experiences of the Implementation of Education

The teachers´ experiences of implementation of education were divided into four subcategories: 1) The variation in the demands of the study courses, 2) The work-life relevance of the studies, 3) Student-centred studies, 4) Commitment to joint development.

The variation in the demands of the study courses related to the misalignment between learning objectives and course content, as well as variation in the workload of students during the courses. Moreover, the respondents sought to ensure that the courses meet the learning requirements of EQF Level 6. Respondents described the relevance of the courses to the world of work as students were able to use the methods they had learned and apply the knowledge in their work with colleagues. The subcategory 'student-centred studies' included expressions describing the possibility for students to choose courses relevant to their learning needs, student-oriented guidance and proactive and clear information about their studies. In the subcategory 'commitment to joint development', the respondents described the differences between teachers in participating in their involvement in the development of the specialisation education and the need to update the course contents to meet the demands of constantly evolving digital developments.

3.2   Teachers' Experiences of Learning in Educational Development

The teachers' experiences of learning in educational development were divided into four sub-categories: 1) Learning together, 2) Enabling self-regulated and systematic learning, 3) Applying effective pedagogical solutions, 4) Development of the studies and course offerings.

The respondents contemplated learning from their own and students point of views. The applicable skills for working life consist of respondents' statements describing how students apply the content and methods of the courses in their own work during their studies. These descriptions were particularly related to the implementation of service design and development tasks. Respondents described collaborative learning as a dialogue involving students in specialisation education and professionals in working life. Teachers´ own learning occurred in collaborative teamwork and in examining the learning tasks and used pedagogy. The category "Development of the studies and course offering" describes the evaluation of the curriculum and the development of structures in specialisation education to make the education more student-centred.

Table 1. Teachers' experiences of implementation and development of specialisation education

Main category	Subcategory	Statement examples
Teachers' experiences of the implementation of the specialisation education	The variation in the demands of the study courses	"The high learning objectives of the studies, which the contents of the study courses do not reach. Variability between study courses; the level of requirements and the workload for students vary significantly from one to another. The EQF6 level needs to be re-evaluated in all study modules."
	The work-life relevance of the study courses	"The development task has proven to be a good method for applying and strengthening the accumulated skills. Particularly pleasing has been the observation of enthusiasm and commitment to development and collaboration with the client of the development task. Development tasks carried out for one's own employer have been motivating. Through the development work, some students have been attached to new job tasks."
	Student-centred studies	"In my opinion, the selection of elective studies should be guided more effectively for students, for example, advising them on what they should choose based on their interests. There should be a greater emphasis on the role of the tutor in this regard." "There is a lot of room for improvement in student/user-centeredness when examining the student administration in higher education institutions. "
	Commitment to joint development	"Some teachers were more committed to the development of study modules than others. In the field of social and health care digitalisation, things are changing rapidly, so study modules should be constantly developed and updated." "Within the universities, the allocation of resources was very different. In some schools, there is a lot of staff, and for some, there may be only limited hours available for the actual implementation. Universities of applied sciences have different practices in general operating procedures."

(continued)

Table 1. (*continued*)

Main category	Subcategory	Statement examples
Teachers' experiences of learning in educational development	Learning together	"The dialogue brought about by the development task with various parties clearly strengthens competence. Additionally, the work done in small groups has proven to be fruitful even in various challenging situations." "Partner universities of applied sciences have learned a tremendous amount along the way. In hindsight, the division of labor could have been further clarified from the beginning."
	Enabling self-regulated and systematic learning	"It's great that a student can choose courses they feel they need for developing their skills and assemble their expertise like a puzzle." "In my opinion, guidance for the selection of elective courses should be even more detailed for students, advising them on what they should choose based on their interests. Emphasis should be placed more on the role of the tutor in this process."
	Applying effective pedagogical solutions	"The large number of students affected the types of learning and assessment methods that could be used in the courses. "
	Development of the studies and course offerings	"Clear structures and operating methods are important, as well as reaching agreements together. It's also crucial to consider whether specialisation courses could be divided into components, from which those specializing can accumulate credits within a specific timeframe." "Clarity and simplicity, especially from the customer's perspective, regarding what the entity consists of what to choose, how to enroll, etc."

4   Discussion

The purpose of this study was to find out, through responses of teachers and project actors, how the respondents have experienced the implementation of the specialisation education and how they describe the implementation and multiprofessional cooperation of the specialisation education. The overall results show that teachers and project actors demonstrate a strong commitment to producing and developing student-centred and work-life-centred online specialisation education [1]. Many students in the specialisation education had long working experience [11]. Teachers were willing to develop curricula from a student perspective. The curricula of the Multidisciplinary digital health and social care service specialisation education is based on nationally described competencies [12]. The results showed that the study management, study guidance and student´s study paths and evaluation were important tools to make students lifelong learning more flexible with working life. In Finland, each University of Applied Sciences (UAS) is an autonomous organisation. UAS´s have different processes for managing and guiding students. There are national level standards and classifications to transfer data stored in the national repository for higher education institutions [19], but there are not common processes for student management [14], which is also reflected in the answers of project actors and teachers involved.

The quantitative data results aligned with the findings of the qualitative analysis upon review. No significant changes were observed when considering the statistical differences between the 2021 and 2023 responses. Based on the qualitative data, the study courses seemed to support working life and developed applicable competencies for the students. Among the courses, the development task and service design courses stood out positively. These courses were positively perceived as offering opportunities for collaboration and dialogue with different partners. "The development task course offers the opportunity for co-development using the concepts learned in the service design course." Earlier research [3] has shown that there arc also many positive ways in digital education to engage students in their studies, allowing them to participate when it is convenient for them, and providing the possibility to combine study and work.

Limitations: The research sample is small, and results are directional.

Disclosure of Interests. There were none.

References

1. Lin, J., Lin, H.: User acceptance in a computer -supported collaborative learning (CSCL) environment with social network awareness (SNA) support. Australas. J. Educ. Technol. **35**(1), 100–115 (2019). https://doi.org/10.14742/ajet.3395
2. Männistö, M., Mikkonen, K., Kuivila, H.M., Virtanen, M., Kyngäs, H., Kääriäinen, M.: Digital collaborative learning in nursing education: a systematic review. Scand. J. Caring Sci. (2019). https://doi.org/10.1111/scs.12743
3. Stover, S., Holland, C.: Student resistance to collaborative learning. Inter. J. Shcolarship Teach. Learn. **12**(2), 8 (2019)
4. Männistö, M.: Hoitotyön opiskelijoiden yhteisöllinen oppiminen ja sosiaali- ja terveysalan opettajien osaaminen digitaalisessa oppimisympäristössä. Acta Universitatis Ouluensis, Väitöskirja, D1554. Oulun yliopisto (2020)
5. Redecker, C.: European framework for the digital competence of educators: DigCompEdu. JRC Working Papers JRC107466, Joint Research Centre (Seville site) (2017)
6. European Comission: European Education Area. Quality education and training for all. European Credit Transfer and Accumulation system (ECTS) (2023). https://doi.org/10.2766/87192
7. Europass.: Description of the eight EQF levels. European Union. https://europa.eu/europass/en/description-eight-eqf-levels
8. Rauhala P, Urponen H.: Selvitys korkeakoulutettujen erikoistumiskoulutuksesta [Report on professional specialisation education for postgraduates, in Finnish]. Opetus- ja kulttuuriministeriön julkaisuja 2019:17. Opetus- ja kulttuuriministeriö (2019) http://julkaisut.valtioneuvosto.fi/handle/10024/161577

9. OECD. Continuous Learning in Working Life in Finland, Getting Skills Right. Paris: OECD Publishing (2020). https://doi.org/10.1787/25206125
10. OECD Skills Outlook 2021: Learning for Life, OECD Publishing, Paris (2021). https://doi.org/10.1787/0ae365b4-en
11. Ahonen, O. M., Sanerma, P., Heinonen, J., Rauha, A., Männistö, M.: Multidisciplinary students' self-evaluated competence at the beginning of studies in digital health and social care service specialisation education. Finnish J. EHealth and EWelfare **15**(1), 23–39 (2023). https://doi.org/10.23996/fjhw.122719
12. Tiainen, M., Ahonen, O., Hinkkanen, L., Rajalahti, E., Värri, A.: The definitions of health care and social welfare informatics competencies. Finnish J. EHealth and EWel-fare 13(2), 147–159 (2021). https://doi.org/10.23996/fjhw.100690
13. Act 932/2014.: Act for University of Applied Sciences. Accessed 14th Nov 2014
14. Digivisio Homepage. https://digivisio2030.fi/en/frontpage. (Accessed 19 Jan 2024)
15. IBM Corp. IBM SPSS Statistics for Windows, Version 28.0. Armonk, NY: IBM Corp (2020)
16. Paired t-test: https://libguides.library.kent.edu (Accessed 19 Jan 2024)
17. Kyngäs, H.: Qualitative Research and Content Analysis. In: Kyngäs, H., Mikkonen, K., Kääriäinen, M. (eds.) The Application of Content Analysis in Nursing Science Research. Springer, Cham (2020)
18. Polit, D.F., Tatano, C.: Beck. Nursing Research: Generating and Assessing Evidence for Nursing Practice. 9. edn. Wolters Kluwer Health/Lippincott Williams & Wilkins, Philadelphia (2011)
19. Act 884/2017.: Laki valtakunnallisista opinto ja tutkintorekistereistä

Supporting Sense of Meaningful Life and Human Dignity in Digitally Assisted Physiotherapy Environment – Qualitative Secondary Research with Thematic Analyses and Inductive Synthesis

Tuulikki Sjögren[1]([⊠]) [iD] and Hilkka Korpi[1,2] [iD]

[1] Faculty of Sport and Health, University of Jyväskylä, Jyvaskyla, Finland
tuulikki.sjogren@jyu.fi
[2] Oulu University of Applied Sciences, OAMK, Culture and Welfare, Oulu, Finland

Abstract. The goal of this secondary research was to create a model that aims at increasing the sense of meaningful life and human dignity in physiotherapy by utilizing remote and digital rehabilitation technologies, focusing on people with cerebrovascular accident (CVA) and multiple sclerosis (MS). The results of this qualitative research effort have been obtained using thematic analyses and inductive synthesis. Our primary research, which provides materials for the secondary analysis, is based on qualitative systematic literature reviews and a meta-synthesis of the perceived meaningfulness of physiotherapy. The outcome of the secondary analysis is a research-based model, which combines rehabilitees´ experiences and expectations towards physiotherapy, professionals' competence needs, and the technological prerequisites for using digital rehabilitation technologies with CVA and MS rehabilitees. Maintenance of human dignity and promotion of the sense of meaningful life, and various issues related to them, were most meaningful for the rehabilitees. The essential prerequisites of meaningful use of re- mote and digital rehabilitation technologies in physiotherapy were enabling identification of the rehabilitees' own current functioning, needs and goals, supporting their motivation and commitment, choosing relevant and meaningful activities, creating safe and variable environments, and enabling social interaction and relationships. As far as we know, this is the first model which combines neuro- logical rehabilitees' experiences of physiotherapy with remote and digital technology's potential. In the future, the usefulness of our novel research-based holistic and biopsychosocial physiotherapy model should be tested in real life situations.

Keywords: Human dignity and sense of meaningfulness · Digitalization · Remote physiotherapy · Modelling physiotherapy

1 Introduction

Countries worldwide face challenges linked to population ageing. This demographic trend, coupled with increasing chronic diseases and mental problems poses significant social challenges. Both the active-age and senior citizens' health and functional ability

© The Author(s) 2024
M. Särestöniemi et al. (Eds.): NCDHWS 2024, CCIS 2083, pp. 371–386, 2024.
https://doi.org/10.1007/978-3-031-59080-1_27

need to be supported to lessen the growth in health care costs and thus to ensure the economic and social sustainability of societies. Therefore, there is an increasing need for effective physiotherapy measures, firstly using early rehabilitation before individuals experience debilitating problems, and secondly to alleviate the inevitable later symptoms and functional capacity problems [1–3].

The tendency toward digitalization and greater role of remote techniques in rehabilitation requires new approaches on rehabilitation research. Compared to traditional face-to-face rehabilitation remote rehabilitation, relying to a greater extent on digital technologies, increases the significance of rehabilitees' own commitment and technological skills. This type of change in the rehabilitation paradigm calls for a deeper understanding of those factors which support the rehabilitees' sense of purpose in their efforts to work towards recovery and thus trigger intrinsic motivation. Consequently, the scope of the current mainstream rehabilitation research should be supplemented with more research on broader biopsychosocial, cultural, environmental, or artistic aspects of the rehabilitation process. Typical rehabilitation studies focus on testing the outcomes and short-term effectiveness of a single rehabilitation technique and some- times just on one group of rehabilitees suffering from a single functionality impairment [4–6].

Even in the most recent policy reports, which cover activities in rehabilitation, the medical aspects have the primary role [7–9]. The organization of health and social services are currently at a watershed moment in Finland. In 2023, the organization of health and social services have been transferred from the responsibility of municipalities to 21 wellbeing services counties [10]. As part of this extensive change, it is important to research and develop the use of digitalization and remote technologies even in physiotherapy, and in such a way that individuals' sense of human dignity and meaningful life is preserved during the rehabilitation process.

In future we urgently need an open-minded approach to new technologies to ensure human resources, develop more personalized services, maintain sound public finances, alleviate sustainability crisis, and all-in-all respond to the variable challenges posed by ageing societies [11]. It is important to develop digital solutions which are useful, efficient and sustainable. During the process, rehabilitees' and rehabilitation staffs' attitudes and opinions should be taken into consideration [12, 13]. For example, our recently published study indicated that, 75% of Finnish physiotherapists reported that they used mainly conventional physiotherapy, and remote physiotherapy is still minimally used as the primary working method at different stages of the physiotherapy process [14]. According to physiotherapists, remote rehabilitation techniques are least suit- able for neurological rehabilitees [15], even though they are a group of rehabilitees who are in most need of very intensive therapeutic training as well as guidance, counselling and support in their everyday life [5, 16–18]. Development of rehabilitation platforms, rehabilitation applications, telemedicine solutions and even digital twin solutions are rapidly increasing [19]. There is a lack of digital and remote technology solutions which are rehabilitee-centered, holistic and reflect the biopsychosocial model of rehabilitation for use in neurological physiotherapy. For example, the main contents of commercial models for MS rehabilitees are still narrowly focused on medical care [19, 20], medical aspects of self-care [19, 21], physical activity [19, 22, 23], or self-management [19, 24].

Non-compliance with various therapies and treatments in chronic diseases is a worldwide problem of striking magnitude, making this a critical issue in population health both from the perspective of life quality, and health economics as well as of health system effectiveness [1]. The same problem concerns also home exercise that shows low adherence (as low as 50%), potentially having detrimental effects on clinical outcomes. Some studies highlight that well-designed health technologies provide us with the opportunity to better support both the patient and clinician. Of significance is a data-driven approach that incorporates features designed to increase adherence to exercise, such as coaching, self-monitoring and education, as well as the ability to re- motely monitor adherence rates more objectively [25]. However, a recently published meta-analysis showed that technology assisted self-rehabilitation (remote coaching, self-monitoring, education, and adherence) did not appear to have a significant effect on the outcomes [26]. So, as far as we can conclude, commitment and adherence in self-rehabilitation context is still an unresolved problem in remote physiotherapy [25–28].

The goal of this research was to create a rehabilitation model that aims at sustaining the sense of meaningful life and human dignity in physiotherapy, potentially having positive effects on rehabilitees´ commitment and adherence when using remote and digital rehabilitation technologies. The focus was on people with cerebrovascular accident (CVA) or multiple sclerosis (MS).

2 Materials and Methods

CVA and MS rehabilitees are very suitable study populations for the purpose of this study. CVA and MS have an impact on persons' physical, psychological, social, and cognitive functioning, affecting their daily life activities, participation, and quality of life. In addition to the affected individuals, CVA and MS also place a considerable burden on their families, caregivers, and in overall on the entire society [29, 30]. Since 1990, the prevalence of CVA has increased over 70% worldwide in less than 30 years [31]. Each year, approximately 1.1 million Europeans suffer a stroke, and in 2020 there were an estimated 9.5 million stroke survivors in Europe [32, 33]. By 2030, the stroke prevalence is expected to rise by 35% [34]. An increasing trend can also be seen in people with MS showing a 30% increase from 2013 to 2020 worldwide [35].

This study is a secondary analysis using thematic analyses and inductive synthesis of detected meanings in the materials [36], considering both the results of rehabilitee experiences of meaningful physiotherapy and the results of the experiences in using rehabilitation technology. The primary analyses have been produced as part of our previous line of research using two extensive systematic literature reviews (publication dates extending from Jan. 2001 to Nov. 2017), the first one focusing on CVA rehabilitees and the second one on MS rehabilitees.

The reviews included 50 qualitative studies in total (711 rehabilitees) [16, 17]. The literature search of qualitative studies was conducted from the Cumulative Index to Nursing and Allied Health Literature (CINAHL), the National Library of Medicine (Ovid MEDLINE), and the Education Resources Information Center (ERIC). In addi- tion, the searches were supplemented with manual and reference searches. According to the qualitative PICoS framework, the inclusion criteria were adult CVA and MS rehabilitees (age ≥ 18 years) (P = population or problem, i.e. patient). Our focus of interest was on rehabilitees' views, perceptions, and experiences of physiotherapy (I = interest). In the literature search, the content of physiotherapy was not limited, and different methods, practices and operating environments of physiotherapy used in Finnish physiotherapy were accepted (Co = context). All original studies conducted using a qualitative research design (S = study design) were included. Studies published in English, Swedish, German and Finnish were accepted as data.

The original idea of the study was to use the literature reviews to investigate reha- bili- tee experiences of meaningful physiotherapy. The analysis of the systematic litera- ture (CVA/MS) review data was conducted in five phases: 1) Classifying and summa- rizing the study results according to the PICoS criteria and main results, 2) narrative synthesis of the results [cf.37], 3) constructing lower and upper themes of meaningful experi- ences [cf. 38], 4) metasynthesis of qualitative research results by rehabilitee-specific (CVA/MS) groups, and 5) combining both rehabilitee groups [cf.38]. The stages of the analysis were carried out as triangulation by two pairs of researchers [16, 17].

The results of our primary research have been published in Korpi et al. 2022 [16], Sjögren et al. 2022 [17, 18]. These results have served as the materials for our secondary analysis, which we have divided into three phases. For the first phase of the analysis, we have focused on the rehabilitee experiences of meaningful physiotherapy and re- classified the findings in such a manner that we can create a coherent synthesis (i.e., phase three) when combined the outcomes with the outcomes of the second phase. For the second phase, the sense of meaningfulness in physiotherapy was examined from the perspective of rehabilitation technologies, including remote technologies. Technology use in rehabilitation was not a specific issue in our primary study, but it frequently had come up as part of the experiences tackled by the rehabilitees. These data were analyzed following a standard thematic content analysis process [cf.38]. For the third phase, we have integrated the main results of the previous secondary analysis phases to create a theoretical model as a synthesis of this study. The model is expected to provide tools for sustaining the sense of meaningful life and human dignity in physiotherapy for CVA and MS rehabilitees, particularly when using digital rehabilitation technologies and techniques of remote physiotherapy.

The key concepts used throughout this study are human dignity and sense of mean- ingful life. Human dignity has generally been identified as a concept or phenomenon intertwined with human rights [39] or defined in several various ways [40]. From the perspective of physiotherapy science or rehabilitation we have not tied the concept of human dignity with any single human characteristic (e.g., gender, functional ability) or operational environment (e.g., clinical work). Our perspective is more linked to the general idea that every individual holds a special value that is tied with their humanity. In our research context, human dignity means that during physiotherapy rehabilitation rehabilitates should be treated in such manner that their individual human value and basic human rights, needs and wishes are consistently respected. The sense of meaningful life, in turn, can be associated with, e.g., safety, dependency, flexibility and one's physical and social world [41].

The entire process of secondary analysis was carried out using researcher triangula- tion conducted by the authors. At first, the researchers worked independently by adding the relevant factors of a meaningful physiotherapy process and the use of technology in the same context to the framework originating from the primary analysis ("meaningful experiences of physiotherapy"). Secondly, the researchers formed a consensus over the results by discussing as well as by forming the principal essential prerequisites for meaningful physiotherapy, also focusing on the use of digital and remote technologies.

3 Results

Our secondary analysis confirmed that the most fundamental generic elements in physiotherapy, based on the interpretation of the rehabilitee feedback (mostly interviews), should be preservation of meaningfulness in life and maintenance of human dignity. These elements were primarily reinforced by treating the rehabilitees as individuals, respecting their independence and freedom of choice, promoting their participation in ordinary life, and ensuring that they could preserve faith and hope for the future (see the middle sections in Fig. 1).

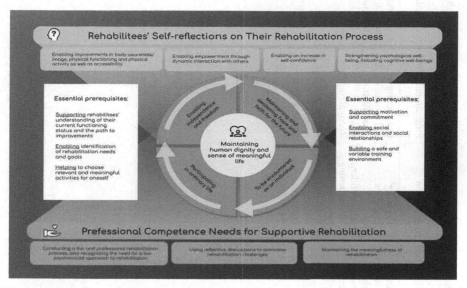

Fig. 1. Technology assisted personalized physiotherapy model: The Human Dignity Centered Rehabilitation approach

Striving for the above listed goals requires a physiotherapy model, which takes into account the following seven factors related to the content of physiotherapy treatment:1) Improving self-confidence, 2) strengthening psychological and cognitive wellbeing, 3) maintaining the meaningfulness of rehabilitation, 4) using reflective discussions to overcome rehabilitation linked challenges, 5) conducting a fair and professional rehabilitation process, also recognizing the need for a holistic biopsychosocial approach to rehabilitation, 6) enabling improvements in body awareness/image, physical functioning and physical activity as well as accessibility, and 7) enabling empowerment through dynamic interaction with others. Table 1 is a concise presentation of all these factors, which have been derived from the systematic literature review data using the applied qualitative analysis approach.

Table 1. Rehabilitees´ experiences in physiotherapy focusing on the elements of human dignity and sense of meaningful life.

Themes supporting human dignity and sense of meaningful life	Rehabilitees self-reflections on their rehabilitation process			Professional competence needs for supportive rehabilitation		
	Enabling improvements in body awareness/image, physical functioning and physical activity as well as accessibility	Enabling empowerment through dynamic interaction with others	Enabling increases in self-confidence Strengthening psychological wellbeing, including cognitive wellbeing	Conducting a fair and professional rehabilitation process Recognizing the Need for a biopsychosocial approach to rehabilitation	Using reflective discussions to overcome rehabilitation challenges	Maintaining the meaningfulness of rehabilitation

(continued)

Table 1. (*continued*)

	Rehabilitees self-reflections on their rehabilitation process			Professional competence needs for supportive rehabilitation		
	Physical functioning and perceived benefits: Physical functioning and participation in society	Social support and relevance of networks: Support from the peers, physiotherapists, friends, and relatives	Psychosocial wellbeing: Mood, psychosocial functioning, and faith in the future	Physiotherapeutic professional competencies, role and significance: Professional skills and experience, positive and considerate attitude, rehabilitation support, individualized therapy and support	Challenges and conflicts in the rehabilitation process: Disappointments, frustration as well as failure to acknowledge individuality, autonomy, accessibility and equality	Experiences of motivation, rehabilitation process requirements and participation: Meaningfulness of exercises, commitment to training, rehabilitation environments and facilities Illness and functional capacity as an individual experience Experience of autonomy, sustainable physiotherapy, participation and use of rehabilitation services Active role in the operating environment, as early and continuous participation as possible positive experiences and hope, individuality and personal wishes regarding physiotherapy, maintenance of hope
People with cerebrovascular accident (CVA) Korpi et al. 2022 [16]						
People with multiple sclerosis (MS) Sjögren et al. 2022 [17]	Body awareness and body functions, physical activity (capacity), physical functioning in everyday life (performance), self-rehabilitation	Working together, being understood, obtained support from physiotherapy	Self-confidence, positive emotions, active everyday life	Good rehabilitee-therapist relationship, diverse and wide-ranging guidance skills, specialized expertise related to the disease, therapeutic permanence	Decreasing physical functioning, failure to reconcile the needs with provision, experiences of failure	Taking into consideration individual autonomy, goal-oriented actions and processes as well as diverse operating environments

Table 2. Examples of rehabilitees' experiences focusing on rehabilitation technology assisted physiotherapy.

Themes Reflecting perceived essential prerequisites for technology assisted physiotherapy	Supporting motivation and commitment	Enabling social interactions and social relationships	Building a safe and variable training environment	Helping to choose relevant and meaningful activities for oneself	Enabling identification of rehabilitation needs and goals	Supporting rehabilitees' understanding of their current functioning status and the path to improvements
Perceived meaningfulness of physiotherapy (CVA) Korpi et al. 2022 [16]	Nintendo Wii game console was experienced to be easy to use and fun Gaming was seen as a new and challenging method of rehabilitation The rehabilitees encouraged their peers to try this method [44] Games were found entertaining and fun and were also regarded to facilitate adherence to rehabilitation [44]	Rehabilitees brought up the idea of developing a rehabilitation app for smartphones, and many of them emphasized that telephone could be a very effective way to maintain contact with their personal physiotherapist [45] Remote communication with their physiotherapist encouraged rehabilitees to become engaged in activities [45] The opportunity to use text messaging was especially beneficial for people with aphasia [45]	Weekly contact by phone was more important for those rehabilitees who could not leave their home due to poor physical mobility or who, for any reason, spent most of their time alone [46]	Digital gaming improved one's possibilities to exercise and recuperate, following one's own preferred schedule [44] Rehabilitees were annoyed by the lack of alternative modes of physiotherapy and exercises in the public sector They proposed Nintendo Wii game console or something similar, which could diversify the available modes of exercising, either independently at home or as part of a structured exercise program [44]	Technology assisted training could help in maintaining hope and therefore encourage the rehabilitees to continue practicing until the desired and valued activity level has been reached [45] Rehabilitees appreciated that digital games gave them instant feedback using metric scores, which helped them to measure their personal development [46]	Digital gaming (e.g. Nintendo Wii game console) had positive effects on cognition. Gaming required concentration and simultaneously exercised both the hand and brain [44] Digital gaming (e.g. Nintendo Wii game console) was perceived challenging. However, gaming was considered good for hand rehabilitation Overcoming the challenges took the rehabilitee to the next level [46] Rehabilitees considered conventional physiotherapy more like physical training whereas virtual reality games were considered demanding in terms of mental and precision exercises [47]

(continued)

Table 2. (*continued*)

Themes Reflecting perceived essential prerequisites for technology assisted physiotherapy	Supporting motivation and commitment	Enabling social interactions and social relationships	Building a safe and variable training environment	Helping to choose relevant and meaningful activities for oneself	Enabling identification of rehabilitation needs and goals	Supporting rehabilitees' understanding of their current functioning status and the path to improvements
Perceived meaningfulness of physiotherapy (MS) Sjögren et al 2022 [17]	Rehabilitees experienced that digital technology assisted exercises had positive effects on the sense of independence and helped to regain control of the disease [48] Technology assisted exercises motivated rehabilitees to excel themselves. They wanted to perform exercises which they had not been able to perform previously, or they wanted to perform better in games they already had played [48]	Digital gaming was found to increase the sense of togetherness with one's significant others. The rehabilitees reported that they played games together with their children, family members and friends [48, 49] Rehabilitees perceived that digital games (e.g. games using the Microsoft Kinect motion controller) could assist in opening a window to the outside world. They could enhance connections beyond one's own living sphere, e.g., communicate with other rehabilitees elsewhere and establish new social relationships [48]	Technology assisted exercises made it possible to challenge balance and body control in a safe environment, which also increased one's self-efficacy related to their balance [49] Digital gaming technology enabled effective, challenging, safe [49] and flexible [50] way to do exercises at home It was particularly important for those who lived far from the city center [48, 50] Technology assisted training was an alternative to outdoor physical training when the weather was bad, or if one had not much time for training [49]	Technology assisted exercises supported rehabilitation processes because the progress was monitored by physiotherapists [50] Men in particular were satisfied with technology assisted training at home because they found group training embarrassing [50]	Rehabilitees were satisfied with the instant feedback given by digital games regarding the time spent and positive results of exercises [49] Rehabilitees appreciated that the gameplay gave them the opportunity to compare their previous performances and set their own goals The possibility of moving to the next level was also perceived as positive [49]	Rehabilitees who had reached higher scores when using digital games did not experience that their everyday activities had correspondingly improved [49] Rehabilitees experienced that gamified exercises were both physically and cognitively unexpectedly demanding, and some of the rehabilitees felt that they needed to rest after the exercises [49]

Keeping in mind the key generic elements of rehabilitation, the process should sup- port the sense of meaningful life and respect rehabilitees' human dignity, even when conventional physiotherapy is supplemented with remote and digital physiother- apy technologies. Such technologies pose obvious challenges, particularly in terms of pro- fessionals' competence requirements, but our results show that digital and remote technologies can also open a window for new opportunities, supposing that the techno- logical solutions are innovative and fit for people facing various disabilities (see Table 2). Such technologies could enable rehabilitees' self-management, ensuring their autonomy, flexibility, and progressive ownership of the rehabilitation process. Rehabilitation tech- nologies could also offer opportunities for equal dialogue, easy communication and fast contact with rehabilitation professionals thus empowering an equal, professional, comprehensive, and fair rehabilitation process. The important elements of (digital) tech- nology assisted physiotherapy consist of the following issues: 1) Motivation and com- mitment support, 2) enablement of social interactions and social relationships, 3) design of safe and variable training environments, 4) flexibility in choosing relevant and mean- ingful activities for oneself, 5) identification of rehabilitation needs and goals, 6) support for rehabilitees to understand their current functioning status and the appropriate paths to improvement (see the left and right edge in Fig. 1).

4   Discussion

The goal of this secondary analysis was to create a practical model for implementation of physiotherapy treatment which support the maintenance and reinforcement of the sense of human dignity and meaningful life among physiotherapy rehabilitees, particu- larly when using remote and digital techniques in physiotherapy. Based on our primary research [16, 17] human dignity and sense of meaningful life appeared to be the most fundamental generic elements in aspired physiotherapy, based on the interpretation of the rehabilitee feedback. This central finding was reinforced by our secondary analysis, which also increased our understanding of the key factors which are considered essen- tial in the content of physiotherapy treatment, both in conventional and remote/digitally supported physiotherapy. The results also gave ideas about the plausible advantages of digital rehabilitation techniques as well as the challenges related to the use of such techniques, the latter being largely linked with current competence requirements of the physiotherapy professionals.

We believe that our rehabilitee-oriented model emphasizing the essential role of in- dependence and freedom of choice, promoting social interactions, participation in the society and in ordinary life, and preservation of faith in the future, all of which help to promote the sense of human dignity and meaningful life, enables stronger adherence to physiotherapy as well as positive effects on biopsychosocial functioning and quality of life among rehabilitees. Rehabilitees´ strong commitment to their rehabilitation process is likely to become even more important in the future, because due to population ageing and cost pressure on public expenditure it is unavoidable that digital services are becom- ing more significant across all sectors of the society, including medical and rehabilitation services [4, 6]. Digitalization of rehabilitation services is likely to increase the role of remote activities in physiotherapy, a central topic in our research effort. This will be a huge paradigm change because, so far, physiotherapy services have mostly been offered as face-to-face treatment [14, 15].

From this perspective, our study approach is valuable, because so far scientific research has largely reflected the traditional rehabilitation research paradigm of quantitative effectiveness studies [e.g., 4]. The expected new physiotherapy and rehabilitation paradigm calls for new approaches to rehabilitation research. To our knowledge, this kind of modelling we have carried out in this paper has not been done before in physiotherapy, at least not among people with CVA and MS rehabilitees.

Our secondary analysis is linked to authors' previous study efforts, in which the goal has been to evaluate effectiveness of physiotherapy and increase understanding of the meaningfulness of physiotherapy among CVA and MS rehabilitees [see 5]. The strength of the study and created physiotherapy model is that it is based on extensive and comprehensive research data (50 studies, 771 rehabilitees) [16, 17] and supported by the authors' long-term experiences in the field of physiotherapy and their intensive researcher triangulation working method extending over all the phases of the research process. During the entire development process (2021–2023) of the model we have also subjected its earlier versions to expert scrutiny at different occasions (conferences, workshops). Expert feedback (researchers, clinicians, teachers) reinforced the view that our research scope focusing on understanding the elements of meaningful physiotherapy, and of even multidisciplinary rehabilitation, in the context of remote and digitally assisted activities is important.

The limitation in our research is that it focuses only on neurological rehabilitees suffering from CVA and MS. Despite the specific disease etiology of CVA and MS, we are quite confident that the generic results of our secondary analysis are generally applicable to physiotherapy. Whatever is causing the limitations in persons' physical, psychological, social, or cognitive abilities, their fundamental desire is to get treatment that makes them feel that they are valued as individuals and promotes their sense of meaningful life, regardless of the degree of improvement in their condition. However, the role of the more practical elements of physiotherapeutic activities can vary depending on what is causing the need for rehabilitation. Therefore, it would be important to study also other rehabilitee groups, e.g. cardiac, chronic pain or dementia patients. Moreover, the study of various rehabilitee groups is essential considering the use of remote and digitally assisted physiotherapy to learn more about how technology can best be utilized with individuals suffering from various health and functionality related issues. All in all, it is important to test our research-based physiotherapy model and future variations of it in real-life settings evaluating the degree of improved adherence and effectiveness of physiotherapy and improved meaningfulness, compared to the results of conventional physiotherapy [cf. 4–6]. The scope of future research should also be extended to the different stages of functioning (primary, secondary and tertiary prevention).

The general opinion appears to be that increased availability of technology, particularly digital technology, is the driving force when societies are moving towards more effective and cost-effective availability of services [42]. However, there are still few studies in rehabilitation that have investigated the cost-effectiveness of technology assisted rehabilitation [cf. 5, 43]. This would be a challenging and complex research topic because one should be able to project simultaneously both short- and longer-term cost effects.

For example, enhancing primary (preventive) rehabilitation may increase spending in the short term but making relevant technology accessible and alluring could decrease future costs in secondary or tertiary rehabilitation. Furthermore, as we have pointed out, factors which strengthen rehabilitees' own commitment to physiotherapy may increase initial costs in physiotherapy but can be of major importance in terms of short- and mid-term effectiveness as well as longer-term impacts. This kind of thinking is crucial in terms of our research approach, and we hope that our research findings will pave the way for developing new modes of rehabilitation services provision. For example, in Finland, people receiving intensive medical rehabilitation has increased from 20000 to almost 40000 individuals in less than 15 years [3].

Countries worldwide are facing similar challenges, at least to some degree. Effective rehabilitation, particularly when extended to preventive rehabilitation, is expected to lessen the burden on health care costs in the long-run and ensure the maintenance of functional capabilities of the working age population. On top of these practical policy issues, we hope that our research and the human dignity and sense of meaningful life centered physiotherapy contribute to the development of theoretical and even philosophical understanding of physiotherapy.

Acknowledgements. Thank you to all who were part of the research project Effectiveness of physiotherapy in multiple sclerosis and cerebrovascular disorder patients' rehabilitation: systematic literature review (In Finnish: Fysioterapian vaikuttavuus vaativassa lääkinnällisessä AVH- ja MS-kuntoutuksessa: järjestelmällinen kirjallisuuskatsaus (2016–22) at the University of Jyväskylä and contributed to this study.

Conflict of Interest Statement. The Authors declare that there is no conflict of interest.

Funding. The authors disclosed receipt of the following financial support for the re- search, authorship, and/or publication of this article: This work was supported by the Social Insurance Institution of Finland (Kela) [Dnro 4212612076].

Data Availability Statement. The data that support the findings of this study are available from the corresponding author, (TS), upon reasonable request.

References

1. Adherence to long-term therapies 2003 Adherence to Long-term Therapies: Evidence for Action. Eduardo Sabaté (Editor). World Health Organization. (2003). ISBN: 92 4 154599
2. Cieza, A., Causey, K., Kamenov, K., Wulf Hanson S., Chatterji S., Vos T.: Global estimates of the need for rehabilitation based on the Global Burden of Disease study (2019)
3. Heino, P., Mäkinen, J., Seppänen-Järvelä, R.: Vaativan lääkinnällisen kuntoutuksen lainmuutoksen vaikutus kuntoutuksen kohdentumiseen. Rekisteritutkimus vuosien 2014, 2016 ja 2017 kuntoutuspäätöksistä. Helsinki: Kela, Sosiaali- ja terveysturvan raportteja 23, (2020). 115 s. ISBN 978–952–284–108–7 (pdf)
4. Rintala, A., Hakala, S., Sjögren, T., (eds.) Etäteknologian vaikuttavuus liikunnallisessa kuntoutuksessa: Järjestelmällinen kirjallisuuskatsaus ja meta-analyysit. Helsinki, Finland: Kansaneläkelaitos. Sosiaali- ja terveysturvan tutkimuksia, 145. (2017). http://hdl.handle.net/10138/180932 Open access

5. Sjögren, T., Rintala, A., Paltamaa, J., Korpi, H. (eds.): Järjestelmälliset kirjallisuuskatsaukset fysioterapian vaikuttavuudesta ja merkityksellisyydestä aivoverenkiertohäiriö ja multippeliskleroosi kuntoutujilla. – Kävelyn ja tasapainon meta-analyysit sekä koetun fysioterapian merkityksellisyyden metasynteesit. Sosiaali- ja terveysturvan tutkimuksia, 145. Kansaneläkelaitos (2022)

6. Ilves, O., Korpi, H., Honkonen, S., Aartolahti, E. (eds.): Robottien, virtuaalitodellisuuden ja lisätyn todellisuuden vaikuttavuus ja merkityksellisyys lääkinnällisessä kuntoutuksessa. Järjestelmälliset kirjallisuuskatsaukset. Kansaneläkelaitos (2022)

7. OKM & STM: Kuntoutuksen koulutuksen ja tutkimuksen kehittämisfoorumi. Kuntoutuksen koulutuksentilannekuva.Väliraportti (2022). https://api.hankeikkuna.fi/asiakirjat/90d774f1-6f16-4b5f-881b-709dac418d75/c739a5b2-7c3a-4887-b454-6d34967bad14/RAPORTTI_20220201061618.pdf

8. OKM & STM: Kuntoutuksen koulutuksen ja tutkimuksen kehittämisfoorumi. Kuntoutuksen osaamis- ja työelämätarpeet. Väliraportti (2022). https://api.hankeikkuna.fi/asiakir-jat/90d774f1-6f16-4b5f-881b-709dac418d75/29698060-f6bf-4041-b776-6d446fb27446/RAPORTTI_20220119114212.pdf

9. OKM & STM: Kuntoutuksen koulutuksen ja tutkimuksen kehittämisfoorumi. Kuntoutuksen tutkimuksen tilannekuva. Väliraportti (2022). https://api.hankeikkuna.fi/asiakirjat/90d774f1-6f16-4b5f-881b-709d

10. Tynkkynen, LK., Keskimäki, I., Karanikolos, M., Litvinova, Y.: Finland: Health system summary (2023). ISSN 2958–9193 (online) ISBN 9789289059398

11. Lehto, P., Malkamäki, S.: The Finnish health sector growth and competitiveness vision 2030. Sitra Publications. Referred 11.10.2023. (2023) https://www.sitra.fi

12. Landi, D., et al.: Patient's point of view on the use of telemedicine in multiple sclerosis: a web-based survey. Neurological Sciences 2021 (43), 1197–1205. (2021). https://link-springer-com.ezproxy.jyu.fi/article/, https://doi.org/10.1007/s10072-021-05398-6

13. Sjögren, T., Anttila, M-R., Kivistö, H., Haapaniemi, V., Paajanen, T., Piirainen, A.: Innovatiiviset etäkuntoutuspalvelut kirjassa Kokemuksia etäkuntoutuksesta. Kelan etäkuntoutushankkeen tuloksia (eds. Salminen A-L & Hiekkala 206–225–225. Kela, Helsinki (2019). 978-952–284–066–0 (nid.) 978–952–284–067–7 (pdf)

14. Hellstén, T. Arokoski, J., Sjögren, T., Jäppinen, A-M., Kettunen, J.: Remote physiotherapy in Finland – suitability, usability, and factors affecting its use. European J. Physiother. (2023). https://doi.org/10.1080/21679169.2023.2233560

15. Hellstén, T., Arokoski, J., Sjögren, T., Jäppinen, A-M., Kettunen, J.: The current state of remote physiotherapy in finland: cross-sectional web-based questionnaire study. JMIR Rehabilit. Assistive Technol. 9(2), e35569. (2022) doi: https://doi.org/10.2196/35569

16. Korpi, H., Lahtio, H., Holopainen, R., Mastola, S., Sjögren, T.: Fysioterapian merkityksellisyys AVH-kuntoutujille. In: Sjögren, T., Rintala, A., Paltamaa, J., Korpi, H. (eds.) Fysioterapian vaikuttavuus ja merkityksellisyys aivoverenkiertohäiriötä ja multippeliskleroosia sairastaville kuntoutujille. Järjestelmälliset kirjallisuuskatsaukset, pp. 116–160. Kela. Sosiaali- ja terveysturvan tutkimuksia 161 (2022). http://urn.fi/URN:NBN:fi-fe2022110163955

17. Sjögren, T., Lahtio, H., Holopainen R., Korpi H.: Fysioterapian merkityksellisyys MS-kuntoutujille, järjestelmälliset kirjallisuuskatsaukset ja metasynteesi (2022). In: Sjögren, T., Rintala, A., Paltamaa, J., Korpi, H. (eds.) Fysioterapian vaikuttavuus ja merkityksellisyys aivoverenkiertohäiriötä ja multippeliskleroosia sairastaville kuntoutujille. Järjestelmälliset kirjallisuuskatsaukset. Sosiaali- ja terveysturvan tutkimuksia, pp. 199–2020. Sosiaali- ja terveysturvan tutkimuksia 161 (2022). http://urn.fi/URN:NBN:fi-fe2022110163955

18. Sjögren, T., Rintala, A., Paltamaa, J., Korpi, H.: Järjestelmälliset kirjallisuuskatsaukset fysioterapian vaikuttavuudesta ja merkityksellisyydestä aivoverenkiertohäiriö ja multippeliskleroosi kuntoutujilla. – Kävelyn ja tasapainon meta-analyysit sekä koetun fysioterapian merkityksellisyyden metasynteesit. In: Sjögren, T., Rintala, A., Paltamaa, J., Korpi, H. (eds.) Fysioterapian vaikuttavuus ja merkityksellisyys aivoverenkiertohäiriötä ja multippeliskleroosia sairastaville kuntoutujille. Järjestelmälliset kirjallisuuskatsaukset, pp. 223–234. Sosiaali- ja terveysturvan tutkimuksia, 145 (2022)

19. Laine, S., Laitinen, A., Leinonen, H., Lähde, S.: eKuntoutus-platform for social-, healthcare- and rehabilitation practices in finland -Unique rehabilitee pathway is the key to meaningfulness (2023)

20. Voig, I., Inojosa, H., Dillenseger, A., Haase, R., Akgün, K., Ziemssen, T.: Digital Twins for Multiple Sclerosis. Front. Immunol. **2021**(12), 669811 (2021). https://doi.org/10.3389/fimmu.2021.669811

21. Van Hecke, W., et al.: A novel digital care management platform to monitor clinical and subclinical disease activity in multiple sclerosis. Brain Sci. **11**(9), 1171 (2021). https://doi.org/10.3390/brainsci11091171

22. Busse, M., et al.: Web-based physical activity intervention for people with progressive multiple sclerosis: application of consensus-based intervention development guidance. BMJ Open **11**(3), e045378 (2021). https://doi.org/10.1136%2Fbmjopen-2020-045378

23. Geurts, E., van Geel, F., Feys, P.: WalkWithMe: personalized goal setting and coaching for walking in people with multiple sclerosis. In: Research Gate: Conference Paper 2019 (2019) https://doi.org/10.1145/3320435.3320459

24. Jongen, P., et al.: The interactive web-based program Msmonitor for self- management and multidisciplinary care in multiple sclerosis: concept, content, and pilot results. Dovepress **2015**(9), 1741–1750 (2015)

25. Argent, R., Daly, A., Caulfied, B.: Patient Involvement with Home-Based Exercise Programs: Can Connected Health Interventions Influence Adherence? JMIR Mhealth **6**(3), e47 (2018). https://doi.org/10.2196/mhealth.8518

26. Matamala-Gomez, M., et al.: The Role of Engagement in Teleneurorehabilitation: A Systematic Review. Front. Neurol. **11**, 354 (2020)

27. Zasadzka, E., Trzmiel, T., Pieczyńska, A., Hojan, K.: Modern Technologies in the Rehabilitation of Patients with Multiple Sclerosis and Their Potential Application in Times of COVID-19. Medicina **57**(6), 549 (2021). https://doi.org/10.3390/medicina57060549

28. Hakala, S., Kivistö, H., Paajanen, T., Kankainen, A., Anttila, M-R., Heinonen, A., Sjögren, T.: Effectiveness of Distance Technology in Promoting Physical Activity in Cardiovascular Disease Rehabilitation: Cluster Randomized Controlled Trial, A Pilot Study JMIR Rehabil. Assist. Technol. 8(2), e0299 (2021). https://doi.org/10.2196/20299 PMID: 34142970PMCID: 8277324

29. Purmonen, T., Hakkarainen, T., Tervomaa, M., Ruutiainen, J.: Impact of multiple sclerosis phenotypes on burden of disease in Finland. J. Med. Econ. **23**(2), 156–165 (2020). https://doi.org/10.1080/13696998.2019.1682004

30. Luengo-Fernandez, R., Violato, M., Candio, P., Leal, J.: Economic burden of stroke across Europe: A population-based cost analysis. Eur. Stroke J. **5**(1), 17–25 (2020). https://doi.org/10.1177/2396987319883160

31. GBD: Stroke Collaborators 2021. Lancet Neurol **20**, 795–820 (2019)

32. Wafa, H.A., Wolfe, C.D.A., Emmett, E., Roth, G.A., Johnson, C.O., Wang, Y.: Burden of stroke in Europe: thirty-year projections of incidence, prevalence, deaths, and disability-adjusted life years. Stroke **51**(8), 2418–2427 (2020)

33. Bejot, Y., Bailly, H., Durier, J., Giroud, M.: Epidemiology of stroke in Europe and trends for the 21st century. Presse Med. **45**(12 Pt 2):e3), ee398 (2016)

34. Norrving, B., Barrick, J., Davalos, A., et al.: Action Plan for Stroke in Europe 2018–2030. European Stroke J. **3**(4), 309–336 (2018). https://doi.org/10.1177/2396987318808719
35. Walton, C., King, R., Rechtman, L., et al.: Rising prevalence of multiple sclerosis worldwide: Insights from the Atlas of MS, third edition. Multiple Sclerosis J. **26**(14), 1816- 1821 (2020). https://doi.org/10.1177/1352458520970841
36. Clarke, V., Braun, V.: Thematic analysis. J. Posit. Psychol. **12**(3), 297–298 (2017)
37. Elliot, A.J.: Using narrative in social research: Qualitative and quantitative approaches. Sage, London (2005)
38. Sandelowski, M., Barroso, J.: Handbook for synthesizing qualitative research. Springer, New York, NY (2007)
39. Göbel, M.C.: Human Dignity as the Ground of Human Rights - A Study in Moral Philosophy and Legal Practice 2018, p. 147. University of Amsterdam (2018)
40. Kadivar, M., Mardani-Hamooleh, M., Kouhnavard, M.: Concept analysis of human dignity in patient care: Rodgers' evolutionary approach. J. Med. Ethics. Hist. Med. **18**, 118; 11:4018). PMID: 30258554; PMCID: PMC6150922
41. Levack, W., Thornton, K.: Opportunities for a meaningful life for working-aged adults with neurological conditions living in residential aged care facilities: A review of qualitative research. British J. Occupat. Therapy **80**(10), 608–619 (2017). https://doi.org/10.1177/030 8022617722736
42. Poon, C.C.Y., Zhang, Y.T.: Some perspectives on high technologies for low-cost healthcare: Chinese scenario. IEEE Eng. Med. Biol. **27**, 42–47 (2008)
43. Sjögren, T., Rintala, A., Hakala, S., Piirainen, A., Heinonen, A.: Yhteenveto: etäteknologia osana liikunnallista kuntoutusta In: Rintala, A, Hakala, S, Ja Sjögren, T. (eds.) Etäteknologian vaikuttavuus liikunnallisessa kuntoutuksessa: Järjestelmällinen kirjallisuuskatsaus ja meta- analyysit, pp. 156–163. Helsinki, Finland: Kansaneläkelaitos. Sosiaali- ja terveysturvan tutkimuksia, 145. (2017). http://hdl.handle.net/10138/180932 Open access
44. Paquin, K., Crawley, J., Harris, J.E., Horton, S.: Survivors of chronic stroke. Participant evaluations of commercial gaming for rehabilitation. Disability Rehabilit. **38**(21), 2144–2152 (2016). https://doi.org/10.3109/09638288.2015.1114155
45. Saywell, N., Taylor, D.: Focus group insights assist trial design for stroke telerehabilitation. a qualitative study. Physiotherapy Theory Pract. **31**(3), 160–165 (2015). https://doi.org/10. 3109/09593985.2014.982234
46. Wingham, J., Adie, K., Turner, D., Schofield, C., Pritchard, C.: Participant and caregiver experience of the Nintendo Wii SportsTM after stroke. Qualitative study of the trial of WiiTM in stroke (TWIST). Clinical Rehabilit. **29**(3), 295–305 (2015). https://doi.org/10.1177/026 9215514542638
47. Lewis, G.N., Woods, C., Rosie, J.A., Mcpherson, K.M.: Virtual reality games for rehabilitation of people with stroke. Perspectives from the users. Disability Rehabilit. Assistive Technol. **6**(5), 453–463 (2011). https://doi.org/ https://doi.org/10.3109/17483107.2011.574310
48. Palacios-Ceña, D., et al. Multiple sclerosis patients' experiences in relation to the impact of the kinect virtual home-exercise programme. A qualitative study. European Journal of Phys. Rehabilit. Med. **52**(3), 347–355 (2016)
49. Forsberg, A., Nilsagård, Y., Boström, K.: Perceptions of using videogames in rehabilitation. A dual perspective of people with multiple sclerosis and physiotherapists. Disability Rehabilit. **37**(4), 338–344 (2015). https://doi.org/ https://doi.org/10.3109/09638288.2014.918196
50. Paul, L., Coulter, E., Miller, L, McFadyen, A., Dorfman, J., Mattison, P.: Web-based physiotherapy for people moderately affected with multiple sclerosis. Quantitative and qualitative data from a randomized, controlled pilot study. Clinical Rehabilit. **28**(9), 924–935 (2014). https://doi.org/10.1177/0269215514527995

Abstracts

Towards 6G Technology Enabled Wearable Patient Monitoring – A Pilot Study in Radiotherapy Treatment Pathway

Teemu Myllylä[1,2,3]($\boxtimes$), Sakari S. Karhula[1,2,4], Daljeet Singh[1],
Jesse Lohela[1,2,4], Sadegh Moradi[3], Kalle Inget[1,2,4],
Vesa Korhonen[1,2,5], Mariella Särestöniemi[1,6], Jarmo Reponen[1,2],
Risto Jurva[6], Tuomo Hänninen[6], Olli Liinamaa[6], Erkki Harjula[6],
and Juha Nikkinen[1,2,4]

[1] Research Unit of Health Sciences and Technology, University of Oulu, Oulu,
Finland
{teemu.myllyla, sakari.karhula, daljeet.singh, jesse.
lohela, kalle.inget, vesa.korhonen, mariella.
sarestoniemi, jarmo.reponen, juha.nikkinen}@oulu.fi
[2] Medical Research Center, Oulu, Finland
[3] Optoelectronics and Measurement Techniques Unit, University of Oulu, Oulu,
Finland
sadegh.moradi@oulu.fi
[4] Department of Oncology and Radiotherapy, Oulu University Hospital, Oulu,
Finland
[5] Department of Diagnostic Radiology, Oulu University Hospital, Oulu, Finland
[6] Centre for Wireless Communications (CWC), University of Oulu, Oulu,
Finland
{risto.jurva, tuomo.hanninen, olli.liinamaa,
erkki.harjula}@oulu.fi

Abstract. Radiotherapy is known as the most effective non-surgical treatment for many cancers, resulting in the elimination of tumor cells by irradiation. Nevertheless, it may cause also side effects particularly in brain cancer treatment, for instance, cognition affecting sub-acutely or chronically and fatigue patients. Many techniques can be employed to detect the adverse pathological changes caused by irradiation, such as, positron emission tomography (PET) and magnetic resonance imaging (MRI). However, possibilities to examine possible changes in the brain function due to the radiotherapy are still limited. For this, easy to use wearable or portable emerging brain monitoring technology that can be used both in hospital and at home could offer new perspectives. Furthermore, wearable technology supported by 6G wireless technology with more advanced cloud and edge computing capabilities may open a new era for the patient monitoring. In brain cancer radiotherapy, it is important to detect in individual level both immediate and long-term effects in brain function. To this end, the basic concepts of the initial pilot in radiotherapy utilizing 6G technology and emerging brain monitoring technology are presented.

Keywords: Patient Monitoring · Brain · Tumor · Cloud Computing

M. Särestöniemi et al. (Eds.): NCDHWS 2024, CCIS 2083, pp. 389–391, 2024.
https://doi.org/10.1007/978-3-031-59080-1

1   Introduction

The 6G technology will be able to accommodate an incredible amount of data with the help of intelligent cloud. The clinical data will be accessible on multiple devices with very strong authentication which will require collaboration among various data stakeholders, like data generation (users/machines), communications to nodes and server storage operations. The processing of such a huge amount of data will require strong artificial intelligence (AI) and machine learning (ML) capabilities in terms of pre-processing, filtering, information retrieval to build smart data-driven applications. Many new healthcare applications have been envisioned or will be created in near future as a result of 6G health technology, and importantly, it also supports the transition of healthcare from hospitals to home [1, 2].

In addition, the collection and transmission of data recorded by wearable sensors is an equally important aspect of smart healthcare permitting network-assisted consultations with medical experts. This will allow early patient discharge from hospitals while health monitoring continues at home. This pilot study aims to respond, using modern technology and research techniques, to the high demand for more optimized treatment strategies for each individual patient with a brain tumor. We investigate potentials to monitor brain cancer patients in their clinical pathway in radiotherapy. Furthermore, based on our previous findings [3], we further study possibilities to measure physiological effects of the treatment by wearable and wireless brain monitoring technology.

2   Materials and Methods

Brain cancer patients typically undergo several radiotherapy treatments, however, possibilities to measure the immediate effects of the treatment on a patient are limited, but the effects of radiotherapy can only be evaluated after the treatment has been completed. Moreover, since the effects of cancer treatment are highly variable, even conventional doses administered to patients can cause long-term side effects in some people [4]. By utilizing 6G enabled brain monitoring technology our goal is to find correlations between the brain data signal trends and treatment effectiveness, see Fig. 1.

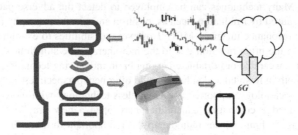

Fig. 1. Clinical data recordings by utilizing 6G wireless wearable brain monitoring technology are performed between multiple treatments to study corresponding brain effects and signal trends caused by the radiotherapy. 6G wireless technology with advanced cloud computing and data management capabilities will enable us to observe in real time brain effects and develop algorithms that we aim to correlate with the radiotherapy effectiveness in individual patients.

We implement wireless and wearable patient monitoring in Oulu University Hospital. In addition, patient questionnaire using DigitalHands remote monitoring solution provided by Siemens Healthineers is used to collect additional information on possible cognitive changes of the patient, which are then compared to brain data findings. The initial study includes up to 20 patients having multiple brain cancer radiotherapy treatments. Brain data recordings are performed before and after each treatment.

3   Discussion

We hypothesize that by combining modern radiotherapy and wearable brain monitoring technologies supported by 6G technology we may provide better possibilities to control the radiotherapy outcome in brain cancer. This will eventually allow patients to retain their functionality and improve their quality of life and prognosis while minimizing unnecessary treatments.

Currently, over a thousand primary central nervous system (CNS) tumors are diagnosed yearly in Finland, and the numbers are only increasing. In the future, the burden will become crucial for health care when more patients require surgical, radiotherapeutic, chemotherapeutic, or a combination of these treatment modalities. Our project offers new approaches for diagnosis-making, treatment planning, and monitoring treatment responses to ease this increasing pressure. To our knowledge, we are the first group targeting optimization to this extent.

Acknowledgments. This work is supported by the Academy of Finland Profi6 programme: 6G-Enabling Sustainable Society (6GESS) and 6G Flagship programme, and Business Finland 6GBRIDGE - Next generation healthcare and wearable diagnostics utilizing 6G project (11146/31/2022).

Disclosure of Interests. Authors have nothing to disclose.

References

1. Nayak, S., Patgiri, R.: 6G communication technology: a vision on intelligent healthcare. In: Patgiri, R., Biswas, A., Roy, P. (eds.) Health Informatics: A Computational Perspective in Healthcare. SCI, vol. 932, pp. 1–18. Springer, Singapore (2021). https://doi.org/10.1007/978-981-15-9735-0_1
2. Nasralla, M.M., Khattak, S.B.A., Ur Rehman, I., Iqbal, M.: Exploring the role of 6G technology in enhancing quality of experience for m-health multimedia applications: a comprehensive survey. Sensors **23**(13), 5882 (2023)
3. Myllylä, T., et al.: Cerebral tissue oxygenation response to brain irradiation measured during clinical radiotherapy. J. Biomed. Opt. **28**(1), 015002 (2023)
4. Barazzuol, L., Coppes, R.P., van Luijk, P.: Prevention and treatment of radiotherapy-induced side effects. Mol. Oncol. **14**(7), 1538–1554 (2020)

Considering the Potential Use of Oura Ring for Remote Monitoring at Home: The Perspective of Ageing Neurological Patients

Melika Azim Zadegan[1]($\boxtimes$) (iD), Rosa Sahlström[2] (iD), Eeva Aromaa[1],
Tero Montonen[1] (iD), Päivi Eriksson[1] (iD), and Ville Leinonen[3] (iD)

[1] Business School, University of Eastern Finland, Kuopio, Finland
melika.azim.zadegan@uef.fi

[2] Neurosurgery, Institute of Clinical Medicine, University of Eastern Finland,
Kuopio, Finland

[3] Department of Neurosurgery, NeuroCenter, Kuopio University Hospital
Neurosurgery, Kuopio, Finland

Abstract. This study involves structured interviews with ten elderly patients (aged 64–79) at the Kuopio University Hospital, exploring their perceptions and expectations of using the Oura ring for Digital Remote Monitoring (DRM) in suspected idiopathic Normal Pressure Hydrocephalus (iNPH) cases. With ethical approval, the interviews focused on demographics, current technology use, and views on the Oura ring's potential application. Most participants, experienced with digital health devices, were positive about DRM's home use, highlighting the importance of user-friendly design, privacy, accuracy, and perceived usefulness. Concerns and expectations also extended to healthcare professionals' roles in ensuring real-time health tracking and support. The study underscores patients' desire to actively manage their health and the role of family in this process, reflecting on the empowerment and safety that informed, timely data can provide. It highlights the evolving patient-caregiver dynamic in the context of home-based health monitoring technologies.

Keywords: Digital Remote Monitoring · Expectations · Oura Ring

1 Introduction

Digital Remote Monitoring (DRM) employs telemonitoring devices in patients' homes to electronically link their health data to clinical sites. This promising health intervention supports home-based care by enhancing patients' ability to manage their health [1] and improving patient satisfaction and quality of life [2]. While healthcare innovations such as telemedicine receive mixed reviews—with some emphasizing their potential and others highlighting adoption challenges [3]—the increasing involvement of patients in DRM raises questions about potential challenges and the effectiveness of these approaches [4]. Previous studies have largely focused on evaluating patient experiences with digital wearables during or after adoption. Yet, understanding patients' expectations of digital monitoring and specific wearables before implementation is crucial [5]. The Oura ring, a compact and lightweight consumer wearable

M. Särestöniemi et al. (Eds.): NCDHWS 2024, CCIS 2083, pp. 392–394, 2024.
https://doi.org/10.1007/978-3-031-59080-1

designed for everyday monitoring, tracks a range of physiological health metrics, including heart rate, respiratory rate, heart rate variability, sleep parameters, and physical activity intensity through photoplethysmography, acceleration, and body temperature sensors. Although previous research on Oura ring has examined user experiences, studies on patient expectations prior to adoption for healthcare purposes are lacking. Embracing diverse perspectives is essential when adopting new healthcare technologies [6]. For the ageing population, certain medical conditions necessitate continuous home monitoring. This study aims to explore idiopathic Normal Pressure Hydrocephalus (iNPH) patients' perspectives and expectations of the Oura ring as a prospective monitoring device, offering insights into patient-centric approaches in adopting new healthcare technologies.

2 Materials and Methods

This study is grounded in structured interviews conducted by a healthcare professional with ten consented patients (aged 64–79, comprising five men and five women) who visited the Kuopio university hospital neurosurgery outpatient clinic for suspected iNPH diagnosis between Dec 2022 and Oct 2023. The first part of the interview focused on demographic information and everyday technology use, and the other on expectations for the potential use of the Oura ring in DRM. Designed for consistency and minimal patient burden, the interviews gained approval from the Research Ethics Board of the Northern Savo Hospital District. Data from the interviews were inductively coded into categories, themes, and aggregate theoretical dimensions.

3 Results

Among the participants, eight had experience with digital health devices such as blood pressure and glucose monitors and showed positivity towards DRM at home. Two expressed reservations about using digital wearables, including the Oura ring, for DRM. The study identified four key themes on patients' expectations: user-friendly design, privacy and data accuracy, a user-friendly monitoring process, and perceived usefulness. It also sheds light on healthcare professionals' expectations that underlined real-time physiological tracking, prompt communication and care, and support in using the Oura. Furthermore, the results illuminate the expectations of patients and their family caregivers regarding engagement, adherence to remote monitoring, self-management, and caregiver involvement in the process.

4 Discussion

For home-based remote monitoring like that for iNPH, wearable acceptance and patient commitment are vital. It necessitates an understanding of patient needs, perceptions, and expectations from such technologies in pre-implementation. This exploration into iNPH patient expectations regarding the Oura ring, enriches the dialogue on patient-centric healthcare. The findings suggest that patients envisage an active role in DRM, resonating with studies that highlight the importance of patient empowerment and active health management [7]. Our results underscore the potential of DRM to empower patients through enhanced disease knowledge, early assessment, improved self-management, and facilitated shared decision-making [2]. We also suggest that the anticipated safety, security, and motivational benefits from the Oura ring data could foster patient engagement. Finally, the active involvement of spouses and relatives [8], is found in our data as crucial in supporting the patient's health needs with DRM offering reassurance to family members and caregivers.

Acknowledgements. This study was conducted in cooperation with the Doctoral Programme in Neuro-Innovation (MSCA co-fund number 101034307), University of Eastern Finland Business School, Kuopio University Hospital VTR fund (grant number 5252614), Academy of Finland (grant number #339767), Sigrid Juselius Foundation (no specified grant number), and the Strategic Neuroscience Funding of the University of Eastern Finland.

Disclosure of Interests. None.

References

1. Hanley, J.A., Fairbrother, P., McCloughan, L., et al.: Qualitative study of telemonitoring of blood glucose and blood pressure in type 2 diabetes. BMJ Open **5**(12), 99–110 (2015)
2. Walker, R.C., Tong, A., Howard, K., et al.: Patient expectations and experiences of remote monitoring for chronic diseases: systematic review and thematic synthesis of qualitative studies. Int. J. Med. Inform. **124**(2019), 78–85 (2021)
3. Nicolini, D.: The work to make telemedicine work: A social and articulative view. Soc. Sci. Med. **62**(11), 2754–2767 (2006)
4. Piras, E.M., Miele, F.: On digital intimacy: redefining provider-patient relationships in remote monitoring. Sociol. Health Illn. **41**(S1), 116–131 (2019)
5. Kurtz, S. M., Higgs, G. B., Chen, Z., et al.: Patient perceptions of wearable and smartphone technologies for remote outcome monitoring in patients who have hip osteoarthritis or arthroplasties. J. Arthroplasty, **37**(7) (2022)
6. Rand, L., Dunn, M., Slade, I., et al.: Understanding and using patient experiences as evidence in healthcare priority setting. Cost Effectiveness Resour. Allocation **17**, 1–13 (2019). https://doi.org/10.1186/s12962-019-0188-1
7. Vallo Hult, H., Hansson, A., Svensson, L., et al.: Flipped healthcare for better or worse. Health Inform. J. **25**(3), 587–597 (2019)
8. Sahlström, R., Azim Zadegan, M., Aromaa, E., et al.: Patients' and Caregivers' Expectations and Acceptance of Digital Remote Monitoring at Home: The Case of Idiopathic Normal Pressure Hydrocephalus (2024)

Intergenerational Learning and Managerial Approaches for Fostering Digital Competence in Health Care – A Qualitative Study

Mira Hammarén[1]([⊠]) [iD], Tarja Pölkki[1,2] [iD], and Outi Kanste[1,2] [iD]

[1] Research Unit of Health Sciences and Technology, University of Oulu, Oulu, Finland
mira.hammaren@oulu.fi

[2] Medical Research Center Oulu, University Hospital and University of Oulu, Oulu, Finland

Keywords: Digital competence · Health care · Inductive content analysis · Interview

1 Introduction

In the evolving landscape of health care and undergoing rapid digitization [1], the imperative to enhance digital competence among professionals has become increasingly pronounced. Intergenerational learning has emerged as one solution to avoid the increasing stress caused by the new technologies, especially among older professionals [2]. Intergenerational learning aims to create cooperative learning were experienced professionals and newer generations exchange knowledge and digital competence [3]. There is limited evidence of how intergenerational learning can be utilized to promote digital competence in health care and how management can provide support for this [4]. The objective of this study is to describe managers' and professionals' views on intergenerational learning and managerial approaches supporting it to foster digital competence in health care.

2 Material and Methods

The study used a qualitative descriptive design. Participants were managers (n = 22) and professionals (n = 12) from public and private health care organizations including basic and specialized health care services in Finland. Managers included frontline leaders, middle or top managers. Professionals were legal health care professionals. Data were collected through semi-structured individual interviews conducted remotely via Microsoft Teams from February to May 2022. Upon reaching data saturation, interviewee recruitment and data collection were concluded. An inductive content analysis approach was applied to analyze the data [5].

M. Särestöniemi et al. (Eds.): NCDHWS 2024, CCIS 2083, pp. 395–397, 2024.
https://doi.org/10.1007/978-3-031-59080-1

3 Results

Intergenerational learning was perceived to impact professional development of both older and younger professionals. Mutual learning between older professionals and younger generations created exchange of tacit knowledge and digital competence. Intergenerational learning was seen to ensure that both experienced and newer professionals contribute to utilizing digital tools for improved health care outcomes. Managers were recognized to have an important role in supporting intergenerational learning by providing resources, freeing up work, and creating opportunities for interaction. Management was perceived to facilitate the formation of diverse-age teams, pair individuals from different generations, and establish mentoring relationships to connect professionals. Managers' role extended to bridging communication gaps, fostering a conversational culture, and promoting intergenerational interaction to prevent misunderstandings.

4 Discussion

The findings highlight the value of intergenerational knowledge exchange, emphasizing the mutual learning between experienced professionals and their technologically adept colleagues. Intergenerational knowledge exchange enhances collective digital competence in healthcare teams. Effective management involves diverse-age team facilitation, thoughtful pairing, and mentoring. Managers play a crucial role in fostering an environment that encourages meaningful interaction, supporting a comprehensive approach to workforce development that leverages each generation's strengths.

In conclusion, effective management is pivotal in fostering intergenerational learning, integrating the wisdom of experienced professionals with the innovation of the younger generation. This collaborative learning environment not only broadens the overall digital competence within the health care team but also contributes to improved patient care through the effective utilization of technology.

References

1. Ahsan, M.M., Siddique, Z.: Industry 4.0 in healthcare: a systematic review. Int. J. Inf. Manage. Data Insights 2(1), 100079 (2022)
2. Kuek, A., Hakkennes, S.: Healthcare staff digital literacy levels and their attitudes towards information systems. Health Inf. J. 26(1), 592–612 (2020)
3. De Leeuw, J.A., Woltjer, H., Kool, R.B.: Identification of factors influencing the adoption of health information technology by nurses who are digitally lagging: in-depth interview study. J. Med. Internet Res. 22(8), e15630 (2020)

4. Hammarén, M., Jarva, E., Mikkonen, K., Kääriäinen, M., Kanste, O.: Scoping review of intergenerational learning methods for developing digital competence and their outcomes. Finnish J. eHealth eWelfare **14**(4), 364–379 (2022)
5. Kyngäs, H., Mikkonen, K., Kääriäinen, M. (eds.): The Application of Content Analysis in Nursing Science Research. Springer, Cham (2020). https://doi.org/10.1007/978-3-030-30199-6

Healthcare Professionals' Digital Competence in Healthcare Settings – An International Comparative Study

Erika Jarva[1(✉)], Anne Oikarinen[1], Boris Miha Kaučič[2],
Zhou Wentao[3], Miyae Yamakawa[4], Janicke Andersson[5],
Olga Riklikienė[6], Marco Tomietto[7], Flores Vizcaya-Moreno[8],
Giancarlo Cicolini[9], Benjamin Ho[10], Aneta Grochowska[11],
Piret Paal[12], Andrea Egger-Rainer[12], André Fringer[13], Kadri Suija[14],
Xiaoyan Liao[15], Petra Mandysova[16], Megan Liu[17],
Tove Aminda Hanssen[18], Nopporn Vongsirimas[19], Younhee Kang[20],
Rita Ramos[21], and Kristina Mikkonen[1]

[1] University of Oulu, Oulu, Finland
erika.jarva@oulu.fi
[2] College of Nursing in Celje, Celje, Slovenia
[3] National University of Singapore, Singapore, Singapore
[4] Osaka University, Osaka, Japan
[5] Halmstad University, Halmstad, Sweden
[6] Lithuanian University of Health Sciences, Kaunas, Lithuania
[7] Northumbria University, Newcastle upon Tyne, UK
[8] University of Alicante, Alacant, Spain
[9] University of Bari "Aldo Moro", Bari, Italy
[10] The University of Hong Kong, Pok Fu Lam, Hong Kong
[11] University of Applied Sciences in Tarnow, Tarnów, Poland
[12] Paracelsus Medical University Salzburg, Salzburg, Austria
[13] Zurich University of Applied Sciences, Winterthur, Switzerland
[14] University of Tartu, Tartu, Estonia
[15] Southern Medical University, Guangzhou, China
[16] University of Pardubice, Pardubice, Czech Republic
[17] Taipei Medical University, Taipei, Taiwan
[18] University Hospital of North Norway, Tromsø, Norway
[19] Mahidol University, Bangkok, Thailand
[20] Ewha Womans University, Seoul, Korea
[21] University of the Philippines Open University, Los Baños, Philippines

Keywords: Competence · Digital health · Healthcare professional ·
International

1 Introduction

The rapid development of digital technologies in healthcare has been recognised to require new competencies from the healthcare professionals. Global and regional digitalisation strategies have pursued to create digital health networks and structures

M. Särestöniemi et al. (Eds.): NCDHWS 2024, CCIS 2083, pp. 398–400, 2024.
https://doi.org/10.1007/978-3-031-59080-1

that promote the utilisation of various digital technologies that would allow the ethical, safe, reliable, sustainable and equitable healthcare delivery [1]. Previous research has explored healthcare professionals' digital health competencies for example by conducting profile analysis in a national level [2], yet an international outlook and assessment of the current situation on healthcare professionals' digital competencies is still lacking. The purpose of the study is to describe the perceptions and factors that affect healthcare professionals' digital competence internationally. The aim of the study is to recognise the issues that are associated with healthcare professionals' digital competence to increase the adoption of digital health tools and services.

2 Materials and Methods

The study entails the linguistic and cultural validation of two instruments and a cross-sectional study which investigates healthcare professionals' digital competence internationally. Data collection takes place in up to 21 countries from healthcare professionals (min n = 300/country), including primary and specialised healthcare organisations. The instruments used in data collection include Digital Health Competence (DigiHealthCom) instrument which entails 5 factors and 42 items to measure the professional's perceived digital competence and Aspect Associated with Digital Health Competence (DigiComInf) instrument which entails 3 factors and 15 items to measure the perceived factors that are associated with digital competence [3]. The factors relating to healthcare professionals' digital competence will be explored by conducting a binary regression analysis. The attributes contributing to digital competence will be identified by conducting a K-mean cluster algorithm when identifying different competence profiles of healthcare professionals. The ethical/research permissions have been requested from each participating organisation undertaking the study according to each country's standard practices. The research follows the ethical principles as stated in Declaration of Helsinki [4]. The societal benefit of conducting the study was acknowledged by each participating country to validate the ethical treatment of the research participants [5].

3 Results

The expected findings suggest that majority of healthcare professionals evaluate their digital competence at a good level but country and digital competence area level differences persist. A variety of factors relating to the professional's professional and personal background and organisational and educational aspects support or inhibit digital competence and digital competence development. Yet, the exact results are presented in the conference in May 2024 after data collection and analysis have been completed.

4 Discussion

The results from this study and the validated instruments to measure digital competence and factors associated with it can be further employed in evaluating and developing healthcare professionals' digital competence in different healthcare contexts in a global scale. Individual and systematic digital competence evaluation and development does not only improve professionals' readiness to adopt and use the necessary digital technologies in their work but also supports individuals and organisations' transformation (change readiness, work engagement and well-being) in the digital shift and ensures high quality patient care.

Disclosure of Interests. The authors have no competing interests to declare that are relevant to the content of this article.

References

1. World Health Organization (WHO). Global strategy on digital health 2020–2025. World Health Organization, Geneva (2021)
2. Jarva, E., et al.: Healthcare professionals' digital health competence profiles and associated factors: a cross-sectional study. J. Adv. Nurs. Early View (2024)
3. Jarva, E., et al.: Healthcare professionals' digital health competence and its core factors; development and psychometric testing of two instruments. Int. J. Med. Inform. **171**, 104995 (2023)
4. World Medical Association Declaration of Helsinki. Ethical Principles for Medical Research Involving Human Subjects. J. Am. Med. Assoc. **310**(20), 2191–2194 (2013)
5. Stang, J.: Ethics in action: conducting ethical research involving human subjects: a primer. J. Acad. Nutr. Diet. **115**(12), 2019–2022 (2015)

Developing National Medical and Dental Education: From Digital Leap to Digital Marathon

Tiina Salmijärvi[1]([✉]) [iD], Petri Kulmala[1,2] [iD], Henri Takalo-Kastari[1] [iD],
and Jarmo Reponen[1,2,3] [iD]

[1] Faculty of Medicine, University of Oulu, Oulu, Finland
{tiina.salmijarvi,petri.kulmala,henri.takalo-kastari,
jarmo.reponen}@oulu.fi
[2] Medical Research Center, Oulu University Hospital, Oulu, Finland
[3] FinnTelemedicum, Research Unit of Health Sciences and Technology,
University of Oulu, Oulu, Finland

Abstract. The MEDigi project, aimed at harmonizing and digitalizing medical and dental basic education, was conducted from 2018 to 2021 through collaboration among Finnish medical faculties. The project's goal was to harmonize curriculum components by identifying common core contents and digitalize teaching practices by providing new tools and knowledge. The project has successfully transitioned into everyday practices in participating universities. This study examined the evolution of this process during and after the project period.

Keywords: Higher Education · Medical Education · Development of Education

1 Introduction

In 2017–2018 the Finnish Education Evaluation Centre (FINEEC) carried out an evaluation of basic medical education, the main result of which was that graduating doctors and dentists must have nationally common basic competencies, knowledge and skills [1]. In accordance with this recommendation, the national MEDigi project in 2018–2021 focused on the harmonization and digitalization of basic medical and dental education [2]. Digitalization has changed the operating methods of educational organizations in Finland in a multidimensional way throughout the 21st century. Changes in the organization of teaching were further accelerated by the COVID-19 pandemic, when distance education was widely switched to on a fast schedule [3].

M. Särestöniemi et al. (Eds.): NCDHWS 2024, CCIS 2083, pp. 401–403, 2024.
https://doi.org/10.1007/978-3-031-59080-1

2   Materials and Methods

During the MEDigi project in a nationwide collaboration, universities defined the core contents of all medical and dental disciplines in 46 specialty-based workgroups. Additionally, a special workgroup identified learning themes for e-Health. These workgroups created shared teaching and examination materials and initiated the development of a national teaching material repository for medical and dental sciences, capable of handling sensitive files. Special emphasis was placed on creating learning materials for teachers to utilize with new methods during the COVID-19 pandemic. In the MEDigi project, the aim was not only to harmonize learning, create new teaching material, and learn new skills but also to seek extensive change and reform in teaching. In addition, the goal was to support teachers and students in continuous learning [4].

The continuity of the MEDigi work was ensured through an agreement between the universities and by hiring a coordinator. The continuity has been guaranteed also structurally. The coordinator is responsible for the organization of activities at the national level. Each higher education institution has a MEDigi contact person. The work is guided and led by a steering group consisting of deans of medical faculties and an executive management group consisting of education program managers. This has ensured that the work continued uninterrupted after the project. Current efforts are guided by the jointly developed and approved MEDigi action program for 2023–2027.

3   Results

Most workgroups have continued their national collaboration beyond the project period. By the end of February 2024, users of the national repository increased to 450, up from 190 at the project's conclusion. The repository now contains 236 sets of digital learning materials. Additionally, universities use two different digital patient simulation environments, along with some joint exams and a radiology teaching database. New learning games have been introduced, and regular webinars and meetings are a vital part of this collaboration. Based on the information received from the workgroups, the core content analyzes produced during the MEDigi project have now been actively implemented. This means that the contents of the teaching have been harmonized nationally and there is a consensus on the priorities of the teaching.

Virtual patient cases, learning games, podcasts, simulations, systems simulating real systems (e.g. an electronic medical record system) and common exam banks increase and support the flexibility of teaching and learning in medicine and dentistry. With the help of these tools, the student can, for example, independently strengthen their skills by practicing the diagnostic problem-solving process central to the work of doctors and dentists or practice different procedures virtually [5]. New ways of organizing teaching also respond to students' growing need to study regardless of time and place. Specific eHealth courses including collaborative work in videoconference platforms were arranged to final year medical and nursing students and a pioneering net course discussing the of Basics in eHealth was organized as a cross university studies for all participating faculties. Furthermore, the progress is investigated by scientific research [6].

4   Discussion

Higher education should be built on strong pedagogical competence and cooperation, which ensures that education produces top-level competence and expertise for society's needs. The content and implementation of the training must be based on up-to-date researched information and new innovations must be introduced based on scientific evidence. MEDigi national cooperation has supported and helped medical and dental teachers in this important quality assurance work. Finnish medical and dental education has significantly advanced in digitalization via MEDigi. The work continues by establishing the teaching use of digital systems and continuing cooperation between universities.

Acknowledgments. The MEDigi project (2018–2021) received support from the Finnish Ministry of Education and Culture (grant record no. OKM/270/523/2017).

Disclosure of Interests. Authors TS, PK and JR are members of the MEDigi executive management group. Author HT-K has nothing to disclose.

References

1. Mäkelä, M., et al.: Educating doctors for the future – Evaluation of undergraduate medical education in Finland. Finnish Education Evaluation Centre. Publications 14:2018 (2018). https://www.karvi.fi/en/publications/educating-doctors-future-evaluation-undergraduate-medical-education-finland
2. Levy, A.R., et al.: National MEDigi project: systematic implementation of digitalization to undergraduate medical and dental education in Finland. Finnish J. EHealth EWelfare **11**(4), 357–361 (2019). https://doi.org/10.23996/fjhw.83309
3. Näpänkangas, R., Tuukkanen, J., Auvinen, J., Kaarteenaho, R., Kulmala, P.: Etäopiskelu lukuvuonna 2020–2021: Ensimmäisen vuoden lääketieteen ja hammaslääketieteen opiskelijoiden kokemukset. Yliopistopedagogiikka **29**(2), 9 (2022)
4. Levy, A., Reponen, J. (eds.): Digital transformation of medical education: MEDigi project report. University of Oulu (2021). https://urn.fi/URN:ISBN:9789526232454
5. Hytönen, H., et al.: Pelit oppimisprosessin rikastajina – kolme esimerkkiä. Games as enrichment of the learning process. In Finnish with an English summary. Finnish Med. J. **78**, e38307 (2023). http://www.laakarilehti.fi/e38307
6. Veikkolainen, P., et al.: EHealth competence building for future doctors and nurses – attitudes and capabilities. Int. J. Med. Inform. **169**, 104912 (2023). https://doi.org/10.1016/j.ijmedinf.2022.104912

Healthcare Professionals' Perceptions of Digital Counselling – A Qualitative Descriptive Research

Kaihlaniemi Juulia[1,2]($\boxtimes$) (iD), Kääriäinen Maria[1] (iD), Kaakinen Pirjo[1] (iD), and Oikarinen Anne[1] (iD)

[1] Research Unit of Health Sciences and Technology, University of Oulu, Oulu, Finland
juulia.kaihlaniemi@oulu.fi
[2] Wellbeing Services County of North Ostrobothnia, Oulu, Finland

Keywords: Digital counselling · Healthcare professionals · Semi-structured interview

1 Background

Digital counselling, or using text-based and video-mediated, interactive applications in counselling, has increased in healthcare. It is suitable for supporting self-management and healthy lifestyles, which have a significant impact on the health of the population [1]. Nevertheless, there is no clear definition of digital counselling in previous research. Thus, the purpose of this research was to describe the healthcare professionals' (HCPs) perceptions of digital counselling.

2 Materials and Methods

HCPs working in Digital Care Pathways (n = 12) were recruited to individual semi-structured interviews using convenience and snowball sampling. Transcribed data was analysed using inductive content analysis [2].

3 Results

According to the perceptions of HCPs, digital counselling is (1) advising on using the digital service; (2) involving the patients in the treatment of the illness; (3) holistic consideration of the patient's situation; (4) aiming for mutual understanding with patient and (5) making decisions about treatment.

© The Author(s) 2024
M. Särestöniemi et al. (Eds.): NCDHWS 2024, CCIS 2083, pp. 404–405, 2024.
https://doi.org/10.1007/978-3-031-59080-1

4 Conclusions

Digital counselling enabled patients' involvement in self-management through interactive means and counselling materials. It was implemented in a patient-oriented way, patients' needs were considered, and they were supported in self-management through discussions and with concrete advice. Mutual understanding was sought through empathy, clear communication and by ensuring understanding of the patients. Nevertheless, digital counselling is not suitable for all situations. It is essential to assess the need for treatment, consult other professionals and use available information. Moreover, it is important to identify patients, who need support to digital counselling and if necessary, offer an opportunity to face-to-face counselling.

References

1. Golinelli, D., et al.: Adoption of digital technologies in health care during the covid-19 pandemic: systematic review of early scientific literature. J. Med. Internet Res. **22**(11) (2020)
2. Elo, S., Kyngäs, H.: The qualitative content analysis process. J. Adv. Nurs.Nurs. **62**(1), 107–115 (2008)

Patients' Experiences of the Digital Counselling Competence of Healthcare Professionals – A Qualitative Descriptive Study

Petra Suonnansalo[1(✉)], Juulia Kaihlaniemi[1], Outi Kähkönen[1,2], and Anne Oikarinen[1]

[1] Research Unit of Health Sciences and Technology, Faculty of Medicine, University of Oulu, Oulu, Finland
petra.suonnansalo@oulu.fi
[2] Department of Nursing Science, University of Eastern Finland, Kuopio, Finland

Abstract. This study aimed to describe the experiences of patients using digital services on the digital counselling competence of healthcare professionals.

Keywords: Competence · Digital Counselling · Patient · Semi-structured Interview

1 Introduction

The digitalization of healthcare services challenges the counselling competence of healthcare professionals. With the shift to digital counselling environments [1], professionals are required to have new kinds of counselling competence to provide high-quality and patient-centered counselling [2]. Patient satisfaction with the care they receive has been shown to influence treatment outcomes and self-care adherence [3]. Limited research has been conducted on patients' experiences of health professionals' digital counselling competence.

2 Materials and Methods

The study aimed to describe the experiences of patients using digital services on the digital counselling competence of healthcare professionals. Data were analyzed in Finland in spring 2023 through individual semi-structured interviews with 11 participants who had received video-mediated counselling in healthcare. Microsoft Teams was used to carry out the interviews. The interviews followed a set of main and ancillary questions [4]. Inductive content analysis was used to analyze the data [5].

© The Author(s) 2024
M. Särestöniemi et al. (Eds.): NCDHWS 2024, CCIS 2083, pp. 406–407, 2024.
https://doi.org/10.1007/978-3-031-59080-1

3 Results

Patients' experiences of healthcare professionals' digital counselling competence consisted of five areas of competence: (1) preparing for video-mediated counselling, (2) digital competence in implementing the video-mediated counselling, (3) interacting with the patient during the video-mediated counselling, (4) supporting the patient's self-management in video-mediated counselling and (5) self-development as a digital counsellor. According to patients' experiences, video-mediated counselling is routine for healthcare professionals, but the limited experience of providing video-mediated counselling is also transparent to the patients. Healthcare professionals need to pay particular attention to the encounters and interactions in the digital counselling situation. In addition, patients stressed the importance of healthcare professionals' mastery of technology as part of smooth digital counselling. Before every digital counselling session, healthcare professionals should ensure that the technical and technological elements are in place and familiarize themselves with the patient's background. Patients felt that it was important for healthcare professionals to involve the patient in digital counselling, for example by sharing screen and using a variety of counselling materials.

4 Discussion

The results of this study suggest that healthcare professionals need a wide range of counselling competencies when counselling patients via video. Our findings set the basis for future research on patients' experiences of healthcare professionals' digital counselling competence. Future research should focus on developing the digital counselling competence of HCPs, as this has a significant impact on the effectiveness of digital services.

References

1. Paalimäki-Paakki, K., Virtanen, M., Henner, A., Nieminen, M.T., Kääriäinen, M.: Effectiveness of digital counseling environments on anxiety, depression, and adherence to treatment among patients who are chronically ill: systematic review. J. Med. Internet Res. **24**(1), e30077 (2022). https://doi.org/10.2196/30077
2. Kaihlaniemi, J., Liljamo, P., Rajala, M., Kaakinen, P., Oikarinen, A.: Health care professionals' experiences of counselling competence in digital care pathways - a descriptive qualitative study. Nurs. Open **10**(7), 4773–4785 (2023). https://doi.org/10.1002/nop2.1729
3. Ramaswamy, A., et al.: Patient satisfaction with telemedicine during the COVID-19 pandemic: retrospective cohort study. J. Med. Internet Res. **22**(9), e20786 (2020). https://doi.org/10.2196/20786
4. Polit, D.F., Beck, C.T.: Generating and assessing evidence for nursing practice, 10th edn. Wolters Kluwer Health, Philadelphia (2017)
5. Elo, S., Kyngäs, H.: The qualitative content analysis process. J. Adv. Nurs.Nurs. **62**(1), 107–115 (2008). https://doi.org/10.1111/j.1365-2648.2007.04569.x

Hybrid Intelligence – Human-AI Co-evolution and Learning in Multirealities (HI)

Sanna Järvelä[1], Guuying Zhao[2], Janne Heikkilä[2], Hanna Järvenoja[1],
Kristina Mikkonen[3(✉)], and Satu Kaleva[1]

[1] Faculty of Education and Psychology, University of Oulu, Oulu, Finland
[2] Faculty of Information Technology and Electronic Engineering,
University of Oulu, Oulu, Finland
[3] Faculty of Medicine, University of Oulu, Oulu, Finland
kristina.mikkonen@oulu.fi

Abstract. The presence of Artificial Intelligence (AI) is growing in all areas of life. However, current data-driven AI is still too narrow to help humans, as it is lacking in social and emotional intelligence, and being restricted by reality. By placing the emphasis on mutual understanding and learning from each other, our research programme aims to combine the strengths of both humans and machines in their co-evolutionary processes. We propose to build the idea of a metaverse by combining our physical and virtual realities in a movement towards a multi-reality. HI integrates the University of Oulu's 4 excellence areas, including Emotion AI, learning processes, perceptual engineering, and nursing science, to generate future AI-based solutions for fields such as education and nursing. Overall, HI aims at advancing the well-being of people in different areas of life and improving the quality of life through the integration of innovative technologies. Our programme focuses on international top-level collaborative and multidisciplinary research, which is supported by the unique learning and interaction research infrastructure LeaF.

Keywords: Hybrid Intelligence · AI · Learning · Multirealities

1 Introduction

Hybrid Intelligence (HI) combines the strengths of both humans and machines to collaborate to learn from and reinforce each other [1]. This is the key difference to AI, which is designed to work independently to perform tasks that normally require human intelligence, such as perception and learning [2]. The fundamental difference between HI and human-centered AI is that HI involves both humans and machines in the loop, emphasizing mutual understanding and learning from each other in their co-evolution.

2 HI Research Programme Themes

HI research programme covers four multidisciplinary research themes (HI1–4) and two cross-cutting themes to facilitate deep data and ethical discussions (H5):

© The Author(s) 2024
M. Särestöniemi et al. (Eds.): NCDHWS 2024, CCIS 2083, pp. 408–410, 2024.
https://doi.org/10.1007/978-3-031-59080-1

Data and algorithm assisted HI (HI1) develops advanced data processing and computing technology for assisting humans and machines to understand each other. It includes new machine learning methods for interpreting human emotions, intentions, preferences and decision making by analysing facial and body behaviours, and physiological signals; endowing machines capabilities of expressing emotions with advanced interactive behaviour synthesis algorithms; and helping humans to understand machines by visualizing and explaining the internal states and status of data, algorithms and models with multi-modality for mixed-reality interfaces. RQ: How to facilitate the information exchange and mutual learning between AI and humans with new data processing methods, computational models and VR/AR approaches?

Understanding humans in/for AI interaction (HI2) strives for understanding human learning and interaction processes to build HI systems that augment rather than replace human intelligence, systems that leverage our strengths and compensate for our weaknesses. This theme will utilize the multimodal data based on the HI.3 multi-reality platforms and the "human-machine understanding" of HI.1 to train, work and collaborate with humans and AI and then transfer of responsibility to humans. HI may need new human skills which also need to be understood. RQ: How can human learning mechanisms be used to adapt and interact in dynamic Hybrid systems?

Extended human mind in multirealities (HI3) investigates AI-methods for extending and changing human perception by means of digital spaces and realities that co-exist with our physical world. Virtual, mixed and augmented reality technologies enable interaction with various degrees of virtual content in cyber- and metaverses seamlessly integrating human senses with multiple concurrent realities, whereas intelligence augmentation can enhance the cognitive abilities of humans with virtual assistants and provide capabilities that go beyond the normal perception. Solutions will be developed to demonstrate how multi-realities and AI together can boost and bring human capabilities to the next level. RQ: How do humans learn, interact, work and collaborate in HI setting and what is the added value of multiple realities, possibly on multiple tasks in complex environments?

Emerging sustainable effects of HI to quality of life (HI4) investigates the ways HI can impact wellbeing and utilize technology in new areas for quality of life, e.g., to improve health care with enhancement of augmented care and development of advanced continuous education. This theme will work with various underserved people and stakeholders to develop adaptive platforms implementing HI. It provides feedback to HI1-HI3 via cyclic processes which helps to push forward positive effects and mitigate negative ones in future development. The 6G connectivity expertise will facilitate the developments. RQ: What are the opportunities offered by HI with multiple realities and how related knowledge and concepts can be utilized to different applications, covering health, education, work-place teams, HCI and for enhancing quality of life?

The Ethics Forum and the Data Forum (HI5) are cross sectional parts of HI1-H4. Various aspects of AI can be seen as intrusive and vulnerable to the purposes of control by both private and public actors. The Ethics Forum will facilitate new research and discussion in ethics, values and societal concerns of HI. The Data Forum will facilitate responsible use, open sharing and storage of data and provide methods and technological basis on responsible and productive data usage in HI. A short-term goal is to host data scientist who give practical guidance to HI research. A long-term goal is to build a network for training, tutorials, forums, etc., with other universities with similar infrastructures.

3 Implications

HI provides better understanding of human-human and human-machine interaction, which, in turn, facilitates novel solutions in areas of crucial societal importance, such as education, aging and care, global population changes, future work and skills [3, 4]. For example, HI is well aligned to offer novel educational methods by blending AI-driven learning technologies and human interactive and creative skills, developing new AI-enabled multi-reality technologies and digital solutions for well-being and health, health care education and distant human-centred care [5]. HI will target the digital divide by addressing how these problems will be affordable and actively engage with policy makers. It will pave the way for a new paradigm of HI-aided services in, e.g., healthcare and education, especially for people with difficulties, thus promoting equal prospects for well-being, enhancing quality of life and for human's effects in environment and resources.

Acknowledgments. This program is funded by Research Council of Finland and University of Oulu.

Disclosure of Interests. The authors have no competing interests to declare that are relevant to the content of this publication.

References

1. Järvelä, S., Nguyen, A., Hadwin, A.: Human and AI collaboration for socially shared regulation in learning. Br. J. Educ. Technol. **54**, 1057–1076 (2023)
2. Russell, S.J., Norvig, P.: Artificial Intelligence: A Modern Approach, 3rd edn. Prentice Hall, Upper Saddle River (2010)
3. European Commission. Digital Education Action Plan (2021–2027) (2020)
4. UNICEF. Policy guidance on AI for children (2021). https://www.unicef.org/globalinsight/reports/policyguidance-ai-children
5. Ahuja, A.S., Polascik, B.W., Doddapaneni, D., Byrnes, E.S., Sridhar, J.: The digital metaverse: applications in artificial intelligence, medical education, and integrative health. Integr. Med. Res. **12**(1), 100917 (2023). https://doi.org/10.1016/j.imr.2022.100917

Digital Health Exemplars: Service Delivery Transformation Through Digital Innovation

Lena Kan[1]([✉]), Patricia Mechael[1], Smisha Agarwal[1], Shivani Pandya[1], and Binyam Tilahun[2]

[1] Johns Hopkins University, Baltimore, USA
lkan5@jhu.edu
[2] University of Gondar, Gondar, Ethiopia

Abstract. Despite increases in primary healthcare (PHC) investments globally, access to and use of PHC services remains challenging. Digitization can advance PHC systems in low- and middle-income (LMIC) countries, and various contextual and implementation factors related to digital governance, training of healthcare workers, interoperability of digital systems, and human-centered design, among others, are critical to effective scale and the effectiveness of digital health interventions (DHIs). The Digital Health Exemplars, a collaboration between the Center for Global Digital Health Innovation (CGDHI) at the Johns Hopkins Bloomberg School of Public Health, eHealth Lab Ethiopia at the University of Gondar, and other partners, aims to evaluate the successful strategies that can advance the integration of digital into PHC systems for improved downstream population-level health outcomes for 5 high-performing countries (India, Brazil, Rwanda, Ghana, and Finland) identified by the project. Following a comprehensive theory of change and a set of primary research objectives, the project will undertake a mixed-methods study design to better understand the digital healthcare landscape in each Exemplar country, as well as the specific digital health interventions and their health impact at national and sub-national levels. Exemplar country inception workshops are underway, and primary and secondary data collection activities will begin in March-May of 2024. The overall study design as well as any potential pre-liminary data from select countries will be ready for presentation by the conference date.

Keywords: Digital health · Primary healthcare · Digital innovation · Health service delivery · Digital transformation · Digital health interventions · Health impact · Mixed-methods design

1 Introduction

Despite increases in primary health care (PHC) investments globally, access to and use of PHC services remains a challenge. Suboptimal financing schemes, an under-resourced health workforce, fragmentation of public and private systems, and low engagement of community health workers are a few of the barriers that have limited effective PHC service delivery. Digitization can advance PHC systems in low- and middle-income (LMIC) countries. The recent WHO guidelines on "digital systems for health systems strengthening" recommended a range of digital strategies that could be

M. Särestöniemi et al. (Eds.): NCDHWS 2024, CCIS 2083, pp. 411–413, 2024.
https://doi.org/10.1007/978-3-031-59080-1

employed to strengthen health systems [1], with an acknowledgment of the critical "implementation" and "contextual" factors that need to be in place to facilitate the effective scale of digital interventions. Several contextual and implementation factors related to digital governance, training of healthcare workers, interoperability of digital systems, and human-centered design, among others, are critical to effective scale and the effectiveness of digital interventions. The Digital Health Exemplars project is a collabo- ration between the Center for Global Digital Health Innovation (CGDHI) at the Johns Hopkins Bloomberg School of Public Health, eHealth Lab Ethiopia at the University of Gondar, and partners including Bill & Melinda Gates Foundation, Gates Ventures, World Bank, and the McKinsey Health Institute. The project aims to understand the pathways countries take to- wards a mature digital ecosystem, and the necessary implementation and contextual factors that must be addressed, across a range of health system settings, to achieve effective and scalable digitization of PHC services. The project has identified 5 high-performing countries that have leveraged digital health transformation towards improving PHC service delivery, including India, Brazil, Rwanda, Ghana, and Finland.

2   Materials and Methods

The project aims to evaluate the successful strategies that can advance the integration of digital into PHC systems for improved downstream population-level health outcomes for all 5 exemplar countries. Following a comprehensive theory of change and a set of primary research questions developed by the study research team on the digital transformation of PHC, the Digital Health Exemplars project aims to assess the digital healthcare landscape in each country in terms of policy program implementation, and health impact at a national level with state-level granularity. The primary research objectives include assessing: 1) the enablers of digital transformation of PHC in the country as well as the effective strategies for engaging key stakeholders for mobilizing resources for and facilitating the adoption of digitization at the national and sub-national levels, 2) the primary pathways to scaling and sustaining digital interventions, and 3) the impact of scaled digital interventions on health coverage, access, quality, and health outcomes. Utilizing a mixed-methods study design and leveraging a set of core conceptual frameworks including the WHO ITU framework [2], the Digital Health Exemplars project aims to better understand the pathways and driving factors of suc-cessful digital health implementations and ecosystems for each core research question and objective. Through a comprehensive initial review of the status of the digital health landscape in each country context and conversations with topical experts, the study research team has compiled a list of scaled digital health interventions (DHIs) and programs in each exemplar country, including national health information systems, mobile health (mHealth programs), or remote health services interventions. A set of primary and secondary data collection activities leveraging qualitative research meth-ods and robust quantitative data analysis will be administered to facilitate compre-hensive data and knowledge generation about the selected DHIs and the overall digital health ecosystem. Specific study methods will include administering in-depth inter-views and focus group discussions with key informants, including key national and sub-national level policy makers and sectoral experts, digital health program implementers, as well as providers and clients interfacing with digital health interventions, and any other key stakeholders engaged PHC and/or digital transformation. Key informants will be recruited through study inception workshops, leveraging in-country research partners and networks (snowball sampling), as well as utilizing peer-reviewed and grey literature. Thematic analysis will be used to analyze qualitative transcripts and secondary program data will be analyzed quantitatively to capture longitudinal time trends of service coverage to evaluate the impact of DHIs while adopting an equity lens. Leveraging a health systems approach, an impact analysis of the selected DH program(s) on health outcomes and a cost-effective analysis will also be conducted for each Exemplar country. Triangulation of qualitative and quantitative data will be performed to reap the benefits of a mixed-methods design and answer all research questions to the best of our knowledge and scientific evidence.

3   Results

Exemplar country inception workshops are currently underway, and primary and secondary data collection activities are anticipated to start in March-May of 2024. Preliminary data from Brazil and Finland are expected to be collected by the conference date. Thus, the primary aim of this abstract submission is to present the overall study approach and design of the digital health exemplars project, along with the potential preliminary data collected for select Exemplar countries.

4   Discussion

The project's goal is to generate robust evidence to advance the integration of digital health into PHC systems for improved downstream population-level health outcomes which can inform overall digital health policy and practice. Key les-sons learned based on cross-country analyses and synthesis will be disseminated with country partners and more broadly.

References

1. Recommendations on digital interventions for health system strengthening. (n.d.). Accessed 12 Mar 2024. https://www.who.int/publications-detail-redirect/9789241550505
2. National eHealth Strategy Toolkit. (n.d.). Accessed 12 Mar 2024. https://www.who.int/publications-detail-redirect/national-ehealth-strategy-toolkit

Measurement Applications of Smartphone with Extended Optical Capability

Jarmo Hietanen[✉]

Measurement Technology Unit, University of Oulu, 87400 Kajaani, Finland
jarmo.hietanen@oulu.fi

Abstract. The objective of the study was to outline application areas and applications that could be exploited the extended light wavelengths (UV–VIS–IR) of smartphone camera technology. The study identified nearly 200 applications. Common observation needs were related to microbial growth, material identification, temperature, and the determination of water contaminants. The underlying needs were related, for instance, to self-monitoring, which could trigger timely standardized laboratory measurements.

Keywords: Smartphone · Optical Measurements · Applications

1 Introduction

Future mobile phones will incorporate even more a higher-end sensor matrix as standard, making applications built around them available for everything from specialized instrumentation to citizen sensing. The global market potential of fast detection responses using new communication solutions and edge computing make them particularly attractive. Several application areas have already been identified from the remote health care services and monitoring to the spread of plant diseases due to climate change.

In this context, NIR and spectral camera applications were considered. Of particular interest were the new business opportunities for small spectral camera modules for smartphone applications. The lower cost of these modules will attract new entrants.

2 Methods

The methods used in this study were workshops, commercial databases, and interviews. In the workshop part, potential measurement targets for cameras were identified through technology research and available tacit knowledge. The workshop identified, developed, and grouped potential applications through a brainstorming process to form a coherent vision. Commercial application data was obtained from a database maintained by Frost & Sullivan, for instance [1–7]. The applications and their industries as well as the technology used, operating companies, and commercial potential were of primary interest. The feasibility and commercialization of the identified application areas were explored in the interview part.

M. Särestöniemi et al. (Eds.): NCDHWS 2024, CCIS 2083, pp. 414–416, 2024.
https://doi.org/10.1007/978-3-031-59080-1

3   Results

The applications were grouped into larger entities for clarity. Figure 1 shows the possible measurement needs of the applications. The outer circle presents the large groups, which were industrial measurements, environmental measurements, primary production measurements and consumer measurements with details. The middle area illustrates the attributes related to the above topics. The inner area describes specific measurement needs that may be related to the attributes. The keywords and their grouping model in this figure are indicative since this diagram can be outlined very many ways.

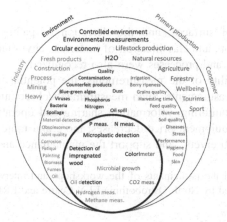

Fig. 1. Possible measurement needs. On the outer ring, there are large business entities. In the outermost area, the sectors of industry are shown. In the middle area, attributes related to the topics are presented. In the innermost area, the measurement needs possibly related to the attributes are presented. The color coding in the innermost area is indicating that same need can be associated with several attributes.

Figure 2 shows another view to gathered data. The diagram presents the sectors where the identified applications could be applied (left), sorted by activity (middle), and listed by the measurement opportunities (right).

4   Discussion

Here, the measurement application areas of the extended wavelength range (UV–VIS–IR) of the smartphone camera were investigated using workshops, database surveys, and business interviews. According to the concept, the key features of the device would be widespread camera technology for the IR and UV ranges, a common and affordable smartphone platform, edge and/or cloud computing, ease of use, and global availability.

In total, almost 200 applications were identified. By combining the results, clear areas of application could be extracted. These included the detection of microbial growth, gases from industrial processes, discontinuities or contamination on or in the

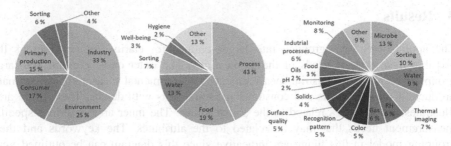

Fig. 2. Measurement applications possibilities of smartphone with extended optical capability by industry (left), activities (middle), and measurement needs (right).

immediate vicinity of surfaces, and the detection of pathogens or diseases. The detection, identification, and classification of materials, environmental emissions, food quality, water supply, and processes were also recognized.

Regarding the ability of the measurements, the potential was seen in indicative rather than precise measurements. Such measurements/observations can be used in the organization's self-monitoring, information sharing and operational development. In other words, as the equipment price decreases, more and more employees can easily become "additional observers" and support the maintenance and quality organization.

Acknowledgments. All the participants of the workshops and interviews are acknowledged. This study was supported by North Ostrobothnia ELY Centre and ERDF (A78617).

References

1. Smart Electronics and Spectral Imaging to Transform End-to-end Food Traceability and Safety, TechVision Analysis DA44 Chemicals, Materials & Nutrition, 24 February 2022. F&S
2. Innovations and growth opportunities in diagnostics, implantables, wearables and medical imaging, TechVision Opp. Eng. D862/29 Healthcare, 25 February 2022. F&S
3. Global Sustainable Agriculture Growth Opportunities, Growth Opportunities PC99 Chemicals, Materials & Nutrition, 9 March 2022. F&S
4. Global Naval EO/IR Competitive Landscape and Growth Opportunities, Growth Opportunities Aerospace & Defense. 11 February 2022. F&S
5. Growth opportunities in oil & gas infrastructure monitoring, oil spill remediation, and digitalization of the oil & gas industry, TechVision Opp. Eng. D998/38 Energy & Power Systems, 21 August 2020. F&S
6. Image Sensors: R&D Portfolio and Opportunity Analysis, TechVision Analysis D8EB Automotive & Transportation Healthcare Measurement & Instrumentation, 30 December 2019. F&S
7. Innovations in Wastewater Treatment, Catalysts, Sustainable Compounds, Waste Management, Hydrogen Production, Food Freshness Detection, Bio-based Sealants, Bioplastics, and Biocomposites, TechVision Opp. Eng. D768/A5 Env. & Building Techn. 4 January 2019. F&S

Use of Digital Technologies in Nursing Homes at a Rural Area of Northern Finland

Pekka Kilpeläinen$^{(\boxtimes)}$, Meira Mankinen, Veijo Sutinen, and Vesa Virtanen

Unit of Measurement Technology, University of Oulu, Kajaani University Consortium, Kehräämöntie 7, 87400 Kajaani, Finland
pekka.t.kilpelainen@oulu.fi

Abstract. Representatives of fifteen nursing homes in Kainuu region were interviewed for use and need of digital technologies at the end of Covid-19 pandemic. The digital technologies were used mostly in drug supply management, activation of elderly persons and already for longer time in personal security of the tenants. The most often presented needs for further or improved technologies were related to professional communication and exchange of data with public health care. Surprisingly, needs for improved health monitoring tools were little mentioned apart from devices or applications for assessment of functional capacity of home-living elderly persons.

Keywords: Nursing home · Elderly care · Remote communication · Health monitoring · Activating technology

1 Introduction

Kainuu region in the Eastern corner of Northern Finland belongs to European regions with the lowest population density (3,5 pers./km^2) and the oldest population. Over 30% of the persons living in Kainuu are 65 years or older. It is expected that in 2030 nearly 20% of the population will be 75 years or older. The elderly care is mainly organized by a public health care system, but nursing home services are often outsourced from private companies or foundations. There are ~ 20 nursing homes offering also intensified care for 24 h per day in Kainuu region. Finnish health care system is under extensive reorganization and pressure to reduce costs. Digital technologies and remote services are widely seen as one of the central tools in cost reduction. To be able to develop and increase utilization of digital technologies, it is essential to know current situation and gather experiences and needs of health care professionals from all levels of professional hierarchy.

2 Material and Methods

We interviewed 15 nursing homes that offer also intensified care in assisted living for 24 h per day and enquired about the use and need of digital technologies and experiences & attitudes related to digital technologies. The interviews were done at the end

M. Särestöniemi et al. (Eds.): NCDHWS 2024, CCIS 2083, pp. 417–419, 2024.
https://doi.org/10.1007/978-3-031-59080-1

of Covid-19 pandemic giving insights also on how the pandemic had affected use of technologies.

When interviews were agreed, the nursing homes were provided with a list of topics and main questions that were to be dealt with in the interview. The nursing homes were instructed to discuss the questions with all their nursing staff to collect opinions widely (7 of 15 homes did this). Persons interviewed as representatives of nursing homes, were senior professionals having education and experience either in nursing or health sciences. An exception was one nursing home where the interviewed person had management experience, but no experience in health care work. The nursing homes were offered an opportunity to take into the interview more than one person, but this option was rarely used. The interviews were carried out remotely and recorded using MsTeams. Although there was a list of questions, the interviewees were allowed to take up also other topics. Afterwards the interviews were transcribed and summarized. The summaries were sent to the nursing homes for further comments and checking that they represented original opinions.

3   Results

3.1   The Main Observations in Different Technology Categories

Health Status Monitoring. Surprisingly, there was no perceived need for new technologies for health status monitoring in units providing housing services, instead the nurses' assessment and blood tests and other traditional surveys were felt to be sufficient. However, a few nursing homes mentioned that e.g. a quick CRP device would be convenient. Some nursing homes send wound images to the wound care nurses in public health care using Com-mitWeb application3, WhatsApp, by picture message or some other connection, e.g. by an e-mail. Patient information was not included in the messages if e.g. WhatsApp was used to send images. Secure data channel for wound care nurses was mentioned as a need, and the public health care had also plans to progress this issue. Those nurses who also worked in home care, mentioned need for technologies related to the assessment of functional capacity of home living elderlies.

Drug Supply Management. Depending on their needs, care units of different sizes had either a nurse handing out the medicines or a pharmacy's dose distribution service in use. No one had or needed a separate drug delivery robot. All but three nursing homes had electronic medicine ordering for the pharmacy, the last three ones were planning to set it up in the following autumn.

Remote Communication. Several nursing homes expressed, some stronger and some weaker, a desire for a digital connection to public health care systems. In this case, the tenants' laboratory results and, more generally, the nursing home's care supply orders would travel between the care unit and public health care more securely and smoothly.

Family Communication. In addition to regular phone calls, the most common way to contact relatives was the use of free messaging services and video calls (WhatsApp, MS Teams, Skype). In a few interviews, it emerged that there was a need for further development. For example, the need for a communication method which would allow the client to talk with relatives independently and confidentially without the presence of the nurse was mentioned.

Activating Technology. Many nursing homes used free internet services (e.g. You-Tube) to watch remote gymnastic instructions or concerts. For others, traditional puzzles, close-ups and CDs were enough and did the trick. The need for an activating technology/content service was mentioned in those nursing homes that did not yet use free internet services or otherwise needed special support for activity. More serious activating technologies or contents aimed at people with memory problems or the disabled.

Personal Safety. The majority felt that they had no technology needs for the subject area. Either safety bracelets or alarm mats were already in use - or the nursing home was home-like and the nurses were always nearby, in which case there was no need for technology. The night guards had a connection with a security company.

For a presentation, an update of current situation with expressed needs will be added.

4   Discussion

Evidently, Covid-19 pandemic brough communication technologies to nursing homes, although most of them used conventional software not meant for professional use in health care. The remote communication was used widely between tenants and their family members, but also between nursing home staff and family members of tenants. Likewise, the use of various activating technologies had likely become more common partly due to isolation brought about by the pandemic.

The digital on-line technologies were used in nearly all nursing homes for drug supply management which was not surprising, since drug prescriptions have been electric in Kainuu region since year 2013. Pharmacies have strongly supported implementation of digital drug supply management and provided training for it. Interestingly, nurses working regularly with drug supply were not completely pleased with the change and told that they have lost contact with pharmacists.

Main need for digital technologies mentioned by nursing homes, was for communication with public health care, both with doctors, laboratories, databases and other information systems. Understandably requirements set by legislation for health data privacy and safety have to be complied with. This slows development and does systems more expensive to develop and to take in use.

Nursing homes did not have perceived additional needs for health monitoring. They had professional staff and typically good connections with public health care. The very few needs mentioned were connected to devices that exists, and it may be difficult even for professionals to name needs requiring technologies that do not yet exist.

Disclosure of Interests. The authors have no competing to declare that are relevant to the content of this article.

Developing Opportunities with Digital Transformation Challenges in Hospital at Home Services

Terhi-Maija Isakov[1]([✉]) [iD], Henna Härkönen[1,2] [iD], Piia Hyvämäki[1] [iD],
Miia Jansson[1,2,3] [iD], and on behalf of the research group

[1] Research Unit of Health Sciences and Technology, University of Oulu, Oulu,
Finland
terhi-maija.isakov@oulu.fi
[2] MRC Oulu, Oulu University Hospital and University of Oulu, Oulu, Finland
[3] RMIT University, Melbourne, Australia

Keywords: Digital technology · Home care services · Hospital-at-home

1 Background

The prevalence of hospital at home services has been increasing in recent years to avoid adverse effects on health and functionality related to hospital admissions, especially among older people living at home. With limited healthcare resources especially in rural areas, and the rapid growth of elderly population with multimorbidity, the opportunities of digital transformation could ensure cost-efficient, accessible, and high-quality hospital at home services. This qualitative study explored what are the service providers' challenges and opportunities in digital transformation of hospital at home.

2 Materials and Methods

A total of 25 semi-structured interviews were conducted in September–October 2023 in all Finnish well-being services counties (n = 21), city of Helsinki (n = 1), and private health service providers (n = 3). The participants were service providers, and a convenience sampling was used. The data were analyzed using inductive content analysis.

3 Results

The analysis revealed challenges and opportunities in digital transformation of hospital at home services, which related to 1) Health information exchange; 2) Management; 3) Logistics and 4) Service provision. Furthermore, digital accessibility and digital competence including both service providers' digital competency and patients' digital skills were related to challenges.

M. Särestöniemi et al. (Eds.): NCDHWS 2024, CCIS 2083, pp. 420–421, 2024.
https://doi.org/10.1007/978-3-031-59080-1

4   Conclusions

Digital transformation of hospital at home services is currently challenging, but opportunities are emerging. Digital transformation might add value by increasing workflow efficiency and communication in hospital at home services. But to achieve this, attention must be paid to the development and implementation of accessible, applicable, and data-driven digital services, with support for the digital competency of both health care professionals and patients.

Robots in the Care of Older People: Robot Literacy Required

Päivi Rasi-Heikkinen[1]([✉]), Susanna Rivinen[1], and Aino Ahtinen[2]

[1] University of Lapland, Yliopistonkatu 8, 96300 Rovaniemi, Finland
`Paivi.Rasi-Heikkinen@ulapland.fi`
[2] Tampere University, Kalevantie 4, 33100 Tampere, Finland

Keywords: Robot Literacy · Older People · Healthcare · Social Care

The last decade has marked a growth in the interest and development of robots in healthcare and social care, particularly in older people's care contexts. The development has been accelerated by the global trend of aging and technological innovations. Care robots are used to assist older people in their daily tasks, such as cleaning, eating, dressing, bathing, social interaction, entertainment, and medication taking. Robots can also provide instructions for the activities of daily life and safety, help monitor older people's behavior and health, and provide companionship and health-related advice.

The uptake of robotics in the care of older people is not, however, without its problems, but raises concerns related for example to equality, acceptability, accessibility, ethics, and agency. From a learning perspective, adopting robots in care processes requires new kinds of digital literacies from both older patients and care professionals.

Robots function as providers of information and services, requiring older people to have *robot literacy*, which is a novel concept in media literacy research. We define robot literacy through seven skill sets: 1) awareness of robots, 2) communication with robots, 3) understanding and evaluating the information provided by robots, 4) promoting safety and privacy when interacting with robots, 5) programming of robots, 6) ethical reflection, and 7) supporting and guiding others in questions related to robotics.

This presentation discusses the uptake of robotics in older people's healthcare and social care through two ongoing projects. *MediaRoboLit 65+* research project addresses learning media and robot literacies as a lifelong process and extends the theoretical understanding by adding robot literacy as a subset of media literacy. The project builds on a strengths-based outlook and identifies older people's capabilities as users of media and technologies instead of focusing only on deficits and barriers. The second, *ArcticRoboWelfare* -project aims to strengthen the data-based utilization of robotics in the digital transformation of the Finnish Lapland region in renewing the operating models of welfare services. Together, these projects highlight the robot literacy needed in the uptake of robotics in older people's healthcare and social care.

Acknowledgments. MediaRoboLit 65+ project is funded by the Academy of Finland (355 063) and Arctic RoboWelfare -project is partly funded by the European Regional Development Fund.

Disclosure of Interests. The authors have no competing interests to declare that are relevant to the content of this abstract.

M. Särestöniemi et al. (Eds.): NCDHWS 2024, CCIS 2083, p. 422, 2024.
https://doi.org/10.1007/978-3-031-59080-1

The Needed Skills and Competencies for Healthcare Providers to Use Technology for Patients with Pain

Johanna Soini[1(✉)], Héctor Beltrán-Alacreu[4],
Asuncion Ferri-Morales[4], Ingrid Jepsen[2], Andrea Kuckert[3],
Katriina Kuhalampi[1], Andreas Kűnz[3], Anna Marie Lassen[2],
Cristina Lirio-Romero[4], Sanna Luoma-aho[1],
Daniel Ramskov Jørgensen[2], Diana Schack Thoft[2],
Diego Serrano-Muñoz[4], Alison Themessl-Huber[3],
and Tobias Werner[3]

[1] Seinäjoki University of Applied Sciences (SeAMK), Seinäjoki, Finland
johanna.soini@seamk.fi
[2] University College Northern Denmark (UCN), Aalborg, Denmark
[3] Fachhochschule Vorarlberg GmbH University of Applied Sciences (FHV),
Dornbirn, Austria
[4] Universidad de Castilla-La Mancha (UCLM), Ciudad Real, Spain

Abstract. Tech2Match project aims to better match and use technology with patients with pain in the future. To achieve the goal, there is a need for understanding elements needed for the future healthcare professionals to be able to use technological solutions. This background study gathered data from previous literature, focus group interviews and Higher Education Institute curriculums.

Keywords: Pain · Technology · Telehealth · VR · Education

1 Introduction

Technology is an indispensable part of healthcare. However, research indicates that healthcare professionals' skills may not be updated to accommodate how to use technologies in cooperation with patients [1]. There are positive results relating to the use of technological solutions with patients [2], but still a lack of knowledge how to implement the technology [3]. Studies have also identified many barriers that may hinder successful integration of digital interventions into practice [4, 5]. The objective of the TECH2MATCH project is to develop a 5 ECTS course to strengthen and increase advanced digital skills and technological competencies among future healthcare professionals within nursing, physiotherapy, occupational therapy, and midwifery to better match and use technologies for patients with pain (PwP). The aim of this background study is to identify and analyze the technological skills and competencies in the current healthcare education, and the skills and competencies needed for the future healthcare system.

© The Author(s) 2024
M. Särestöniemi et al. (Eds.): NCDHWS 2024, CCIS 2083, pp. 423–425, 2024.
https://doi.org/10.1007/978-3-031-59080-1

2 Materials and Methods

For this background study, three different methods were used. The literature search was performed from Cinahl Ebsco, Cochrane database, PubMed- Medline, Psychinfo, Education source and Embase databases from years 2018 - 2023. The search terms were Pain AND Health care AND ("Augmented Reality") OR ("Virtual Reality") OR telemedicine OR telehealth OR ("mobile application") OR "mobile app" OR wearables OR technology) AND report OR policy OR classification OR standard OR law OR "white paper" OR summary. The literature review was conducted using the Covidence review tool to handle the scientific data (n = 476). Each partner participated in the study by summarizing relevant data. Approved data (n = 56) included scientific articles about pain and selected technologies including VR/AR-technology, telehealth, mobile apps and monitoring.

Another part of this background study included focus group interviews in each partner country. The aim of these interviews was to gather information about challenges in health education, needed skills and the use of technology. Focus groups included people with pain and their next of kin, professionals, teachers, and students. In addition, an investigation of each partner's Higher Education Institute (HEI) curriculums about technology use in education was also performed to find the current situation in education with technology. Ethical review was carried out and the approval for the study was received by the Ethical committees of each organization.

3 Results

Based on the literature review, the technological skills and competencies required for healthcare personnel are specialized expertise, knowledge of technology, and technical know-how. Examples of the needed skills in each technology are provided in Table 1.

Table 1 Examples of needed skills for healthcare providers based on literature review

Technology	Needed skills	Pay attention to
Telehealth	Technical literacy, knowing how to use the technology	Patient safety and identification
Mobile apps	Appropriate apps to recommend to patients, contact without jargon, knowledge of the application technology	Possibilities to customize the application based on the patients' needs and interests
VR/AR	Guidance competence for health care professionals for VR treatment. Explaining the VR application to patients and a positive attitude can strengthen the trust in patient - nurse relationship	Available VR glasses, personnel education, technical infrastructure, and support are necessary

The results of the focus group interviews highlighted that healthcare professionals should have sufficient competencies and skills to use technology for pain management. In addition, healthcare professionals need to have knowledge about individual pain management, the ability to guide the patient, and the ability to use technologies to manage pain. To improve the quality of life of PwP, interaction - and social skills were found to be important personal competence requirements for healthcare professionals.

The curriculum analysis emphasized that technology in HEI's was defined in broad terms, which means that a clear definition of technology and its content is currently missing. The teaching of technology depends a lot on the competencies and knowledge of the individual teacher.

4   Discussion

This background study supports that there is a need for knowledge and more technology-oriented courses for students in health care. Future healthcare professionals need more tools, but also skills, to be able to use different technologies to guide patients and improve the quality of life for PwP.

Acknowledgements. The project 'TECH2MATCH' has received funding from Erasmus+ under Form ID: KA220-HED-A7C7B68D.

Disclosure of Interests. The authors have no competing interests to declare that are relevant to the content of this article.

References

1. Hascalovici, J., et al.: The pain medicine fellowship telehealth education collaborative. Pain Med. **22**(12), 2779–2805 (2021)
2. Martínez de la Cal, J., et al.: Physical therapists' opinion of e-health treatment of chronic low back pain. Int. J. Environ. Res. Public Health **18**(4), 1889 (2021)
3. Schreiweis, B., et al.: Barriers and facilitators to the implementation of eHealth services: systematic literature analysis. J. Med. Internet Res. **21**(11), e14197 (2019)
4. Safari, R., Jackson, J., Sheffield, D.: Digital self-management interventions for people with osteoarthritis: systematic review with meta-analysis. J. Med. Internet Res. **22**(7), e15365 (2020)
5. Varsi, C., et al.: Health care providers' experiences of pain management and attitudes towards digitally supported self-management interventions for chronic pain: a qualitative study. BMC Health Serv. Res. **21**, 275 (2021)

Adoption of a Clinical Decision Support Tool for Capacity-Building of Community Health Workers: A Longitudinal Case Study Using the NASSS Framework

Anton Elepaño[1](✉) ⓘ, Regine Ynez De Mesa[2] ⓘ, Catherine Pope[1] ⓘ,
and Antonio Miguel Dans[3] ⓘ

[1] University of Oxford, Oxford OX2 6GG, UK
anton.elepano@phc.ox.ac.uk
[2] Johns Hopkins University, Baltimore, MD 21205, USA
[3] University of the Philippines, 1000 Manila, Philippines

Abstract. Introduction: Community health workers (CHWs) in rural Philippines are compelled to provide basic clinical care to support overstretched healthcare professionals, yet they struggle due to a lack of capacity-building opportunities. To address this, the Philippine Primary Care Studies (PPCS), a policy advisory group, piloted the use of a commercially available clinical decision support (CDS) tool (UpToDate, Wolters Kluwer) for CHWs in two municipalities.

Materials and Methods: In this study, the NASSS (non-adoption, abandonment, scale-up, spread, and sustainability) framework was used to evaluate the technology's implementation from 2019 to 2023 using a multimethod analysis of interviews (48 CHWs across eight focus group discussions), multi-stakeholder meetings and reports, and usage logs.

Results: Adoption of the technology by CHWs was facilitated by social influence and availability of offline content, but marred by infrastructural barriers, particularly poor Internet access. PPCS led a policy push for scale-up, championing an executive order for satellite telecommunications services in disadvantaged areas and the integration of the CDS within the national practice guidelines program. The low marginal cost of spreading the technology presented a value proposition for the service provider to offer complimentary access to CHWs, tied to a nationwide subscription for government physicians. Complexities arose due to precarious job security resulting from volatile political climate, nascent regulatory standards, and unintended consequences related to misinterpretation of technical clinical information.

Discussion: This study provides recommendations to navigate these complexities and contributes insights on the use of the CDS in resource-limited settings, especially those with a maldistribution of health workers.

Keywords: Community Health Workers · Clinical Decision Support · Health Systems Research

M. Särestöniemi et al. (Eds.): NCDHWS 2024, CCIS 2083, p. 426, 2024.
https://doi.org/10.1007/978-3-031-59080-1

Patients' Experiences of the Digital Counselling Competence of Healthcare Professionals – A Qualitative Descriptive Study

Petra Suonnansalo[1]([⊠]), Juulia Kaihlaniemi[1], Outi Kähkönen[1,2], and Anne Oikarinen[1]

[1] Research Unit of Health Sciences and Technology, Faculty of Medicine, University of Oulu, Oulu, Finland
petra.suonnansalo@oulu.fi
[2] Department of Nursing Science, University of Eastern Finland, Kuopio, Finland

Abstract. This study aimed to describe the experiences of patients using digital services on the digital counselling competence of healthcare professionals.

Keywords: Competence · Digital Counselling · Patient · Semi-structured Interview

1 Introduction

The digitalization of healthcare services challenges the counselling competence of healthcare professionals. With the shift to digital counselling environments [1], professionals are required to have new kinds of counselling competence to provide high-quality and patient-centered counselling [2]. Patient satisfaction with the care they receive has been shown to influence treatment outcomes and self-care adherence [3]. Limited research has been conducted on patients' experiences of health professionals' digital counselling competence.

2 Materials and Methods

The study aimed to describe the experiences of patients using digital services on the digital counselling competence of healthcare professionals. Data were analyzed in Finland in spring 2023 through individual semi-structured interviews with 11 participants who had received video-mediated counselling in healthcare. Microsoft Teams was used to carry out the interviews. The interviews followed a set of main and ancillary questions [4]. Inductive content analysis was used to analyze the data [5].

© The Author(s) 2024
M. Särestöniemi et al. (Eds.): NCDHWS 2024, CCIS 2083, pp. 427–428, 2024.
https://doi.org/10.1007/978-3-031-59080-1

3   Results

Patients' experiences of healthcare professionals' digital counselling competence consisted of five areas of competence: (1) preparing for video-mediated counselling, (2) digital competence in implementing the video-mediated counselling, (3) interacting with the patient during the video-mediated counselling, (4) supporting the patient's self-management in video-mediated counselling and (5) self-development as a digital counsellor. According to patients' experiences, video-mediated counselling is routine for healthcare professionals, but the limited experience of providing video-mediated counselling is also transparent to the patients. Healthcare professionals need to pay particular attention to the encounters and interactions in the digital counselling situation. In addition, patients stressed the importance of healthcare professionals' mastery of technology as part of smooth digital counselling. Before every digital counselling session, healthcare professionals should ensure that the technical and technological elements are in place and familiarize themselves with the patient's background. Patients felt that it was important for healthcare professionals to involve the patient in digital counselling, for example by sharing screen and using a variety of counselling materials.

4   Discussion

The results of this study suggest that healthcare professionals need a wide range of counselling competencies when counselling patients via video. Our findings set the basis for future research on patients' experiences of healthcare professionals;' digital counselling competence. Future research should focus on developing the digital counselling competence of HCPs, as this has a significant impact on the effectiveness of digital services.

References

1. Paalimäki-Paakki, K., Virtanen, M., Henner, A., Nieminen, M.T., Kääriäinen, M.: Effectiveness of digital counseling environments on anxiety, depression, and adherence to treatment among patients who are chronically ill: systematic review. J. Med. Internet Res. **24**(1), e30077 (2022). https://doi.org/10.2196/30077
2. Kaihlaniemi, J., Liljamo, P., Rajala, M., Kaakinen, P., Oikarinen, A.: Health care Professionals' experiences of counselling competence in digital care pathways - a descriptive qualitative study. Nurs. open **10**(7), 4773–4785 (2023). https://doi.org/10.1002/nop2.1729
3. Ramaswamy, A., et al.: Patient satisfaction with telemedicine during the COVID-19 pandemic: retrospective cohort study. J. Med. Internet Res. **22**(9), e20786 (2020). https://doi.org/10.2196/20786
4. Polit, D.F., Beck, C.T.: Generating and Assessing Evidence for Nursing Practice, 10th edn. Wolters Kluwer Health, Philadelphia (2017)
5. Elo, S., Kyngäs, H.: The qualitative content analysis process. J. Adv. Nurs.Nurs. **62**(1), 107–115 (2008). https://doi.org/10.1111/j.1365-2648.2007.04569.x

Author Index

Printed in the United States
by Baker & Taylor Publisher Services